The
COMPLETE BOOK
of
MEDICAL TESTS

The
COMPLETE BOOK
of
MEDICAL TESTS

Mark A. Moskowitz, M.D.

Michael E. Osband, M.D.

W · W · NORTON & COMPANY
New York   London

Copyright © 1984 by Mark A. Moskowitz and Michael E. Osband
Published simultaneously in Canada by Stoddart, a subsidiary of General Publishing Co.
Ltd, Don Mills, Ontario.
Printed in the United States of America

The text of this book is composed in 11/13 Palatino, with
display type set in Palatino. Composition and
manufacturing by The Maple-Vail Book Manufacturing Group.
Book design by Nancy Dale Muldoon

First Edition

Library of Congress Cataloging in Publication Data

Moskowitz, Mark A.
The complete book of medical tests.

Bibliography: p.
Includes index.
1. Diagnosis.   2. Consumer education.   I. Osband,
Michael E.   II. Title.
RC71.3.M68   1984   616.07′5   83–27473

ISBN 0-393-01794-X

W. W. Norton & Company, Inc., 500 Fifth Avenue, New York, N.Y. 10110
W. W. Norton & Company Ltd., 37 Great Russell Street, London WC1B 3NU

1 2 3 4 5 6 7 8 9 0

To Debbie and Barbara
for their love and support

Contents

PART III
The Use of Medical Tests on Healthy Patients

PART IV
The Use of Medical Tests in Special Situations

PART V
The Use of Medical Tests in Illness

PART VI
Medical Tests You Can Do Yourself

EPILOGUE
Recent Advances in Medical Testing   349

APPENDICES

Acknowledgments

THE writing of this book was possible only because of the help of many people. We would like to take this opportunity to thank them:

Gennaro Carpinito, M.D., who coordinated our x-rays and photograph sessions;

Cathryn King Norton, who was very generous with her time and helped us in many ways throughout the preparation and writing of the manuscript;

Reuven Miller, who coordinated our artwork, took the photographs throughout the book, met our unreasonable deadlines and, most importantly, is a dear and special friend;

Paul Palefski, M.D., who made us appreciate the care, concern, and medical knowledge of an expert radiologist;

Deborah L. Shipman, M.D., who, in addition to juggling three careers as a pediatrician, mother, and "lab rat," showed us great skill as an editor.

In addition, we have been blessed throughout our careers with many colleagues who are both teacher and friend. Many of them offered freely of their time and expertise in reading the manuscript and pointing out our mistakes with the perfect mixture of face-saving kindness and thought-provoking candor: Jack Ende, M.D., Richard Krikorian, M.D., and Benjamin Siegel, M.D.

We also want to thank everyone in Michael's lab who was forced to put up with countless pieces of manuscript lying around, lost time on the computer in the name of word processing, and yet still gave us their understanding, patience, and support; Caroline Peyser and Rochelle Walter, who contributed to the proofreading and preparation of the manuscript; Mary Cunnane, our editor at Norton, who has been a continual source of guidance and encouragement, our skillful copyeditor, Florence Kurzman, and our proofreader, Millie Susser.

Finally, but certainly most important, this book was accomplished only because of the understanding, love, and support given us by our wives and by our beloved children—Elliot, Rachel, and Philip; and Yardaena, Mechael, and Noam.

Introduction

FROM the time we were medical students together, the two of us have enjoyed discussing our professional experiences. Even though our paths have diverged—one of us is an internist, the other a pediatrician—throughout the years we have periodically met to share with each other ideas and thoughts about our patients. A few months ago, late one night, we were sitting around and talking about the kinds of questions patients and their families ask us most frequently. After listing a variety of different questions we had been asked that week, we both came to the conclusion that the most common topic brought up by patients concerned medical tests. To test that theory, we decided that over the next few days we would each write down the various questions patients asked us about medical tests, and the next time we saw each other, compare our lists. When we met a few weeks later, we were amazed to find that on our lists the same kinds of questions kept coming up again and again:

"What is the purpose of this blood test (or electrocardiogram [EKG] or x-ray or other medical test)?"

"How are they done?"

"What risks are there to x-rays and other tests?"

"How much do various medical tests cost?"

"If the test results are normal, can I be sure I am healthy?"

"What preparation must I make for various tests?"

Two things were clear to us: first, that patients have numerous questions and real concerns about medical tests; and, second, that there is little opportunity for them to get the answers they seek. Most doctors don't have the time to discuss these kinds of issues in great detail. In addition, many patients first think of their questions only after they have left the doctor's office and are embarrassed to call their doctor with their concerns. Finally, we made a thorough search of our local libraries and could not find any reference books about medical tests that we could enthusiastically recommend to our patients. It was not long before we had come to the obvious conclusion that there were many patients who would benefit greatly from having a book about medical tests available to them. Our decision to write this book then became an easy one: our experiences taking care of patients had identified a real need and we wished to fill it.

The translation of that idea into reality, however, was more difficult, as we had to decide carefully what material—out of a vast body of scientific and medical knowledge at our disposal—should be included in the book and what could be safely excluded.

Most importantly, we wanted a book for you that would be useful. So our primary criterion for putting something into the book was: "Would you—the reader—be able to put the information to use?" Second, and nearly as important, we wanted a book that is interesting. We love our work and we wanted to convey to you some of the excitement and spirit that we feel in the practice and teaching of medicine. So our task was clear.

The first decision we had to make was what tests to include. We decided to describe in the book every medical test that we use with any kind of routine frequency. In addition, we have included parts on the proper use of medical tests for healthy people of all ages as well as the use of tests for common symptoms and diseases.

It is our hope that this book will become a valuable resource for you, answering your many questions about medical tests and explaining them in a manner that will enable you to work more effectively with your doctor and get the most out of them. We wish to emphasize however that this book is not meant to be a substitute for medical care by a competent physician nor should it be used by you to interpret the results of medical tests that he may order.

We'd like to mention a couple of additional points before letting you go on and get into the book itself. The English language needs a personal pronoun that is neither male or female. Until such time as one is evolved, we are forced to make choices that are less than wholly satisfactory. Strictly as a convention, whenever we refer to a physician, we have used the male pronoun: he, him, or his.

This is nothing more than a convenience.

We would enjoy hearing from you with your comments and suggestions about this book. We wrote it for you, and we want to know which parts were especially useful and interesting and which were not. We would be delighted to receive your comments about the use of medical tests in general as well as your reactions to this guide: how it helped you and what could be included in the book to make it even more useful.

PART I

The Basic Information You Need to Know

1

How and Why to Read a Book about Medical Tests

COME make rounds with us as we see our patients on the wards of a large medical center where we work in Boston. We'll start off on the surgical service. The first patient we see is Barry P., a 38-year-old attorney who was admitted to the hospital yesterday because he is experiencing abdominal pain and passing black stools. Today he is scheduled to have a gastroduodenoscopy, and an upper GI (gastrointestinal) series is booked for tomorrow. He is very worried and anxious—both about his health and about the tests that are to be done. He tells us that he doesn't know how the tests will be done, what problems might arise with them, and what preparation he must undergo for them to be done correctly.

In the next room is Louise F., a 45-year-old woman and mother of four children who was seen by a doctor for her regularly scheduled complete physical, which included a mammogram. When her doctor examined her breasts he did not find any problems, but the mammogram revealed the presence of a small tumor in her left breast and she has been admitted to the hospital for a biopsy. She is very confused and asks us how it is possible that the physical examination could be normal but the mammogram showed a possible tumor. In addition, she tells us that she is uncertain why the biopsy is being done and what it might reveal.

Finally, we visit Jeff D., a 22-year-old law student who was admitted to the hospital just this morning for elective surgery to repair the hernia he developed while lifting weights. As part of his work-up in the hospital, he has had a chest x-ray, EKG, complete blood count (CBC), an SMA-12 (a battery of 12 different blood-chemistry tests performed on a machine called the Sequential

Multiple Analyzer), a blood typing (a test done to determine the patient's blood group in case a blood transfusion is necessary), a prothrombin time, a partial thromboplastin time, and a bleeding time. (The last three tests are designed to test if his blood will clot normally during the surgery.) In total, he has had medical tests costing over $500. Not surprisingly, because he is an otherwise healthy young man in good condition, all the tests were normal, and he will have his surgery done tomorrow morning as scheduled.

Leaving the surgery ward, we walk over to the medical service. In the first room is Susan W., a 46-year-old woman who has had diabetes for over 25 years. Even though she has diabetes she works full time as an elementary school teacher and maintains an active and full life. She monitors her own blood and urine sugar levels at home; she called her doctor a couple of days ago when her blood glucose level was consistently elevated beyond what it had been for the past several months. Her physician admitted her to the hospital to reevaluate her insulin dose and monitor its use for a few days and, in general, make sure that her diabetes is under control.

In the same room with her is Jane S., an elderly woman who lives in a nursing home. She began vomiting two days ago and when she was admitted to the hospital this morning, her tests showed that her blood was very low in potassium, a mineral that is critical for many bodily functions. Outside the room her family is waiting to discuss these results with her doctor. They do not know the significance of this low potassium level and, in addition, want to know why it had never been previously detected. They think the nursing home should have done the test more frequently if it was that important.

From the medical service we go over to the pediatric wards where we see one of our own patients—Sean P.—a two-month old infant who last night developed a fever and became very irritable. When we saw the baby in the emergency room last night we thought it possible that the baby had meningitis, and we did a spinal tap to see if this was the case. In order to understand what happened to Sean, it is important to know that there are two kinds of meningitis. One, caused by a virus, will get better by itself and rarely results in any long-term complications. The other kind is caused by bacteria and requires immediate treatment with antibiotics. If this isn't done, serious complications, and even death, can occur.

The results from the tap showed that Sean probably did have meningitis, but, fortunately, it appeared to be the kind that is caused by a virus. Even so, we ordered that Sean receive antibiotics until other tests come back confirming for certain that this is not a case of bacterial meningitis.

Just before leaving the hospital we go to the delivery room in the obstetrical wing. There, Alice G., a 39-year-old business executive, is giving birth to her first child. When she was four-months pregnant, Alice had an amniocentesis performed to make sure that the baby did not have a genetic disease, like Down's syndrome. Now, at the time of delivery, her obstetrician is worried because she has been in labor for over 24 hours. He decides to monitor the labor to be sure that the fetus is in no danger. To do so, he attaches an electrode to the fetus's scalp to check on its heart rate, and, in addition, he takes a small amount of fetal blood to see if the fetus is getting sufficient oxygen during this difficult delivery. Outside the delivery room door we meet Alice's husband. He is confused and frightened. No one has explained to him what is happening, and all he hears from the hospital personnel walking by are a few fragmented phrases with such words as "pH," "arterial blood gas," and "late-phase deceleration," all of which are mysterious and unknown to him.

From the hospital we stop by the outpatient clinic to see two patients who have been referred to us by other doctors. Karen F. is an 18-year-old woman on a track scholarship at one of the local colleges where she is majoring in primary school education. She trains daily, frequently running over 5 miles. The physician at the college health service did a routine physical and discovered that the level of two enzymes in her blood—SGOT and LDH—was elevated. He thought she might have hepatitis and referred her to us for evaluation. After examining her carefully and doing some more tests, we are able to tell Karen that elevations of these enzymes—which can, in fact, be a sign of hepatitis—also occur in people who exercise rigorously, and that she is perfectly healthy. Although she is relieved and happy at the good news, she stays and talks to us for another half hour before returning home, trying to find out how hepatitis and exercise can cause a similar pattern in blood enzyme levels.

The last patient we see this day is Fred S., a 35-year-old account executive at an advertising agency. Although he used to play tennis three times a week when he was younger, he hasn't touched his racket in over 10 years. Now he has joined a local tennis club and wants to begin playing again. He and his wife are concerned that maybe, after being sedentary for these 10 years, he would suffer a heart attack when he starts this exercise program. One of his friends at the tennis club is a doctor who thought he should have an exercise stress test performed to be sure that his heart can withstand the tennis program Fred envisions. His friend did not tell Fred, however, that getting a stress test in this circumstance may do more harm than good. After we explain to Fred why this is so, he goes home—reassured that he can start to play tennis again—but without having had the stress test done.

The one thing all the patients we saw today share in common in their health care is the use of medical tests. In some instances the tests were ordered properly; some of the tests were inappropriate and unnecessary. In all cases the patients or their families had numerous concerns and questions about the medical tests that were being performed and on which their medical care would so heavily depend. Medical tests are only one facet of health care, but a unique one because they often are seen as mysterious and are not well understood.

Blood is taken and sent away—hours or days later the doctor refers vaguely to the results from "the blood tests." Or perhaps this has happened to you: the doctor orders a test, maybe mentioning the name to you, or maybe not. Either way, you go to a room and a nameless technician places electrodes on your body, connecting them to a sophisticated piece of electronic equipment filled with dials, switches, and flashing lights. What are these tests that are being done? What is being measured and why? What preparation must be done for them? Will any risks or discomforts accompany the test? Will any medication interfere with the results? How are the results given and what do they mean? The list of questions that patients ask about their medical tests is endless and we have written this book to answer them for you. We hope this book will provide you with all the information you need to understand your medical tests and to relieve unnecessary anxiety and fear.

We doctors cannot work effectively alone. We look to you, our patients, for help in managing your health. As physicians we have come to depend heavily—perhaps too heavily—on the use of medical tests in performing this task. We look to you to work with us in making sure that these medical tests—sometimes helpful but always potentially dangerous—are used with care in an effective way that will benefit you the most.

Let us tell you a little about how the book is arranged so that you can use it in the best manner possible.

Part I contains some basic information that you need to know as well as our plan to get the most out of your medical tests. We don't expect you to read these pages every time you consult the book, but, initially at least, you should read these chapters carefully.

Part II is the core of the book. Over two hundred medical tests are listed and described in full detail using a standardized format with such headings as: Purpose of the Test, Background, How the Test is Done, How the Results are Given, Patient Preparation, Risks and Discomforts, Normal Range of Values, and Cost. In addition, with each test we provide a list (and explanation) of the various symptoms and diseases for which that particular test is commonly obtained.

Part III details our recommendations for the use of medical tests for healthy people. Specific charts are provided—categorized by age and sex—which list the tests that should be performed at each visit to the doctor. Each of these tests is then discussed, providing information as to why it is useful for that particular test to be performed when you are healthy.

Part IV discusses medical tests with regard to three special situations: pregnancy, hospitalization, and an exercise/physical conditioning program.

Part V details the proper use of medical tests in 21 common symptoms and 16 common diseases.

Finally, Part VI describes a series of medical tests that you can do yourself. We give specific information on how to perform and interpret these tests, when to do them, and what they mean.

Appendix 1 to the book presents some information on how certain drugs can interfere with test results; Appendix 2 gives an example of a medical test diary that we recommend you and members of your family maintain; Appendix 3 contains a bibliography that will help the reader obtain more information about medical tests; Appendix 4 contains a list of abbreviations that are commonly found in medical tests.

The book is structured in a manner that allows you to look directly in Part II for any test about which you want detailed and comprehensive information. In addition, information is grouped within various settings (health, illness, pregnancy, hospitalization) in which medical tests are frequently performed. Since it is likely that you will find yourself looking in more than one location in the book to get information, we have provided extensive cross-referencing between the various parts.

As we have mentioned before, one important part concerns the use of medical tests for healthy patients. At first glance you may think that the use of medical tests when you are healthy is obvious and simple. But, in fact, it is when you are healthy that medical tests are most abused and their use more controversial. For example, should patients have a stress test done at their annual physical? But even that question is premature because it is not certain that your regular checkup should be annual. Perhaps a complete physical every two, three or five years would be just as good. How often should a woman have a Pap smear or mammography done, and what is the harm if these tests are performed too often? In fact, it is our experience that choosing the right tests for healthy patients is more difficult than choosing the right ones for sick patients. It is our hope that this book will provide guidelines that will enable you to work with your doctor in reaching these sometimes difficult decisions.

Other parts of the book focus on medical tests that should be obtained when one has certain common symptoms or a particular disease. We have not only listed the tests, but we have also told you why they are done in these situations and what the doctor hopes to accomplish with their use.

Throughout the book, at the end of every test, we provide a normal value for that specific test. We discuss on p. 13 the entire concept of what a normal value is, and it is critical for you to read that information to understand what a normal value can and cannot be used for, and what it does and does not mean. Unfortunately, one problem with medical tests that the medical profession and health industry must correct is the way in which normal values are described. For many tests there are numerous systems by which the results are given. If you think the metric system and English system of measurement are difficult to keep straight, medical testing by comparison can be mind boggling. For example, results from the blood test that measures for the enzyme alkaline phosphatase can be reported in five different units: the normal range can be expressed as 1.5–4.5 Bodansky units, or 4–13 King-Armstrong units, or 0.8–2.3 Bessey–Lowry units, or 10–15 Shinowar-Jones-Reinhart units, or 0–70 International units (IU). And, what makes it worse, no two hospitals will use the exact same system for reporting test results. Standardization is needed and it is not yet forthcoming. For each test we have listed the results in the measurement system that is most commonly used for that particular test. Your hospital or doctor may use a different measurement system than the one we provide, so before checking your test results against the ones in the book, make sure that the measuring units for that particular test are the same.

Another important piece of information that we want to give you is the cost of specific tests. We struggled for a long time before deciding on the best way to present this information. The range of costs among medical tests is great (e.g., simple blood tests may cost approximately $5 and cardiac catheterization, over $1000.), and, in addition, there is wide variation among hospitals and laboratories throughout the different regions of the country. What we have done, therefore, is to provide the costs that are charged by laboratories in the Boston area where we practice. The costs that we provide are not meant to give you a tight guideline for judging whether your own cost for a particular test is unusually high or unusually low. Instead, we want you to use this information as a relative index for the costs of the various tests.

At times we had to repeat ideas and concepts in different places in the book in order to make certain key points.

One last point: many tests have a number of different names. An electroencephalogram, for instance, can also be referred to as an EEG or brain wave test. If a test is not listed by the name familiar to you, look it up in the detailed index, where it may be found under a different name.

2

The Fifty Most Important Questions about Medical Tests

1. What is a medical test?

Our ability to provide good medical care depends to a large extent on gathering accurate and reliable information from our patients. This process can be divided into three components. First, and perhaps most important, we gather information by listening to what a patient has to say about his health. Based on what the patient tells us, we will ask the patient a series of questions. All the information that results is called the patient's *medical history*, and it is critical to good medical care.

The second component of information gathering is the *physical examination*—giving us the opportunity to observe, touch, feel, and listen directly to the patient's body.

The third and final component of information is the results obtained from *medical tests*. This was not always the case. In the previous century physicians had available only the first two of these three methods of gathering information: the medical history and the physical examination. Over the last one hundred years large numbers of medical tests have been developed that now allow the physician to interpret much more accurately the information that he gains from the medical history and physical examination.

Medical tests, therefore, are performed to aid in caring for the patient. *Medical tests* can be done on specimens obtained from the patient, such as blood and urine, or on the patient himself, such as an electrocardiogram. *Medical tests* can be very sophisticated, such as computerized axial tomography or CT scan (p. 115), or simple, such as a hematocrit (p. 51). *Medical tests* are usually performed by a member of the health care team—physician, nurse, or medical technician—but they are sometimes performed at home by the patient, as in home pregnancy testing or urine and blood testing for diabetes.

The full story about medical tests remains unfinished. Every year new tests are developed and others are eliminated—either discarded by the medical profession because they are replaced by improved techniques or recognized as ineffective at providing useful and important information. Yet one thing remains clear: medical tests have become an invaluable part of the health care system.

2. What are medical tests used for?

All medical tests can be placed into one of four categories: (1) screening, (2) diagnostic, (3) prognostic, (4) monitoring. Medical tests used for *screening* are usually simple, relatively inexpensive, and without substantial risk to the patient. We will use them to see if a particular illness or problem is present in a patient who appears healthy and has no symptoms or complaints. Examples of medical tests that can be used to screen patients in this way are blood glucose (p. 61) and urinalysis (p. 87).

Often, however, we may suspect a specific illness on the basis of the patient's medical history and physical examination. Medical tests that we use in this circumstance are *diagnostic* tests to confirm or deny our clinical impression. For example, we frequently see in our office children complaining of fever and a very sore throat. During the physical examination we often find that the throat is red and the tonsils are covered with pus. When this happens we suspect that the patient has a "strep throat," the name given to those infections of the throat caused by the streptococcus bacteria. In order to confirm our suspected diagnosis, we will order a throat culture (p. 174) as a *diagnostic* test to see if strep—and not another bacteria or virus—is indeed the cause of the sore throat. This is an example of a diagnostic medical test because it is not used on healthy children but is done only on those patients who are suspected of having a strep throat.

A third major use of medical tests is to provide us—when we have already made a diagnosis—with information about our patient's *prognosis.* For example, a 58-year-old woman we saw with a lump in her breast had a biopsy performed that showed breast cancer. Even though we were certain of her diagnosis (breast cancer), we ordered additional tests to determine her specific prognosis. By getting a bone scan (p. 133) and chest x-ray (p. 113), we were able to tell that the cancer had spread to her bones and lungs. The results from those tests helped us to counsel the patient and her family and determine that additional cancer treatment was necessary.

The fourth and final category of medical tests is those that we use to *monitor* or evaluate medical treatment that we have given to our patients. For example, a few months ago a 48-year-old man came to our office complaining of pain and swelling in his right calf. We examined him and found thrombophlebitis—inflamed veins in the leg that are filled with blood clots. This is a serious condition that requires treatment with Coumadin, a drug that prevents the blood from clotting normally. But, as one would expect, the use of Coumadin can be dangerous because if too much of the drug is present in the blood, it will prevent clotting to the extent that unnecessary bleeding may result. There is a medical test called prothrombin time (PT, p. 80) that measures how well the blood clots. Our patient taking Coumadin requires weekly prothrombin times performed to determine whether clotting has been controlled to the right degree and not more.

3. Okay, there are four reasons why medical tests are done. At different times can a single test be used for more than one of these reasons?

Absolutely! And it is important to remember that most tests are done for a variety of reasons. For example, one day we walked into the x-ray reception room at the hospital and found four of our patients waiting to have chest x-rays done—each for a different reason. The first patient, a 62-year-old man in good health, was having the x-ray done as part of his regular physical. The chest x-ray used in this manner is a *screening* test that is done periodically to see if any diseases are present, even though the man has no symptoms or medical problems.

The second patient, a 33-year-old woman, had been coughing for three days, and we ordered the chest x-ray as a *diagnostic* test to see if she has pneumonia.

The third patient was a six-year-old girl who has curvature of the spine. The chest x-ray is being done to find out how severe the curvature is in order to determine if surgery is necessary.

Although we had already diagnosed her problem, the chest x-ray was useful because it provides critical information concerning her *prognosis*.

The fourth patient, a 42-year-old man, was on treatment with penicillin for pneumonia. We ordered the chest x-ray to *monitor* the treatment and see if the pneumonia has disappeared.

4. It is clear that an individual medical test can be used for more than one purpose. Can a person have several medical tests done at a single time for more than one of these reasons?

It is fairly common for this to be the case. Let's take one example and see how this works. Helen P., a 63-year-old woman with diabetes, told us during her regular checkup that for the past two weeks she has had a burning sensation when she urinates. As part of her visit with us, three medical tests were ordered. A blood sugar (p. 61) was obtained to monitor the insulin that she uses to control her diabetes. A hematocrit (p. 243) was done as a screening test, although she has no specific symptoms suggestive of anemia. And finally, a urinalysis (p. 87) was done as a diagnostic test to see if she had a bladder infection.

5. During a conversation with this patient two days later to review the test results, the doctor mentions that her hematocrit is normal. What does a "normal" result mean?

We can only interpret a test result obtained in a particular patient by comparing it to results obtained from identical tests performed in other people. For example, we were able to tell Helen P. that her hematocrit was normal because the value obtained—39%— was within a range of values that has been established as being normal for this particular test. The "normal values" for a particular test have been selected so as to include the values obtained in 95% of healthy people. The normal range for hematocrit in women is 37%–47% because it is within this range that the hematocrit values of 95% of healthy women will fall.

6. Who are the healthy individuals who are used to determine these "normal ranges" for medical tests?

The usual way by which "normal values" have been determined has been to take a population of healthy volunteers and test them. This is usually done by the company that makes the test equipment or occasionally by the laboratory performing the test. The range of test values that includes 95% of these healthy individuals is considered normal. In most instances the healthy volunteers have consisted largely of young males—often medical students at a large medical center where such testing is performed. Are the normal values determined from that group of young males a fair comparison by which to judge the blood test of a 55-year-old woman? Probably not. Ideally, one would like to develop a range of normal values for each patient studied, taking into account specific factors such as age, sex, and race. But that would be an impossible task. So, instead, we live with normal values that are really normal only for one group of patients and try to make sense of comparing that normal range with the specific results in a particular patient. Unfortunately, problems still result.

7. If I have a normal test result, does that mean that I am healthy?
8. And, if I have an abnormal test result, does that mean that I am sick?

The answer to both questions is "no," and that is because medical tests are not perfect. Even if the proper normal range were used to evaluate the test result for an individual patient, medical tests do not always predict accurately who is sick and who is healthy because they are neither specific nor sensitive enough to do so. In fact, even with the best screening tests, it is not unusual that only 30% of those patients with an abnormal result are truly sick.

9. Are there still other reasons why a medical test can give a normal result when I am really sick or an abnormal result when I am healthy?

Yes, and the results have nothing to do with the accuracy of the test itself. Instead, incorrect results are caused by the test being done under erroneous assumptions. There are five such errors that can be made:

Medications: Certain medicines taken by patients can affect the results of medical tests. For example, many drugs can cause an abnormal result in liver function tests (p. 77). Consequently, if your physician does not know that you are taking one of these medications, he may misinterpret an abnormal result to mean that you have infectious hepatitis, when, in fact, the abnormal value resulted from your taking one of these drugs.

Improper patient preparation: Many tests require specific preparation. If this is done improperly, the test results may be impossible to interpret correctly. The most common mistake involves the patient eating or drinking before a test when he has been instructed not to. Many tests require that the patient fast for a specified period of time prior to a particular test being performed. For example, the night before a blood glucose level (p. 61) is to be done, you will frequently be instructed not to eat or drink after 10 P.M. If, however, you forget and eat breakfast before the blood is taken, the glucose level may be very high. Your doctor would be very concerned at this result and perhaps suspect that you have diabetes, when, in fact, you are healthy and the abnormally high glucose level resulted from eating breakfast.

A mistake in the way the test was conducted or the sample was collected: For example, arterial blood gases (p. 183) require that the blood be refrigerated immediately after it is drawn. Sometimes the physician, nurse, or blood technician fails to do this and the sample will measure much less oxygen than is actually there. The abnormal result obtained will be due to a problem with the technique and not any disease in the patient.

Mislabeled samples: The fourth reason for an inaccurate result is that the test sample or x-ray has been mislabeled with the wrong patient's name on it. Although you may think this happens rarely, it is a surprisingly common cause of error.

Lab error: The laboratory may use the wrong chemicals in performing the test or may record the results incorrectly.

10. What can I do as a patient to be sure that my medical tests are accurate?

Think about the reasons for errors and do what you can to ensure that they don't happen. Make sure the doctor knows the name of every medicine and drug—both prescribed and over-the-counter—that you have taken in the recent past. Even if you do not think that it is an "important medicine," be sure that the doctor knows that you have taken it.

Be very certain to follow the directions given to you for the test. And, if you have made a mistake and not followed the preparations exactly, it is important to tell your doctor so that an improper interpretation will not result.

Finally, be certain that you are identified properly when the test is being conducted. Take care that the person doing the test knows your name and that the right test is being done. If you go to the hospital emergency room because you tripped and injured your ankle and the doctor tells you that he wants x-rays, you have every right to ask the technician what is going on if he begins to prepare you for a chest x-ray and not for x-rays of your ankle.

11. *Are medical tests dangerous?*

Because all medical tests have side effects, they should never be done without a specific reason. These risks can be slight, as, for example, a bruise on your arm after a blood test, or life-threatening, such as an allergic reaction to the dye used in an intravenous pyelogram (IVP, p. 121). The specific dangers vary with the type of test, the age, and health of the patient and the reasons for which the test is being done. The risks are described in detail with each specific test in Part II.

12. *Who performs medical tests?*

Like all medical care, medical tests require a team effort. The physician is the person who generally orders the test and must consider: Is it dangerous? Is it a good test? Is it accurate enough to provide information that is useful in the care of this patient? What is the cost? How quickly will I have the answer?

Usually, nurses and technicians play an important role as well. Some tests, such as a blood test or EKG, are often performed entirely by the nurse or technician. More complicated tests, such as bronchoscopy or cardiac catheterization, are performed by the doctor with the assistance of the nurse or technician.

13. *Where are medical tests done?*

It depends on the kind of test. Blood tests, for example, require two steps, each of which is done in a different place. First, the blood is drawn from the patient. This is done in your doctor's office, your hospital room, or in the blood-drawing room of a laboratory. Second, the blood must be sent to a laboratory for processing and for the actual testing. Many doctors have laboratories for doing simple blood tests in their office. All hospitals have laboratories that are capable of much more sophisticated tests. In addition, many doctors and hospitals send blood samples to commercial laboratories if they do not have the equipment to do the test themselves. These commercial laboratories provide a large range of tests, both simple and complex, and are regionally located. It is common, therefore, for blood to be sent many miles—even across the country—for processing and testing. The same is true for urine and other body fluids. All laboratories, whether in a hospital or commercially owned, must be licensed by the local, state, and federal authorities to guarantee that high standards of quality are maintained.

X-rays, as a rule, can be done either in a doctor's office—if he has the appropriate equipment—or in the hospital. Other tests, such as cardiac catheterization, must be done in the hospital.

Blood Tests

14. When I go to the doctor I am frequently told that I need some blood tests. Are all blood tests the same?

There are well over 50 different kinds of blood tests. Each of them measures something different in the patient's blood. Some tests measure the different kinds of blood cells (red blood cells, white blood cells, or platelets); others measure certain minerals (such as sodium, potassium, and calcium); while additional tests measure other substances found in the blood (e.g., uric acid, alkaline phosphatase, or bilirubin). Some tests, like the one that determines the level of glucose in the blood, are done frequently and may be performed on a patient every day during a hospital stay. Other tests are performed less often and will be done only when the doctor is concerned about certain symptoms or is monitoring a particular disease.

15. When my doctor orders blood tests, there seem to be two ways to obtain blood: either by inserting a needle into a vein in my arm or by pricking the tip of my finger to squeeze out blood. What is the difference?

There are two differences between the blood obtained from a finger prick (in newborn infants this prick is often done in the heel and is called a heelstick) and that gotten from a venipuncture (the term used when blood is drawn with a needle from a vein). First is the amount. A finger prick can provide, at most, half a milliliter of blood (about ⅟₆₀ of an ounce), while a venipuncture can furnish as much blood as the doctor needs. Secondly, the blood from a venipuncture is obtained directly from the vein, while that gotten from a finger prick is literally squeezed out through a small hole in the skin. This squeezing often causes the blood to be diluted with other fluid in the skin and can lead to inaccurate results. Therefore, the blood from the vein will usually provide more reliable information. Many patients prefer to have blood drawn from a finger prick because they think it will be less painful than a venipuncture, but the exact opposite is true. A venipuncture hurts only at the moment when the needle is being inserted in the vein, while a finger prick can hurt long after the blood is taken.

16. When my doctor orders blood tests, I have noticed that the blood is collected into tubes with different color tops. What do these various colors mean?

Each of the many different kinds of blood tests must be handled by the laboratory in a special way. The various tubes contain different chemicals that begin processing the blood even before it reaches the laboratory. The person drawing the blood will know what tests are to be performed and will use the appropriate colored tube. For example, blood tests that measure chemicals or minerals in the serum (the liquid portion of blood) are usually drawn in tubes with red or green tops. The following list gives the common tests for which different tubes are used:

Red—tests that measure chemicals, minerals, antibodies, hormones, or drugs.

Lavender (pale purple)—tests that measure the number of the various cells found in the blood, including red cells, white cells, and platelets.

Blue—tests that measure the ability of the blood to clot.

Gray—tests that measure the level of glucose in the blood.

Green—tests that measure the level of minerals or hormones in the blood as well as tests that measure the function of white blood cells.

17. Does it matter what time of day blood tests are drawn?

The levels in the blood of certain chemicals or hormones go up and down during the day. This continual fluctuation is called diurnal variation and must be taken into account when tests are drawn to measure those particular substances. For example, the level of cortisol—a hormone made by the adrenal gland—is highest in early morning and lowest in the afternoon. Similarly, the level of blood sugar is lowest in the morning before breakfast and changes throughout the day after eating. In most hospitals blood is drawn in the morning, soon after the patient has awakened, so that the laboratory can begin processing the blood at the start of the day.

18. How long does it take for blood tests to be completed?

Most blood tests can be completed within a few hours, and in the hospital the doctor has most test results back the same day that the blood is drawn. In your doctor's office it might take longer since the blood first has to be picked up and brought to the laboratory and then the results sent back to the doctor. Even then, if the situation is serious, the doctor can get the results of most tests within a few hours after the blood is drawn in his office. There are a few blood tests, such as certain immune studies, that may take many days to complete, but these are the exception.

19. I am always worried that the doctor takes too much blood for my tests. Why do blood tests require so much blood to be drawn, and isn't that dangerous?

Although it looks like a large amount, the volume of blood that is collected for a standard series of blood tests is not much at all. Generally, when we order a series of blood tests, approximately 1 ounce of blood is taken. This is less than 1% of the blood found in the body of an average adult (5 to 6 quarts). The body will usually replace that small amount of blood within the day, so there is no danger, even to a patient in a hospital where blood is drawn every day.

20. Are there any discomforts or risks to blood tests?

There are only three slight problems associated with blood tests. First is the pain, and while not a "risk" in the sense of posing a threat to the patient's health, it is slightly uncomfortable for a very short time. Second, a venipuncture sometimes causes a bruise at the site where the blood was drawn. Again, this is not a threat to a patient's health but for a short period can be slightly painful, tender, and noticeable. Finally, some patients may feel faint while blood is being drawn, and, although rare, a few may actually "pass out."

21. Is there anything special I should do if I know that I am going to have blood tests drawn?

Your doctor will instruct you if any special preparations are necessary. Sometimes he will require you to fast after dinner on the night before a test. For other tests only certain foods must be avoided for a period of time.

URINE TESTS

22. Why is urine used in medical tests?

For a variety of reasons urine is one of the best specimens that can be collected from the body and studied. First, it can be obtained without much bother—no needles, pricks, pain, bruising, or laboratory technician needed to draw it. Second, it can be obtained in relatively large quantities. Third, virtually no processing is required before it can be analyzed and tested in the laboratory. Finally, and perhaps most important, urine reflects the overall health of the body in general and the specific status of the kidneys and bladder in particular. For all these reasons urine testing is one of the first kinds of medical tests that were ever done. Nearly 2500 years ago, in ancient Greece, Hippocrates recognized that tasting the urine to see if it was sweet from sugar was useful in the detection of diabetes.

23. If urine is such an easy and simple specimen to use in medical tests, why are blood tests done at all? Why not always use urine?

There is one disadvantage to using urine as a test specimen. In order to understand this problem, it is necessary to review what urine is. Urine is the product of the kidneys, the organ whose major job is to filter and cleanse the blood. When working properly, the kidney is extremely efficient. It is estimated that all of your blood (approximately 5 to 6 quarts in an adult) flows through them every 20 minutes—well over 300 quarts a day. And yet, after filtering all that liquid, the kidney "makes" only 1 quart of urine; the rest of the liquid that is filtered is returned to the blood stream. In the urine are found the waste products of the body (urea), certain minerals (sodium, chloride, and potassium), as well as water. So how is that a problem for using urine in medical tests? Most substances found in the blood are not excreted in the urine. Antibodies, hormones, enzymes, albumin, serum proteins, and lipids are just some of the major types of chemicals that are present in blood, yet not in the urine. In fact, of the many substances that are measured in various blood tests, only a few are ever found in the urine. Consequently, urine remains an easy way for a medical test to be done—but only if the substances to be measured or analyzed are present in the urine; and, in fact, few are.

24. For some urine tests the doctor has me clean and wash my genital area before providing the specimen. Other times I simply urinate into a container without any preparation. What is the difference between these two kinds of urine tests?

The first kind of specimen—called a clean-catch urine—is used whenever an infection in the kidneys or bladder is suspected. Cleaning the genital area is necessary because in those circumstances a urine culture (p. 174) must be performed, a test that requires that the urine specimen not be contaminated by bacteria from the skin. For all other urine tests it is sufficient to void directly into the container and the specimen need not be sterile.

25. Sometimes my doctor has me provide a specimen during my visit to his office, while other times he gives me a container and I collect my urine for 24 hours and return it to his office. Why?

There are two ways to collect a specimen for a urinalysis. The first method is to collect from the patient a single urine sample. We use this type of specimen—called a random urine or spot urine—for most urine tests. If we are checking for the possibility of a urinary tract infection, we may request that this random specimen be a clean-catch urine as well. Sometimes, however, it is important to measure over a 24-hour period the excretion of certain chemicals or substances into the urine. In such cases, we will ask you to collect the urine for 24 hours, and the appropriate test is performed on the entire specimen.

26. When I do provide my physician with a 24-hour specimen, he gives me a large container with some liquid in it. What is in the container and how should the urine be collected?

The biggest problem we face with collecting urine over 24 hours is that during the course of the day the substance in the urine to be measured may decompose, often due to the growth of bacteria in the specimen. There are two things to prevent bacteria from contaminating your specimen. First, the container in which the urine is collected may contain a small amount of liquid preservative that will kill any bacteria before they have a chance to do harm. This liquid will also serve to preserve the urine and any substances in it until the test is completed. The other way of decreasing the chance of bacterial contamination is to store the specimen in the refrigerator over the 24-hour period. Each time a patient urinates, he should collect the urine in a small container and then pour the specimen into the large container that is kept in the refrigerator.

27. When I am giving a random specimen and not a 24-hour one, does it matter what time of day the urine is collected?

Since a person does not usually drink any liquid during the night, the first urine voided in the morning is the most concentrated and contains the highest levels of the various chemicals and substances that are normally present. Often, therefore, we will ask for the first morning specimen.

28. Other than washing myself for a clean-catch specimen, is any preparation necessary on my part before a urine test is collected?

Preparation is rarely required for urine tests. Sometimes we will request our patients not to eat or drink the night before a specimen is collected. Occasionally, we will put patients on a special diet for a few days before the test is done. Again, as with all tests, it is your job to ask your doctor if it is necessary for you to prepare in any manner or do anything special before a test is performed.

29. What happens to the urine after the specimen is sent to the laboratory?

It depends on what specific kind of urine test is being performed. In general, there are four different ways to conduct a urine test: (1) dipstick analysis, (2) automated processing, (3) microscopic examination, (4) culture.

Dipstick analysis is the most common. In this kind of urinalysis, the dipstick—a narrow strip of plastic about 4 by ¼ inches—is dipped into the specimen. Depending on the specific dipstick being used, small squares of paper (from one to eight) on the end of the dipstick will change color when exposed to various chemicals or substances in the urine. In this way the presence of blood, acid, protein, and sugar can be quickly and simply determined. *Automated processing* uses laboratory machinery to measure these and other chemicals. Although these measurements are more sensitive than those obtained from a dipstick, a trained laboratory technician is needed to run the expensive equipment. We use *microscopic examination* to visualize any bacteria or blood cells that are present in the urine. Finally, the urine can be tested in a *culture* to detect the possible presence of bacteria.

X-Rays, Computerized Axial Tomography (CT) Scans, Nuclear Medicine, and Ultrasound

30. What are x-rays?

Simply put, x-rays are pictures of the body. All x-rays involve the same basic principle: they have a short wavelength, which gives them a special quality not shared by visible light—they can pass through solid objects, such as patients and walls. But x-rays are similar to visible light in that they cause a chemical change to occur on photographic film from which a picture can be developed.

31. If x-rays pass right through the body, how does a picture result?

Although x-rays pass through solid substances, the actual amount that can pass will vary depending on how dense the substance is. For example, x-rays penetrate and pass easily through feathers, a substance that is not very dense. On the other hand, x-rays virtually do not pass through lead, an extremely dense substance. What would an x-ray picture of a piece of lead inside a bag of feathers look like? The feathers would barely show up on the picture because the x-ray beam would pass right through them, while the piece of lead—which blocks the passage of x-rays—would leave a distinct shadow image on the x-ray film. X-rays are most useful, therefore, in distinguishing between objects of different

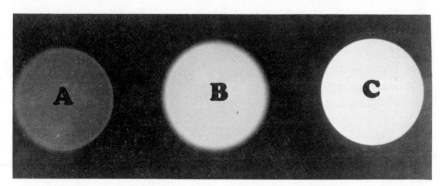

X-ray of glasses containing liquids of different densities. Glass A contains oil, which produces the x-ray density of fat in the body. Glass B contains water, which is the x-ray density of most solid tissues in the body (e.g., heart and liver). Glass C contains barium contrast medium (p. 99), which is the x-ray density of bones. The glasses are surrounded by air, which produces a black x-ray image, as occurs with the lungs. (Courtesy of Dr. Paul Palefski.)

densities. The human body has varying densities within it. Bone is the most dense, because it is composed of calcium and minerals. The lungs—filled mainly with air—are the least dense. Most of the other organs and tissues have a density between these two.

32. *If x-rays are like photographs, why do they look different?*

Although x-rays work on the same principle as photographs, they really look nothing like the pictures you take with your camera. This is true because x-rays are negative prints and therefore will come out the exact opposite of what you would expect. The x-ray image of a bone is white because no x-ray beam passed through it. Conversely, the x-ray image of the air-filled lung is black because all the x-ray beam was able to pass through it.

33. *How many different kinds of x-rays are there?*

There are four major kinds of x-ray pictures. Routine x-rays are the kind taken of the chest or an injured limb. The patient is placed in front of the photographic plate and the x-ray beam is directed through the part of the body to be examined onto the plate. These routine x-rays are called *plain films* or *flat plates.* A second kind of x-ray is *tomography.* In this technique, the x-ray "camera" moves around the patient, as does the photographic film. It allows the beam to focus only on the desired location and lessens the image of the surrounding tissues in the background. A third x-ray technique is called *computerized axial tomography* or *CT scan.* With this method, the "camera" takes hundreds of x-ray pictures from various angles. These images are fed into a computer and analyzed. *Fluoroscopy* consists of moving x-rays that are projected onto a television screen. This permits the doctor to see movement of various parts of the body.

In addition to these four major types of x-rays, there are other types less commonly used. One example is *xerography* (p. 124), which combines the technology of x-rays with that found in photocopying (Xerox) machines.

34. *One time, when I was suffering from chronic indigestion, the doctor had me drink some barium before taking x-rays. What was the barium used for?*

Barium is one of several substances—called contrast agents or dyes—that are used in taking x-rays. Since x-rays depend upon the differing densities within the body, it is sometimes necessary to enhance these differences. For example, the intestines and the abdominal cavity in which they are found have the same general density, somewhere between that of air and bone. Consequently, a plain film x-ray of the abdomen is limited in the amount of information it can reveal because it does not distinguish between the individual organs. If the intestines, however, are filled with a material that is very dense, a contrast in densities is created, allowing for much better detail to be visible in the x-rays that are taken.

Contrast agents can be swallowed (as in the case of an upper GI series, p. 128), used as an enema (as with a barium enema, p. 109), or injected into the vein (as is done with an intravenous pyelogram or IVP, p. 121). Contrast agents have greatly improved the utility of x-rays, and they can be used in conjunction with the other techniques available, such as CT scans. They do, however, have two serious disadvantages associated with their use. First, some people are allergic to them, and, consequently, their use can result in serious, even life-threatening allergic reactions. Thus, patients with a history of previous allergic reactions may not be able to have these kinds of tests done. A second problem is that, because of the chemical nature of the contrast agents, kidney damage can result from their injection into the veins or arteries, especially in elderly patients or those with other medical problems such as diabetes. We often give these patients extra fluids—either orally or intravenously—to decrease the chance of this problem.

35. Are x-rays dangerous?

Yes. It has been proven that the radiation used in taking x-rays can cause birth defects, cancer, and leukemia. But some x-rays are more dangerous than others because they expose the patient to much more radiation. In addition, these risks from radiation are cumulative, and the more often you are exposed to x-rays, the greater is the danger. This does not mean, however, that x-rays should never be taken. What it does mean is that you must do everything you can to lessen their danger. In general, the newer x-ray equipment in use today exposes the patient to less radiation than did the older machines. For a more detailed discussion, see p. 100.

36. What can be done to lessen the danger from x-rays?

It will never be possible to remove all the risk from x-ray exposure, but you can lessen it by remembering the following two points:

1. Don't have x-rays unless they are absolutely necessary, and if x-rays are taken, make sure they are as few as possible. How do you know if an x-ray is necessary? You can start by asking the doctor why the x-ray is being taken. If the doctor cannot give you a good reason, then it should not be done. Also, less is generally better; often, even when x-rays are necessary, fewer pictures may be required then previously thought. For example, it used to be the policy in most hospitals that a child who suffers a convulsion should have an x-ray examination of the skull to see if the seizure was due to the presence of a brain tumor. At one time this resulted in such a patient having a total of six x-rays of the skull. Now we know that one x-ray—taken from the side of the skull—provides as much information as six. Consequently, it has become our policy that children with seizures must still have x-rays, but one instead of six will suffice.

2. Be sure that the radiologist or technician places lead shields over those parts of the body not being x-rayed and likely to be damaged by unnecessary x-ray exposure. Special attention should always be given to protecting the testes and ovaries of children and adults of child-bearing age. For example, an x-ray of the chest should be done only with a lead apron placed over the reproductive organs.

37. Are x-rays riskier for a pregnant woman than for a nonpregnant one?

Definitely yes. A fetus, especially during the first three months of pregnancy, is very susceptible to x-ray damage. Although it is known that x-rays can damage the fetus, it is not at all certain whether one or several x-rays are necessary for this to happen. Therefore, the basic rule here is simple: pregnant women should have no x-rays of any kind (even dental x-rays) unless they are absolutely necessary.

38. Who takes x-rays?

The radiology technician is the person who usually positions the patients, places the film, shoots the picture, and develops the x-ray. The physician specialist, who "reads" and interprets the x-ray, is called a radiologist. Radiologists have M.D. degrees and have completed an intensive and lengthy residency program lasting many years.

39. Why are x-rays so expensive?

The bill for an x-ray covers two costs—the x-ray itself as well as the charge for the radiologist to interpret it. Sometimes these two charges are separate, while other times they will appear as a single amount. X-rays are expensive medical tests because the equipment with which they are done is costly. For example, a CT scanner can cost several hundred thousand dollars. Also, the recent increase in the cost of silver, an important ingredient in the photographic plates used in x-rays, has contributed to the increase in costs.

40. What is nuclear medicine?

Nuclear medicine is a specialized technique that uses radioisotopes—radioactive materials that emit radiation—to detect disease in the body. Various radioisotopes are used for specific parts of the body and will be absorbed differently by healthy tissues than by diseased or abnormal ones. The differences in radioactivity that result between healthy and diseased tissue can be detected by the use of a machine, similar to a Geiger counter, that measures the radioactivity that is continuously emitted by the radioisotope. For example, the radioisotope called technetium phosphate is absorbed by bone. If a bone scan is ordered, the patient will be injected with that radioisotope and the scan will reveal any abnormal distribution of the radioactivity in his bones.

41. Since radioisotopes are radioactive, are such tests very dangerous?

In fact, routine x-rays are more dangerous than radioisotopes since the amount and nature of the radioactivity that these chemicals emit are low-grade. However, as with all radiation, its exposure should be limited to only those circumstances when it is absolutely necessary. And, in fact, there are two circumstances when a nuclear medicine scan should be avoided if possible. Nuclear medicine tests should never be performed on a pregnant woman or a mother who is breast feeding, since many of the radioisotopes are passed through the milk and would be ingested by the nursing infant.

42. What is ultrasound?

Ultrasound examinations—also called ultrasonography or echography—are a way to visualize the internal structures and organs by recording the reflection of ultrasonic waves directed at the body. They are based on the same principle as the sonar found on ships. The reflections of the ultrasonic waves bouncing off the internal organs produce a distinctive pattern that can be recorded on film or an oscilloscope. The actual film tracing that result is called an echogram or a sonogram.

43. *Are ultrasound examinations dangerous?*

They do not involve any radiation or radioactive energy, and as far as we know at this time they cause no harm to the patient. Nevertheless, until they are proven to be fully safe beyond any doubt, they should be performed only when there is a compelling reason to do so.

44. *Why doesn't ultrasound replace x-rays?*

In many instances it has. For example, at one time if we needed to know the location of the fetus's head in the pregnant mother— as might be the case if breech birth is suspected—an x-ray was taken. Today we would use ultrasound instead. But even though the technology is improving, ultrasound does not currently produce pictures with the same detail and clarity as do x-rays. Second, since ultrasound does not penetrate air, it is not useful in the examination of air-filled organs such as the lungs.

45. *All right, the doctor has available many techniques that serve to take pictures—of one form or another—of the inside of my body. How does he decide which technique to use in any situation?*

Although these techniques all view the body, they emphasize different aspects and are most useful under varying circumstances. For example, let us take the case of two patients who came to us complaining of abdominal pain. The first was a 52-year-old man who began to have pain in his upper abdomen that was worse on an empty stomach and was relieved by taking antacids or drinking milk. The second patient was a 45-year-old woman who had abdominal pain on her upper right side, most often after eating fried food. What tests did we order?

Many tests that we have discussed—ultrasound, plain x-rays, contrast x-rays, tomography, CT scans—could have been used to view the various organs of the abdomen. But the doctor does not order all these tests for these patients. For the first patient, in

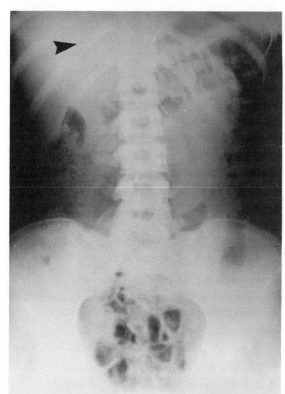

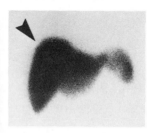

Four different techniques by which a doctor can evaluate a patient's liver, identified in each with an arrow. Top left: abdominal x-ray (KUB, p. 105); top right: liver-spleen scan (p. 141); bottom left: abdominal ultrasound (p. 147); bottom right: abdominal CT scan (p. 115).

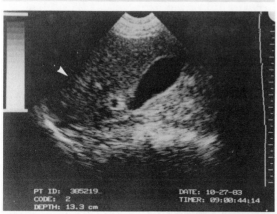

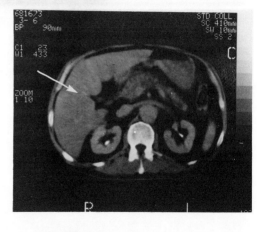

whom we suspected an ulcer, we ordered an upper GI series. For the second patient, in whom gallbladder disease was suspected, an ultrasound was obtained. The same is true of all our patients. Based on the particular symptoms or results of other laboratory tests, we will order one or more of these studies.

Costs

46. How much do medical tests cost?

The easy answer is "too much." Health care is the second largest industry in this country and is growing in fact at a quicker rate than any other. It contributes approximately 10% to the Gross National Product—well over 100 billion dollars a year. Medical tests make up a significant proportion of that amount, with recent studies showing that over 20 billion dollars was spent on medical tests in 1982 alone.

47. Why are medical tests so expensive?

There are many components that add to the cost of medical tests. The following is a list of the various steps involved in the performance of the simplest kind of medical test—a blood test.

1. A technician must draw blood from the patient.
2. The blood must be transported to the laboratory.
3. A technician must process the blood.
4. A machine must be used to analyze the sample.
5. The test results must be recorded and checked for accuracy.
6. The report must be sent to the doctor who requested the test.

Each part of this complex process costs money and increases the expense of the test. Although many blood tests have been automated and results can now be obtained faster than ever before, the machines used are very expensive. This is one example of where modern automation has saved time but not money. Many other tests such as x-rays and electrocardiograms have another aspect that add considerably to the cost: besides the expense involved in performing the test, a second fee is generated because a medical specialist is needed to interpret the results. Finally, still other tests, such as a cardiac catheterization, involve an additional set of costs because the patient must be hospitalized for a few days while the test is being done. During this hospital stay blood tests must be performed before the actual catheterization occurs to make sure the patient is well enough to undergo the testing. These additional preliminary tests together with the hospital stay can be quite costly.

48. Does every laboratory charge the same amount for a specific test?

The price of a specific laboratory test, such as a blood glucose, will vary among the different parts of the country, as well as among the various types of laboratory where the test is performed. A large commercial laboratory that is open from 9:00 A.M. to 5:00 P.M. on weekdays only and limits itself to commonly performed tests may be able to charge much less than a hospital laboratory that must remain open 24 hours every day, holidays and weekends included. Moreover, most hospital laboratories must provide the facilities to do a variety of rarely performed and expensive tests. This also increases the cost considerably. Finally, hospitals sometimes use medical tests as a means of sharing the expenses for items that they cannot explicitly charge the patient (overhead, salaries, maintenance, etc.). Hospitals know that patients (and their insurance companies) will not object to paying large amounts for a battery of sophisticated medical tests. On the other hand, it is much more difficult to charge for the time a nurse spent counseling a dying patient and his family.

Also, it should be made clear that there is little of the competitive pricing for medical tests among laboratories as there is for drugs among pharmacies. This lack of price competition has kept medical test costs high and resulted in widely varying prices for the same test within the same city.

49. Why are twelve blood tests sometimes cheaper than four tests?

In the early 1960s the development of more sophisticated machinery enabled laboratories to perform 12 different blood tests on one tube of blood. Even if only one of these 12 tests was ordered by the physician, the machine ran and obtained results for all 12. Laboratories have continued to encourage doctors to obtain all twelve results even if they want only three or four because special handling is necessary if the machine is not used in the usual fashion. Therefore, since commercial laboratories frequently bill the 12 tests as a unit package, the cost is less than that for the individual tests.

50. Who pays for medical tests?

In most states Blue Cross, Medicare (public assistance for the elderly), Medicaid (public assistance for the poor), or other health insurance plans pay for all or a substantial part of most medical tests that are ordered. Although you may not be actually paying directly, all of us pay for medical tests through increased insurance premiums (in the case of health insurance) and our taxes (in the case of Medicare and Medicaid). Indiscriminate and inappropriate use of tests will increase these costs. We have included a cost figure with each test. We hope that by listing these costs we will all be motivated to use medical tests more effectively.

3

How to Get the Most Out of
Your Medical Tests

BASED on our experiences in taking care of patients, we are convinced that learning about medical tests will make you a more educated patient and one more responsible for your own health care. Throughout the rest of the book, we will provide you with factual information about medical tests—how they are done, when to get them, and how they should properly be used in health and disease. This chapter, however, will not explain any specific test but, instead, will give you a plan to follow in order to get the most out of your medical tests.

One: Understand that even though medical tests are very important, they can never replace a good relationship with your doctor.

There are many different aspects to your health care besides medical tests, including diet, exercise, periodic visits to your doctor, and the proper use of medical treatment when required. Although medical tests will help your doctor to evaluate your health, they are but one small part of this entire process. No matter how accurate and effective these tests are, they can never compensate for a person who is careless about his health, nor can they replace a good relationship with your doctor. The most important part of any visit to your doctor's office is not the EKG, or the blood tests, or the urinalysis, or any test for that matter. It is communicating with your doctor and establishing a comfortable relationship.

Two: Before any test is done, be satisfied that you understand why it is necessary.

33

By establishing a good relationship with your doctor, you will begin to learn how he thinks about problems and approaches their solution, including the proper use of medical tests. When you understand the way your doctor is thinking, you can become actively involved in your health care. Before a doctor considers the use of a medical test in any patient, he will ask himself three questions. It is the answer to these three questions that will ultimately determine if a test is ordered or not.

1. What specific information will this particular test tell me about the patient at this time? No matter what the test, the answer to this question will identify for the doctor the specific facts he can learn by doing this test.

2. What difference will these facts make in the care of the patient? If the test will make no difference at all—in either the diagnosis, prognosis, medical treatment, or approach to the patient—then the test should probably not be done.

3. What risks and discomforts are associated with this test? Only if the benefits gained from the test outweigh the risks and discomforts will the test be done. As a patient you should ask yourself these same three questions before a test is done, and if you are not sure of the answers, do not be afraid to discuss them with your doctor.

Three: Ask your doctor the following questions before any medical test is done:

1. What is the purpose of this test in my particular situation?

2. How is the test actually done?

3. What are the risks and discomforts associated with this test, and what can be done to lessen them?

4. What preparation must I make before the test?

5. Will any medications or drugs that I am currently using interfere with the test results?

6. When will the results be made available to me?

7. Would the results of any previous medical tests that I have taken be useful?

8. How much will the test cost?

Four: Be sure you carry out any preparation that is required on your part for the test, and do all you can to make sure the test will be accurate.

As we have mentioned previously, most tests require some preparation on your part. Be sure that such preparation is done accurately. If a test requires that you fast beforehand, even a small breakfast will invalidate the results. Always ask if a test requires preparation. Many hospital radiology departments have brochures or instruction sheets available that will detail these preparations, especially before tests like a barium enema or upper GI series. If the doctor doesn't mention any specific preparation, check with him or the nurse and consult this book to be sure.

There are many reasons why tests are sometimes inaccurate—and you can help in this area. First, be sure that the test the doctor has ordered is the one that is being done. If you and he discussed doing a chest x-ray, and you get to the radiology suite, where the technicians begin talking about drinking barium and taking pictures as you swallow, it is your right to speak up and question what is going on. If your doctor mentions that a urine culture is required, and the nurse gives you a specimen cup but no swabs or instructions about cleaning yourself, ask why that is the case. In addition, be sure that all x-rays and specimens (blood, urine) are properly labeled with your name so they will not become confused with those from another patient. Most of all, since many medications and drugs that patients take interfere with test results, be sure that your doctor is aware of any medicine you may be taking, even over-the-counter preparations you can buy without a prescription.

Five: Find out the results (as well as their interpretation) of any medical tests that are done.

Many people have a test done and then sit back and wait for someone to contact them with the result. Sometimes the doctor's office will let you know the test result only if it is abnormal or if further testing or treatment is required. It is your right, however, to find out the results of tests that are done, for a normal result will be reassuring to you. In any case, no matter what your results are, be sure to record them (as we will discuss shortly) in a medical test diary.

Although it is important for you to find out your test results, *what you really want to know is the interpretation*, not the actual numbers. For example, suppose your doctor suspects you are anemic and orders a complete blood count as a diagnostic test. The information that should concern you most is not the actual hematocrit (33% for example) but the interpretation: was the hematocrit low and anemia present, or was it normal. Similarly, when an x-ray is performed, the report from the radiologist that gets sent to your doctor has two parts: the upper portion of the report gives his description of what he actually sees on the x-ray, while the lower portion gives his interpretation. Don't be as concerned with what the x-ray actually looked like (e.g., ". . . mucosal surface looked smooth without lesions") as with the interpretation (". . . intestine was normal").

Having just used the terms normal and abnormal, let's review some of the points we have made elsewhere in this book about their use. A healthy patient can receive an abnormal test result, while a sick patient can receive a normal one. Tests are not always 100% accurate and the terms normal and abnormal are not perfect.

Let's look at a couple of examples. We once saw in the office a 42-year-old hard-driving executive who came to us complaining of abdominal pain that used to awaken him during the night. The pain would vanish when he drank milk, and recently he started taking antacids frequently. We made the diagnosis of an ulcer and sent him for an upper GI series to confirm this diagnosis. The test result came back normal. Does that mean that an ulcer is definitely not present? No. It simply means that an ulcer was not seen on that x-ray—a very different conclusion. We then ordered a gastroscopy, which did in fact reveal the presence of a small duodenal ulcer. Was the upper GI series wrong? Yes, to the extent that it failed to detect the ulcer. But we were well aware that this was possible, even though the report from the upper GI series said that the study was normal. Similarly, we once sent off a complete blood count on a nine-month-old baby to screen for the presence of anemia. The blood test came back from the lab with a hematocrit result of 34% and a notation that this is abnormally low. Yet we told the mother that no anemia was present. Why? Because the laboratory result is printed out by a computer that does not differentiate between adults and children. While 34% is low for an adult and would be a sign of anemia, it is not an abnormal hematocrit for a nine-month-old baby.

Six: Remember that every patient is different.

We often lose sight of the fact that every patient is different. What do we mean? Your doctor has ordered a chest x-ray on you, and the only person you know who has had a chest x-ray is your

Uncle Harry who turned out to have tuberculosis when his x-ray was done. Does that mean that the doctor suspects tuberculosis in you? Probably not, because all patients are different, and the same chest x-ray can be ordered in different patients for different reasons. There is very little you can learn by comparing your medical case with that of another person. You are an individual, thus your medical case is unique. Don't bother comparing your tests or their results to those of anyone else, as little good will be gained.

Seven: Keep a medical test diary.

One point we have tried to make throughout the book is that you must share the responsibility with the medical profession for the appropriate and effective use of medical tests. One important way to do this is to keep an accurate and reliable medical test diary. This record should be made available to your doctor, especially when new medical tests are being considered. There are three ways in which this diary will help you.

1. The results of previous medical tests—even those taken months or years in the past—will often help your doctor in his thinking.

2. Many medical tests are most useful for comparison to previous results from the same test. For example, Linda L., a 40-year-old woman, has fibrocystic disease of the breast, a common condition in which benign tumors occur. Because of this problem, Linda had a mammogram done when she was 38. This year, when her doctor felt a new lump, he obtained another mammogram. There was a questionable lesion seen on the x-ray. By comparing the new mammogram with her old one, her doctor was able to assure her that the x-ray finding was not serious and was only one of the benign tumors that occur frequently in this disease. Had the old x-ray report been unavailable, the doctor would have been forced to do a biopsy.

3. Having the results from old medical tests will sometimes obviate the need for taking new ones.

You must remember that a medical test diary is not a substitute for your doctor's keeping good medical records. But today many patients will be under the concurrent care of more than one doctor. The results obtained from tests taken for one doctor will often not be sent or given to another. An accurate medical test diary can do much to alleviate this problem.

In Appendix 2 we give a sample diary and explain our method of how to keep one for you and your family.

Eight: Ask questions.

Perhaps the most important lesson we would like you to take away from this book is that your involvement in your medical care must not be passive. You must be involved—and the best way to do that is to ask questions. Every doctor should conclude his visit with you by asking if you have any questions. If you do, don't be afraid to ask them. If you are not certain why a test is being done, ask the doctor to explain. If you are not sure why a particular medicine is being ordered, question the doctor about it.

Sometimes your doctor will not have the time during that visit to answer all your questions. If so, make an appointment with him to discuss your questions and concerns. We encourage and welcome patients to make what we call in our office "talk appointments," and we spend the entire visit answering their queries.

Remember: the first step toward better medical care is patient education. And the first step in education is asking questions.

PART II

The Most Important Medical Tests

4

Blood Tests

It is a morning in 1674 in Amsterdam. As soon as dawn breaks, Anton van Leeuwenhoek, a young Dutch scientist, pulls himself from his bed and walks to the table positioned near an open window so as to catch the first rays of the sun. Sitting on the table is the project to which he will devote his life's work—the first microscope. Invented by him just a few months before, he has been spending these last weeks using it to examine anything he could place on the microscope slide.

Like many others of his times he is an explorer—not traveling across previously uncharted oceans but moving into a world previously invisible to man's eye. This morning he will use his microscope once more to study something new. He takes a sharpened knife and, wincing slightly, uses it to cut his finger, then collects a drop of his blood on one of his microscope slides. Positioning the mirror of the microscope carefully so as to receive the most sunlight, he places the slide on the microscope and peers through. He is amazed at what he sees. Blood is not a pure liquid at all but instead is composed of millions of small cells floating in the liquid. Most of the cells he sees are red; for this reason blood looks red. Other cells are colorless. Fascinated and entranced, he spends the day without moving, except to write down some notes and draw pictures of what he sees.

We have made tremendous progress in the scientific and careful examination of blood since that day over three hundred years ago. Today, in hospital laboratories, automated microscopes every hour will analyze and interpret the blood from fifty different patients.

It probably seems that whenever you go to the doctor, whether in sickness or in health, blood tests are performed. And there are so many different kinds. Usually your doctor will tell you that in addition to whatever else he has to do he is "going to get a blood test," and he does not go into great detail about what specifically is being measured. In fact, from one tube of blood as many as twenty different chemicals and minerals in the blood can be measured. Before we go into detail about the individual tests, let's review some of the basic information about blood and the way blood tests are done. (Some additional questions about blood tests are discussed on p. 17.)

As van Leeuwenhoek discovered, blood is a mixture of many different substances, and because each one can be measured, there are many different kinds of blood tests. The easiest way to think of blood is to remember that it is composed of two major parts: solid and liquid. The solid portion of blood consists of three different kinds of cells: red cells, white cells (the colorless ones that van Leeuwenhoek saw), and platelets. The liquid portion of blood—called serum if the blood is allowed to clot before the liquid is removed, and plasma if it is not—contains numerous chemicals, minerals, proteins, hormones, antibodies, and other substances found within the blood stream.

The manner in which blood tests are done has changed remarkably within the last few years. As recently as 25 years ago, only a few sophisticated laboratories could perform blood tests, and these took many hours because they were done by hand. Our professors in medical school used to regale us with stories of how they would spend the entire night performing laborious measurements on sick patients who had been admitted to the hospital. Today all that has changed. Nearly all commonly performed blood tests are done automatically on machinery that can process many different blood samples in a few minutes.

Little progress, however, has been made in the standardization of the units in which test results are reported. This is discussed in greater detail earlier in the book (p. 8), but suffice it to say that the current system is very confusing. Because many laboratories use different units, it is difficult to compare results.

There are two methods in which samples of blood for the different blood tests can be obtained:

1. The most common is venipuncture, in which blood is taken from a vein in the arm or occasionally from veins in other parts of the body as well. The person drawing the blood—doctor, nurse, or laboratory technician—ties an elastic band around the upper

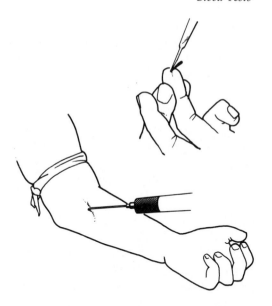

The two ways of obtaining blood from a patient: fingerstick (top) or venipuncture (bottom).

arm. This band, called a tourniquet, is made tightly enough to prevent the flow of blood in the veins, causing them to bulge beneath the surface of the skin. The person drawing the blood will feel for the vein with his finger and then clean the skin over it with alcohol. A needle will then be placed into the vein and the blood collected into a tube or syringe. Once enough blood has been obtained, the tourniquet is released and a gauze pad or cotton ball placed over the needle as it is withdrawn from the vein. The patient is usually asked to place pressure on this gauze to stop the bleeding, and then a small bandage is applied. Sometimes you will hear him say that "his veins are hard to find." And even after the tourniquet is placed, his veins are difficult to feel. He can, however, always point out to the person drawing the blood the site of the vein that had been easiest to find for past blood tests.

2. The other method is by a fingerstick or heelstick, the latter used almost exclusively in newborn infants. Alcohol is used to clean the skin, and a small sharp piece of metal, called a lancet, is used to prick the tip of the finger or the heel. The blood is then squeezed out and either collected in a small glass tube or placed directly on a microscope slide.

With either of these two methods of drawing blood, slight pain or bruising can occur. Very rarely, the patient may become dizzy and even faint momentarily.

Unless otherwise stated in the discussion of a specific blood test, no patient preparation is required for any of these tests, and the sample can be drawn at any time.

ACID PHOSPHATASE

Acid phosphatase is an enzyme that is widely distributed throughout the body but has its highest concentration in the prostate gland. The most common cause of increased acid phosphatase levels is prostate cancer. Recently, a new method has been developed for measuring acid phosphatase levels using an antibody technique that is better able to detect even very small amounts of the enzyme. At one time it was thought that screening healthy men with this test would be very useful for early detection of prostate cancer. In fact, numerous articles were written about the development of the male "PAP" test (*prostatic acid phosphatase*). More recent studies, however, have shown that this is not a reliable screening test in healthy men, and its major use comes in following the clinical course of men who have already been diagnosed as having that disease.

NORMAL RANGE: 0–2 U / L.
COST: approximately $10.

AMYLASE

The starch in our diet must be converted into sugar before our body can use it effectively. This is accomplished by the enzyme *amylase*. It is mainly secreted by the pancreas and salivary glands. If either of these two organs is inflamed, amylase will be leaked into the blood and found there in higher than usual levels. This occurs in pancreatitis (inflammation of the pancreas) as well as other abdominal diseases. Amylase levels will also be elevated in mumps, which causes inflammation of the salivary glands. A variety of drugs can give a falsely elevated level, especially narcotic pain killers, including codeine, Demerol, Talwin, and morphine.

NORMAL RANGE: 5–37 U / L.
COST: approximately $10.

Antinuclear Antibody (ana) and Rheumatoid Factor (rf)

A basic tenet of medicine is that the patient's immune system fights off foreign substances but does not react against the patient himself. In a group of diseases—generally called autoimmune diseases or collagen-vascular diseases—this rule seems to be broken and the patient's immune system begins to attack the body itself. There are many such diseases but the most important are lupus erythematosus and rheumatoid arthritis.

These two tests, *antinuclear antibody (ana) and rheumatoid factor (rf)*, are designed to detect this abnormal reaction of the immune system against the patient. The ana, commonly found in patients with lupus, detects antibodies that attack the patient's own deoxyribonucleic acid (dna) and other parts of the cells, while the rheumatoid factor, usually detected in patients with rheumatoid arthritis, measures abnormal antibodies that attack the patient's own immunoglobulins (proteins important to the immune system). All of these tests are nonspecific. A positive or negative result in any of them does not confirm or rule out any of the various autoimmune diseases, but it suggests to the physician some likely possibilities.

NORMAL RESULT: negative.
COST: RF—approximately $10.
ANA—approximately $25.

Bilirubin

Bilirubin is a product of the body's breakdown of hemoglobin. It is carried by the blood to the liver, where it is chemically processed into a form that can be excreted by the body into the urine and stool. Bilirubin exists in two forms in the body: *Indirect bilirubin,* which has not yet been processed by the liver; and *direct bilirubin,* which has. When a *bilirubin level* is sent to the laboratory, a total bilirubin level—direct and indirect combined—is initially measured. If this is elevated beyond the normal range, further tests are performed on the sample to measure separately the direct and indirect bilirubin levels.

In general, too much bilirubin in the blood results from one of two causes: either the body is making bilirubin at a much greater than usual rate, or it is making the usual amount but excreting it at a less than normal rate. Excessive red blood cell destruction, as can occur in a variety of diseases, is the cause of too rapid a bilirubin production, while liver or gallbladder disease is the usual cause of decreased excretion. If the increased bilirubin level is high enough (hyperbilirubinemia), the patient will appear yellow (jaundiced). Bilirubin levels are frequently done in patients with anemia (p. 309), hepatitis, abdominal pain (p. 285), and anyone who is jaundiced (p. 300). Many drugs can cause elevated bilirubin levels, including a variety of antibiotics, blood pressure pills, oral contraceptives, and narcotic-based pain killers.

NORMAL RANGE: total bilirubin—0.1–1.0 mg / dl.
                  direct bilirubin—0–0.3 mg / dl.
COST: approximately $10.

Blood Typing

The red blood cells of every person carry certain proteins on their surface, called antigens, that can be used to characterize, or type, the cells. There are two major antigen systems and several minor ones. The major antigen systems are ABO and Rh. With regard to the ABO system, every person will fall into one of four categories:

1. Blood type A (A antigen is found on the red cell surface).
2. Blood type AB (both A and B antigens are found on the cell surface).
3. Blood type B (B antigen is found on the red cell surface).
4. Blood type 0 (neither A nor B antigen is found on the cell surface).

With regard to the Rh system (named for the *Rh*esus monkey in whom it was discovered earlier this century), people can be in one of two categories:

1. Blood type Rh positive or (+) (Rh antigen is found on the cell surface).
2. Blood type Rh negative or (–) (Rh antigen is not found on the red cell surface).

Using both systems in combination, a person's blood type can be identified as one of eight: A+, A–, B+, B–, AB+, AB–, O+, O–.

Blood typing is important because blood transfusions should come only from blood donors with matching blood grouping as the patient-recipient. If a blood donor of an inappropriate type is used—called a mismatch—a serious, even life-threatening transfusion reaction can occur.

Blood typing of all potential blood donors and patients is done in the blood bank of a hospital. When a physician orders that a patient receive a blood transfusion, a "type and cross" test is done. First, the patient's blood type is determined and a unit of donated blood in the bank with the appropriate ABO and Rh type is identified. Then that unit is "crossed" or checked with the patient's blood to screen for the possibility of transfusion reactions due to blood antigen differences in systems other than ABO and Rh. If the unit shows no such reactivity against the patient's blood, it is then released from the blood bank for transfusion into the patient.

Blood typing is also important during pregnancy, because if the mother and baby are of two different blood types (as is frequently the case, since the genes that control blood type come from both parents), serious reactions in the baby can occur during pregnancy and at the time of delivery. Blood typing is also useful in paternity testing, although this has been largely replaced by HLA typing (p. 66). Blood types are generally reported as the ABO type— A, B, AB or O—as well as Rh positive or negative.

COST: blood typing only—approximately $15.; the actual cost of transfusion is higher because it involves the use of the blood.

CALCIUM, PHOSPHORUS, AND MAGNESIUM

Calcium is the mineral found in the highest quantity in our bodies. It is necessary for a variety of bodily functions to work properly, including muscle contraction, heart function, blood clotting, and the transmission of nerve impulses. It is also necessary for the formation of strong and durable teeth and bones, where over 98% of the body's calcium is stored. The proper level of calcium is so important for a variety of critical functions that our bodies allow very little fluctuation in the amount of calcium that circulates in the blood.

There are two ways by which the body keeps the calcium level tightly regulated. First, there is a complex series of hormones, the most important of which is parathyroid hormone which works, in part, by controlling the amount of calcium excreted in the urine. Second, the bones act as a storage depot for calcium. If there is too much calcium circulating in the blood, the bones will take up the excess and bring the level down into the normal range. Similarly, if the calcium level in the blood is too low, the bones will send some of their stored calcium into the blood to raise the level to the normal range. If a person were to have no calcium in his diet, the calcium level in the blood would not vary much, but the bones would slowly soften as they excrete stored calcium into the blood stream to maintain the normal level. In addition, the kidneys and vitamin D are important in maintaining a normal calcium level in the blood.

The major symptoms of hypocalcemia (low calcium level in the blood) include muscle twitching and spasm. This condition can be caused by decreased function of the parathyroid glands, low dietary intake or absorption of vitamin D or calcium, as well as kidney disease. Too high a calcium level in the blood (hypercalcemia) can be caused by excessive function of the parathyroid gland, prolonged immobilization (as might happen with a patient recuperating from multiple fractures), and cancer. The symptoms of hypercalcemia are less specific than those of hypocalcemia but include lethargy, headache, loss of appetite, nausea, and vomiting. The level of calcium in the blood can be affected by a variety of drugs that patients might take, especially diuretics and vitamins.

NORMAL RANGE: 8.8–10.8 mg / dl.
COST: approximately $10.

Phosphorus, another important mineral in our body, is closely related to the body's calcium metabolism. In fact, most phosphorus in our bodies is stored in the bone in the form of calcium phosphate. Generally, calcium and phosphorus have an inverse relationship in their blood levels. Those diseases that are characterized by hypercalcemia (too high a blood calcium level) are often associated with hypophosphatemia (too low a phosphorus level). Similarly, those diseases that cause hypocalcemia (too low a calcium level) are usually associated with hyperphosphatemia (too much phosphates in the blood). The most common of these is kidney failure. Phosphorus is necessary for proper growth of healthy bone as well as the metabolism of food and its conversion into energy for the body's use. The measurement of phosphorus and calcium in the blood is almost always done at the same time.

NORMAL RANGE: 3–4.5 mg / dl.
COST: approximately $10.

Magnesium is another mineral that is required for normal body function. It is important in nerve and muscle function as well as in the metabolism of proteins and carbohydrates. The level of magnesium in the blood is related closely to that of calcium. When magnesium is low, calcium almost always is too. In fact, the symptoms of hypomagnesemia (too low a magnesium level in the blood) are similar to those of hypocalcemia (too low a calcium level in the blood). Magnesium is found in almost all foods, so it is difficult for a person eating a normal diet to have a magnesium deficit from nutritional reasons alone. Instead, most cases of hypomagnesemia care caused by liver disease or kidney failure. In addition, alcoholism and the use of diuretics can lead to hypomagnesemia. No special preparation is necessary prior to drawing a magnesium level. Most often, when a patient has blood drawn for a magnesium level, he will have the levels of other minerals (calcium, phosphorus, sodium, potassium) determined as well.

NORMAL RANGE: 1.5–2.4 mEq / L.
COST: approximately $15.

CARBOXYHEMOGLOBIN

When a person breathes carbon monoxide, this gas will combine with the hemoglobin in the red cells and form carboxyhemoglobin, which cannot transport or carry oxygen. This is why breathing carbon monoxide can quickly lead to death. The *carboxyhemoglobin* test measures how much of this substance is present in the blood. Its most important use is not to test for obvious carbon monoxide exposure—such as when a person is found unconscious with the automobile motor running in a closed garage—but, instead, to test for low levels of carbon monoxide that are occurring over an extended period of time.

Symptoms of this problem will include headaches, lethargy, and weakness. Some common causes include occupational exposure to exhaust fumes in factories as well as defective home heating units. This has become especially true with the increase in wood-burning stoves. Often, people who have survived a fire and possibly suffered smoke inhalation will have this test done. As much as 15% of hemoglobin may be poisoned to carboxyhemoglobin in smokers as well. In addition, studies have shown that the car-boxyhemoglobin level in city-dwellers may be much higher than that of their rural counterparts, probably from the continual expo-sure to automobile fumes.

NORMAL RANGE: less than 5% of total hemoglobin.
COST: approximately $30.

CARCINOEMBRYONIC ANTIGEN (CEA)

Carcinoembryonic antigen (CEA) derives its name from the fact that it is a protein found in embryos as well as in tumors (carcinomas) from the gastrointestinal tract of adults. The history of CEA mea-surement is an interesting one. When CEA was first discovered, it was thought that this protein would revolutionize the doctor's ability to detect cancer of the colon. We would simply get this blood test in every patient whom we suspected of having colon cancer, and if his CEA was elevated, we would know the diagno-sis. But these expectations did not last. Although 70% of patients with cancer of the colon do have an elevated CEA level, we now know that this level is commonly increased in patients with malignancies of other organs (e.g., the pancreas) as well as with certain noncancerous diseases of the gastrointestinal tract, such as colitis. Even more confusing is that the CEA is also elevated in patients who smoke cigarettes.

We soon learned that the CEA test—although an important one—has very definite limitations: (1) an elevated CEA level is not an absolute indication of the presence of cancer, (2) normal levels of CEA are not an absolute proof that cancer is absent or permanently cured, and (3) all other tests that are being done to diagnose and manage a patient with a real or suspected malignancy must still be performed even though CEA levels are being done.

A CEA measurement can be useful, especially in following a patient with a known colon cancer in order to monitor therapy and detect if the cancer is recurring. For example, if a doctor finds that the CEA is elevated in a patient with colon cancer and that after surgery and radiation therapy the level has returned to nor-mal, he will probably have repeat levels drawn every three to six months to check that the CEA does not rise again—a likely sign of the cancer returning.

NORMAL RANGE: 0–2.5 ng / ml.
COST: approximately $40.

COMPLETE BLOOD COUNT (CBC)

This test is the most commonly performed blood test. It provides enormous amounts of information about the three different types of cells located in the blood: red cells, white cells, and platelets. Although the most frequent reasons for having a complete blood count done are to check for the presence of anemia (too few red cells) or infection (too many white cells), the complete blood count actually measures more than those two conditions. It is composed of seven different tests performed automatically by a machine (usually called a Coulter Counter, named for the company that developed it). These seven tests are:

Red Blood Cell Tests
1. Red blood cell count
2. Hematocrit (Hct)
3. Hemoglobin (Hg or Hb)
4. Red blood cell indices

White Blood Cell Tests
5. White blood cell count (WBC)
6. White blood cell differential

Platelet Tests
7. Platelet count

In addition, whenever a complete blood count is obtained, a *peripheral smear analysis* is usually performed to examine the various blood cells with the aid of a microscope. Let us look at each of these tests separately to see how and why they are performed.

The most numerous type of blood cell is the red blood cell—an adult may have 30 trillion of them. Approximately 40% of the volume of blood is actually not liquid at all but is made up of these red blood cells. And since there are so many of them, it is not surprising that the color of blood is red. These red blood cells, or erythrocytes (Greek for "red cell"), are remarkably simple cells in that they are little more than packages of hemoglobin, the protein that binds oxygen. The sole function of red blood cells is to transport oxygen from the lungs to all parts of the body.

The *red blood cell count* is an actual measure of the number of red blood cells present. The *hematocrit,* which is the most powerful of these tests, measures the percentage of the blood volume that is made up of red blood cells. A low hematocrit percentage indicates that an anemia is present, but it does not specify the cause. The *hemoglobin* measures the amount of hemoglobin that is present in the blood. The *red blood cell indices* (MCV, MCH, MCHC) measure among other things the actual size of the red blood cells. This measurement is quite a remarkable achievement, considering that the average red blood cell is less than $\frac{1}{3000}$ of an inch in diameter, and is helpful in determining the specific cause of the anemia. Many times doctors obtain the hematocrit separately; in this case, the blood is usually collected from a fingerstick and the test is not done on a Coulter Counter but rather on a centrifuge designed for that purpose.

There are far fewer white blood cells than red cells: for every 1000 red blood cells there is only 1 white blood cell. The major function of white blood cells is to fight infection. The *white blood cell count* will measure the number of white blood cells present in the blood. The most common reason for the white blood cell count to be elevated is the presence of infection, although inflammation can cause an elevation as well. Very high white counts may be a sign of leukemia.

Not all white blood cells are the same, however. There are five different types that are normally found in the blood stream: neutrophils (also called polys), lymphocytes, monocytes, eosinophils, and basophils. In addition to knowing the total number of white blood cells, it is important to know what proportion of the cells is made up of each of these five different types. This information is obtained from the *white cell differential,* which will actually count the number of the five types of white cells and report it as a percentage of the total number of white cells present. The table on p. 54 lists the usual diseases associated with increased numbers of different types of white blood cells. Leukemia is an abnormal number of immature white blood cells; thus, the presence of large numbers of immature white cells will suggest the disease.

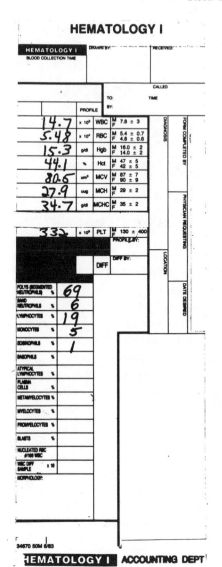

HEMATOLOGY I

PROFILE				
14.7	x 10³	WBC	M/F	7.8 ± 3
5.48	x 10⁶	RBC	M 5.4 ± 0.7 / F 4.8 ± 0.6
15.3	g/d	Hgb	M 16.0 ± 2 / F 14.0 ± 2
44.1	%	Hct	M 47 ± 5 / F 42 ± 5
80.5	um³	MCV	M 87 ± 7 / F 90 ± 9
27.9	uug	MCH	M/F 29 ± 2
34.7	g/d	MCHC	M/F 35 ± 2
332	x 10⁶	PLT	M/F 130 ± 400

DIFF	
POLYS (SEGMENTED NEUTROPHILS) %	69
BAND NEUTROPHILS %	6
LYMPHOCYTES %	19
MONOCYTES %	5
EOSINOPHILS %	1
BASOPHILS %	
ATYPICAL LYMPHOCYTES %	
PLASMA CELLS %	
METAMYELOCYTES %	
MYELOCYTES %	
PROMYELOCYTES %	
BLASTS %	
NUCLEATED RBC #/100 WBC	
WBC DIFF SAMPLE x 10	
MORPHOLOGY:	

34670 50M 6/83

HEMATOLOGY I **ACCOUNTING DEPT**

Coulter Counter (automated blood-cell analyzer) result in a 29-year-old woman with pneumonia. The white blood cell count (WBC) is elevated (14,700) and there is a higher percentage of polys and band neutrophils than usual. The other values on the printout are the red blood cell count (RBC, 5.48 million), hemoglobin (Hg, 15.3 gm/dl), hematocrit (Hct, 44.1%), red blood cell indices (MCV, MCH, and MCHC), platelet count (PLT, 332,000), and white blood cell differential.

Whenever a patient has fever, the white blood count and differential will be performed to determine the cause and to monitor the therapy used to treat the infection.

The function of platelets is to aid in the clotting of blood. A *platelet count* is obtained to see if adequate numbers of platelets are present to insure proper clotting. Excessive bleeding or frequent bruises can be caused by a decreased number of platelets and is a reason to measure the platelet count. Another test—the

PROBABLE CAUSES OF ELEVATION IN THE WHITE BLOOD
CELL COUNT

Increased Percentage of:	Is Usually Associated with:
Neutrophils (polys)	Bacterial Infection.
Lymphocytes	Viral Infection.
Monocytes	Viral Infection.
Eosinophils	Parasitic infection. Allergies. Asthma.
Basophils (rarely elevated)	Chronic Leukemia.

bleeding time (p. 80)—will determine whether the platelets that are present are working properly.

The *peripheral smear analysis* can be used to judge the size of the red blood cells; if any of these red cells have abnormal shapes, as can occur in anemia; the numbers of the different types of white blood cells; and if sufficient numbers of platelets are present. Evaluation of the peripheral smear in someone who has anemia will often help to pinpoint the specific cause of that problem. The normal range for CBC is listed below:

Hematocrit
Adult men: 42–52%
Adult women: 37–47%
Children: 31–41%
Newborns: 44–64%

Hemoglobin
Adult men: 14–18 gm / dl
Adult women: 12–16 gm / dl
Children: 10–15 gm / dl
Newborns: 14–25 gm / dl

Red Blood Cell Count
Adult men: 4.5–6.3 million / mm^3
Adult women: 4.2–5.4 million / mm^3
Children: 3.8–5.2 million / mm^3
Newborns: 4.1–6.1 million / mm^3

White blood Cell Count: 4,000–10,000 / mm³
Platelet Count: 150,000–350,000 / mm³

COST: approximately $10 for all of the tests.

COOMBS' TEST

Whenever a body is exposed to a foreign substance, such as a virus or a transplanted organ, it produces molecules called antibodies to attack these substances. Normally, the body does not have antibodies present that are directed against its own red blood cells. There are, however, three circumstances in which these antibodies might be found: (1) in a patient who received a blood transfusion that was not compatible with his own blood; (2) in an infant whose blood contains antibodies that have crossed through the placenta from a mother of a different blood type; and (3) in a patient with autoimmune hemolytic anemia, a disease in which the person begins to make antibodies against his own blood cells. The *Coombs' test* detects the presence in the blood of antibodies directed against red cells. Results are given as positive (antibody is found) or negative (no antibody is found).

NORMAL RESULT: negative.
COST: approximately $10.

DRUG LEVELS

Many of the medications that patients use daily, including over-the-counter drugs, can have dangerous side effects if present in too high quantities in the blood. But it is not always possible to know how much of a medication will be present in the blood because we cannot predict how quickly it will be absorbed or excreted. Drugs that are taken orally must first be absorbed into the blood stream from the stomach or intestine, and the speed and efficiency with which this happens will not be the same for all patients.

Drug levels are obtained when patients are brought to the hospital unconscious or exhibiting bizarre behavior, and the doctor suspects the use of illegal drugs or improper use of medications. The drug level will be zero (or below a detectable level) in the blood of a person not taking the specific medication being tested.

Patients taking a drug routinely may have a level that is in the therapeutic range (normal range), the toxic range (too-high range), or subtherapeutic range (too-low range). We have included the usual therapeutic range for many of the drugs, but your doctor may want to keep the blood level higher or lower than this range depending upon the specific clinical situation.

Blood levels can be obtained for almost all medications. Some commonly measured ones are:

Theophylline: This medication, which is used to treat asthma, can cause shakiness, abdominal pain, and even seizures if too much is present in the blood. Some people will take only small amounts of this medication and develop high blood levels, while others may take large amounts of this medication and still have low blood levels. Measuring the amount of theophylline in the blood will help guide the doctor as to what dosage of the drug should be taken. The same is true of many other drugs as well.

THERAPEUTIC RANGE: 10–20 mcg / ml.

Alcohol: When patients come to the hospital in coma or exhibiting bizarre behavior, an alcohol level is frequently measured. It is also measured for legal purposes after an automobile accident to determine if a driver is intoxicated. In most states an alcohol level greater than 0.10% is proof that the driver is intoxicated, while a level less than 0.05% is proof that legally he is not intoxicated. Levels between 0.05–0.10% are evidence of recent alcohol ingestion but not high enough for legal proof of intoxication. Most people are concerned with how much alcohol must be consumed before they become intoxicated, but this is not a reliable guide. For example, if a person who weighs 120 pounds takes two shots of whiskey on an empty stomach, he may have a blood level of 0.10%; if a 250-pound obese man drinks the same amount after a large meal, his blood level may be only 0.05%. Thus, it is important to remember that what really correlates with the effect of alcohol on driving and behavior is the blood level, and, as is true with all drugs, it is impossible to predict the level in the blood from the amount ingested.

Antibiotics (e.g., gentamycin): Measuring blood antibiotic levels is useful to determine if adequate amounts are present to treat the infection. In addition, one family of antibiotics, called aminoglycosides, of which gentamycin and tobramycin are examples, can cause serious kidney damage and hearing loss if present at too high a level in the blood. Many hospitalized patients receiving these antibiotics will have levels of these drugs measured to prevent these complications.

THERAPEUTIC RANGE 1 HOUR AFTER RECEIVING THE DRUG: 4–12 mcg / ml.

"TROUGH" LEVEL (AMOUNT IN THE BLOOD BEFORE THE NEXT DOSE OF MEDICATION IS GIVEN): less than 2 mcg / ml.

Barbiturates: When accidental or intentional overdose of these dangerous medications is suspected, blood levels will determine the specific type of barbiturate taken and facilitate appropriate treatment. Barbiturate levels are also obtained to monitor the level of the drug in patients taking it to control seizures (epilepsy).

THERAPEUTIC RANGE FOR PHENOBARBITAL: 15–40 mcg / ml.

Digoxin: This medication, which is helpful in treating heart disease, can cause irregular heart beats, vomiting, and hallucinations if taken in excessive doses. A blood level will determine if a dangerous level is present.

THERAPEUTIC RANGE: 0.8–2.0 ng / ml.

Dilantin: This medication, which is also used to treat seizures, can cause dizziness and irregular heart beats if taken in excessive doses. Measuring a blood level is helpful in order to adjust the dosage of this drug.

THERAPEUTIC RANGE: 10–20 mcg / ml.

Salicylates (aspirin): Aspirin ingestion is the most common cause of accidental poisoning in children. Measuring a blood level can determine whether an overdose has occurred, and, if so, how serious it is. A blood level is also helpful to monitor the dose of the drug in patients with arthritis.

THERAPEUTIC RANGE FOR TAKING ASPIRIN FOR ARTHRITIS: 10–20 mcg / dl.

Although no special preparation is necessary for these drug level tests, it is important to tell the doctor when you last took any medication.

COST: The cost for drug levels ranges, according to the particular drug being measured. Aspirin levels are the least expensive:

approximately $10.; barbiturates and other less commonly used antibiotics are higher: approximately $50.

ELECTROLYTES (SODIUM, POTASSIUM, CHLORIDE, BICARBONATE)

Electrolytes are four minerals—sodium, potassium, chloride, and bicarbonate—found in our body. Three of them—*sodium, potassium* and *chloride*—are involved in maintaining proper water balance in the body. They will be measured whenever it is suspected that the patient has lost too much fluid from the body (dehydration) or has too much water present. In addition, since the most important organ of the body involved in water regulation is the kidney, electrolytes will be measured whenever kidney disease or damage is suspected. Finally, many diuretics (medicines used to treat hypertension) cause too much of these minerals to be excreted, especially potassium, so that patients taking this kind of medication will also have this test performed frequently.

In contrast to the other three electrolytes—whose basic job is to maintain water balance in our body—the primary purpose of *bicarbonate* is to regulate the acidity of the blood. When the level of bicarbonate is elevated, the blood has low acidity (alkaline). The amount of bicarbonate in the blood is controlled by the kidney and the lungs. In addition to measuring bicarbonate from a routine blood test, the bicarbonate level can also be measured when an arterial blood gas (p. 183) is performed.

NORMAL RANGE: Sodium: 134–145 meq / L.
Potassium: 3.5–5.5 meq / L.
Chloride: 96–110 meq / L.
Bicarbonate: 24–30 meq / L.

COST: approximately $15. for all four electrolytes together.

ERYTHROCYTE SEDIMENTATION RATE (ESR)

OTHER NAMES: sed rate, sedimentation rate.

The modern history of the sed rate dates to the early part of this century when Robin Fahraeus, a Swedish doctor, was searching for a test to diagnose pregnancy. One day, after he was finished seeing patients, he walked into the laboratory where the blood samples were stored and noticed—quite serendipitously—that the red cells of his pregnant patients had settled in the test tube to a much greater extent than did those of his nonpregnant patients. He thought his search for a pregnancy test was over. It was only when he began to study the sedimentation rate in a variety of other patients with conditions and illnesses other than pregnancy that he realized that this increased settling time was not unique to pregnancy but a sign of many diseases as well. Interestingly, although Fahraeus was the first "modern" physician to discover the value of measuring the erythrocyte sedimentation rate, he may have only rediscovered something that was known to the ancient Greeks over two thousand years ago.

Most medical historians believe that variations in the sedimentation rate between healthy and sick people led to the Greek theory of the four humors. When blood is withdrawn from a sick person and allowed to stand, the sedimentation rate may be so high that some red cells settle quickly to the bottom, forming a dark red band. Other red cells, not settling as quickly, will form a lighter, pink colored band on top of the dark red one. On top of both of these layers will be a grayish-white layer formed by the white blood cells, often increased in number when disease is present. And, finally, the top layer will be the yellow serum. The Greeks named these four layers (from top to bottom): yellow bile, phlegm, sanguis (or true blood), and black bile (or melancholia). They believed that disease arose from a failure of these four blood humors to mix together. Although we no longer use the sed rate as a test for pregnancy, it is—like temperature or pulse—a good guide to the overall state of health in the body. An elevated *erythrocyte sedimentation rate* is not specific for a particular disease but is often used to measure whether inflammation, chronic infection, cancer, or rheumatoid arthritis is present.

Because the test requires little equipment, doctors frequently perform it in their office. In addition to aiding in the diagnosis of many diseases, this test also monitors the response to treatment for infections and other diseases such as rheumatic fever or rheumatoid arthritis. The test result is reported as the actual distance—in millimeters—that the red cells settle in one hour.

NORMAL RANGE: women—0–20 mm.
                 men—0–10 mm.
COST: approximately $10.

GENETIC SCREENING

Recently, blood tests have been developed that enable doctors to screen for various genetic diseases. These disorders are due to the fetus inheriting an abnormal or defective gene from one or both parents. In most genetic diseases the person will not have the disease unless he carries two defective genes—one from each parent. A person who has only one defective gene is often well and is said to be a "carrier" for that particular disease. Although many genetic diseases can now be screened through a blood test, there are four major disorders.

Sickle cell disease is found primarily in black populations and affects the red blood cells. It is discussed separately in this chapter (p. 82).

Tay-Sachs is a fatal neurological disease. Approximately 1 in 25 Jews of Ashkenazi (Eastern Europe) descent carry the Tay-Sachs gene. These carriers are well and perfectly healthy. However, if two carriers have a child, there is a 1 in 4 chance that the newborn infant will receive the defective gene from both parents, resulting in the actual disease. When two defective genes are present, the children have a total lack of the enzyme hexosaminidase A in their cells, leading to the buildup of a substance called Gm2 ganglioside. When sufficient Gm2 ganglioside is present, the cell will die. Children with Tay-Sachs disease are born healthy but will begin to experience irreversible neurologic degeneration at six to seven months; death is inevitable and occurs at three to four years. Both carriers and children with the actual disease can be detected by testing their blood for the level of this enzyme. The test is used whenever this diagnosis is suspected in a child, or for prospective parents as a genetic screening test during pregnancy (p. 263).

NORMAL RESULT: "enzyme activity is present."
COST: approximately $165.

The *phenylketonuria test* is used to detect infants with a deficiency of the enzyme phenylalanine hydroxylase, which metabolizes phenylalanine, an amino-acid protein building block. If the enzyme is deficient, phenylalanine cannot be metabolized and will accumulate in the body, causing brain damage and severe mental retardation. Fortunately, once detected, the brain damage can be prevented by feeding the baby a specially prepared food that is low in phenylalanine. The test can be performed on both blood and urine. Most states have a law mandating that the blood test be performed on newborn infants before they are discharged from the hospital. In the hospital nursery the specimen is usually obtained from a heelstick puncture.

NORMAL RANGE: 0–4 mg / dl.
COST: approximately $65.

Red blood cells contain a variety of enzymes that are critical to their function. Lack of certain of these enzymes can lead to destruction of the blood cells, resulting in anemia. Many patients with anemia will have a blood test done to measure if these enzymes are present in normal amounts in the blood. The enzyme that is most commonly deficient is glucose 6-phosphate dehydrogenase, or G6PD. A G6PD test checks to see if this enzyme is present. Prior to the test the doctor will often ask the patient if he has taken any aspirin or any other medication since many of these drugs can cause the red blood cell destruction if the enzyme is missing. About 10% of blacks as well as many of Mediterranean descent (Greeks, Italians, Sephardic Jews, Arabs) will have G6PD deficiency, which throughout the world represents the most common genetic disease. In many hospitals newborn babies from these ethnic origins will have a screening test done on their blood (p. 250) to detect this problem as early as possible.

NORMAL RESULT: "normal enzyme activity is present."
COST: approximately $45.

GLUCOSE AND GLUCOSE TOLERANCE TEST (GTT)

OTHER NAMES: blood sugar.

The most important sugar in our bodies is glucose. The body maintains the level of glucose in the blood as constant and steady as possible through a complex network of insulin and other hormones. When a person fasts—even for days—the glucose level in the blood does not drop but is maintained in the correct range as the body produces glucose on its own by breaking down its stores of fat and protein. Glucose is generally formed, however, from the digestion of starches, complex sugars, and other carbohydrates in our diet. After you eat a meal, your glucose level will become temporarily elevated, until insulin and other hormones can work on the newly digested food and bring the glucose back to normal levels. For this reason, however, the *blood glucose* test is frequently done first thing in the morning after overnight fasting. This way, a recent meal will not influence the result and the patient's base-line glucose level can be determined.

There are diseases in which the glucose level is too high, and others in which it is too low. Diabetes mellitus, or "sugar diabetes," is the major disease associated with elevated blood glucose levels; it is usually due to a disturbance in the way insulin is made or is working in the body. Diabetes will be suspected when a patient complains of frequent urination, excessive drinking or eating, or infections that do not heal properly. At the opposite end of the scale, dizziness and light-headedness can be signs of abnormally low levels of blood glucose or hypoglycemia. This condition can occur in some patients without any cause, but it can also be due to excessive alcohol use or strenuous exercise. In addition, hypoglycemia can occur in a diabetic who takes too much insulin. A blood glucose test is ordered by the doctor whenever he suspects that diabetes or hypoglycemia is present. The test is also used to monitor the correct amount of insulin a patient should take to control his diabetes.

Many patients come to us or their own doctors because they suspect they have hypoglycemia. They complain of symptoms including lethargy, irritability, tremors, light-headedness, or dizziness. Generally, hypoglycemia is not the problem. Nevertheless, in these situations we will often obtain a blood glucose level because it is a simple, relatively inexpensive test, and it will tell us whether our patient has hypoglycemia. Often, instead of obtaining a fasting glucose in the morning, we will ask the patient to have the blood drawn at the time he is feeling the symptoms.

Sometimes diabetes will still be suspected in a patient with a fasting blood glucose level that is normal or only slightly elevated. In order to determine if he has diabetes, a *glucose tolerance test* can be done. Normally, when a person eats a meal high in sugar content, the blood glucose level rises for up to one hour after the meal and returns to normal within two to three hours. People with diabetes have a one-hour blood glucose level that is higher than normal and a three-hour level that will not yet have returned to base line.

This test is performed as follows: The patient should eat a diet containing adequate carbohydrates (but no alcohol) for several days prior to the test. No food (though water is allowed) is ingested for 12 hours before the test. Base line blood and urine samples are obtained. Either oral or intravenous glucose is then given to the patient. Blood and urine samples are obtained at 30, 60, 90, 120, and 180 minutes after the glucose is given. The oral glucose tolerance test is more commonly done than the intravenous glucose tolerance test because it is more comfortable and convenient.

NORMAL RANGE FOR A FASTING BLOOD GLUCOSE: 70–110 mg / dl.

COST: glucose—approximately $5.
glucose tolerance test—approximately $30.

HEART ENZYMES

OTHER NAMES: creatine phosphokinase (CPK or CK), serum glutamic-oxaloacetic transaminase (SGOT), lactic dehydrogenase (LDH).

A heart attack is only one of the many causes of chest pain. It is not uncommon, therefore, that when a doctor admits a patient to the hospital with chest pain, he is not certain if the symptoms are due to a heart attack or some other cause. One test that is very useful in these situations is the measurement of the *heart enzymes,* substances that are normally found within the heart cells and leak out into the blood only if a heart attack has occurred. Usually the heart enzymes are tested during the first three days after the patient is admitted to the hospital to see if an actual heart attack has occurred. Although there are three heart enzymes, the diagnosis of a heart attack is not made on the basis of any one enzyme level but on the enzyme levels together with the patient's history and EKG (p. 193)

Creatine phosphokinase (CPK or CK) is an enzyme that is found in brain, muscle, and heart cells and released into the blood within a few hours after one of these organs is damaged. Because the CPK result does not tell whether it came from the brain, muscle, or heart, a special test called *CPK isoenzyme* is performed whenever the CPK is elevated. This test differentiates and measures heart CPK separately from muscle and brain CPK. The CPK level reaches a peak 24 to 36 hours after a heart attack.

NORMAL RANGE FOR CPK (i.e., a person who has not had a heart attack): 0–180 IU / L.
HEART CPK: less than 3% of the total.

Serum glutamic-oxaloacetic transaminase (SGOT), an enzyme also found in heart cells, is released into the blood stream 24 to 48 hours after a heart attack has occurred. It is maximal at 24 to 48 hours after a heart attack and returns to normal in five days. Although the SGOT is also found in the liver, its elevation in association with elevation of the CPK and LDH will be used to diagnose heart cell death.

NORMAL RANGE FOR SGOT: 1–50 IU / L.

Lactic dehydrogenase (LDH) is found in many body organs including red blood cells, heart, liver, and muscle. The LDH becomes maximally elevated at two to three days after a heart attack and does not return to normal until 11 days. In order to determine from which organ the elevated LDH comes, *LDH isoenzymes* can be performed. The LDH coming from the heart can be identified and measured separately from other sources of LDH.

NORMAL RANGE FOR LDH: 90–250 IU / L.
LDH II isoenzyme is normally greater than LDH I, but this is reversed in a heart attack.
COST: CPK　—regular, approximately $10.
　　　　　　isoenzymes, approximately $20.
　　LDH　—regular, approximately $10.
　　　　　　isoenzymes, approximately $30.
　　SGOT　—approximately $10.

Hemoglobin A1c

The glucose that circulates in the blood will combine with hemoglobin and form *hemoglobin A1c*. The test that measures this form of hemoglobin is less than 10 years old but has already become an important tool for doctors. The blood glucose test (p. 61) measures the glucose level in the blood at the particular moment that the blood sample is taken. Recent meals will influence it greatly, and in a diabetic the glucose level will be dependent upon the timing and amount of the most recent insulin injection. When a doctor measures a blood glucose and finds it high in a diabetic, he can only guess whether that level is the only high glucose in the last few weeks or a very representative measurement reflecting a continuous state of high glucose levels.

The hemoglobin A1c test can answer that question. When the glucose level is high, more of the hemoglobin becomes hemoglobin A1c, and it will stay in that form for many weeks. In this way the measurement of hemoglobin A1c does not reflect the glucose level of the moment but is a summary report of the glucose levels of the last three to four weeks. The test is done commonly in diabetics as well as in pregnant women in whom diabetes is suspected. Hemoglobin A1c functions like normal hemoglobin in that it can bind oxygen and can transport it throughout the body.

NORMAL RANGE OF HEMOGLOBIN A1c: 4.0–7.5%.
COST: approximately $25.

HEPATITIS TESTS

OTHER NAMES: Australia antigen, hepatitis-associated antigen (HAA), hepatitis B surface antigen (HBsAg), hepatitis B surface antibody (HBsAb).

Hepatitis is frequently caused by either of two different viruses: hepatitis A or hepatitis B. Hepatitis A (infectious hepatitis) occurs after oral contact with someone who has the virus or after eating certain foods that can contain the virus, like shellfish. This illness is mild and the person recovers completely. A much more serious illness occurs after exposure to hepatitis B (serum hepatitis). The *hepatitis B surface antigen (HBsAg)* was formerly called *hepatitis-associated antigen (HAA)* or *Australia antigen* and is found in the blood of a person two weeks after he is exposed to the hepatitis B virus. It can take as long as 20 weeks after exposure before actual symptoms develop. In most people the HBsAg remains positive for only two to six weeks after symptoms of the virus occur. Some people, however, are permanent carriers of HBsAg after infection with the hepatitis B virus, and others carry HBsAg in their blood even though they may not be aware of having had hepatitis. People who have the HBsAg in their blood are infectious and can easily transmit the virus to others. This test is performed on all blood donated at a blood bank to prevent the recipient from getting hepatitis from infected blood. It is also done on people with jaundice (yellow skin), dark urine, enlarged liver, and itchiness. Antibodies can be measured to determine if a person was ever exposed to hepatitis.

The test for the *hepatitis B surface antibody (HBsAb)* is also used to screen those people at risk for hepatitis B (dentist, doctors, drug addicts, homosexuals). If the HBsAg is negative, then immunization should be done with the hepatitis B vaccine. These tests are done on patients with hepatitis to determine whether they have recovered normally from the infection.

COST: hepatitis antigen (HBsAg)—approximately $20.
hepatitis antibody (HBsAb)—approximately $20.

HLA TYPING

Within the nucleus of human cells are found 23 pairs of chromosomes—46 in all. These chromosomes contain the genes that control all aspects of our development and health. Increasingly, medical research demonstrates the importance of genes to a person's overall health. Besides the most obvious genetic traits (hair color, height, body-build and so on), these important pieces of DNA (or deoxyribonucleic acid, which contains the genetic code) may influence our susceptibility to various cancers, determine behavior, be critical to the development of a variety of different diseases, and be crucial to the body's ability to accept or reject transplanted organs. It would be very useful to do some test that would characterize a person's genes. One test that is available—chromosome analysis and karyotyping (p. 208)—determines the number of chromosomes that are present. Results other than the normal 46 are associated with a variety of diseases, such as Down's syndrome.

Another test—*HLA typing*—provides information about one chromosome pair—the sixth. On this chromosome is located a group of related genes called the Major Histocompatability Region or MHR. Each MHR contains four different gene locations that are identified as HLA A, HLA B, HLA C, and HLA D. Since there are two sixth-pair chromosomes in a cell, each person has two of each of those four gene locations, or eight in all. Each of those eight gene sites can be filled by one of a large number of different genes, of which over one hundred have been identified thus far. These eight HLA genes produce various proteins called antigens, which are found on the surface of white blood cells.

HLA typing involves the task of identifying the specific eight HLA genes that are present by carefully analyzing a person's white blood cells. There is no "normal range" in HLA typing. Instead, the specific genes (identified by a number) at each of the HLA gene sites are identified, so a typical result for HLA typing might be: A2, A12, B4, B8, C2, C4. Since genes are transmitted from parent to child, family members will have similar HLA typing. In fact, all children will have one-half of their HLA genes identical to each parent. There is a 25% chance that any two siblings will have identical HLA typing. On the other hand, the chance of two non-related persons having identical HLA typing is very remote. In homogeneous societies, such as exists in Scandinavian countries where this typing has been well-studied, the chance is 1 in 50,000. In America, which as a "melting pot" is a much more genetically mixed society, the chance is even far less than that. HLA typing is useful for three situations:

1. Organ transplant: If an organ is transplanted from a donor that is HLA similar—or ideally, identical—to the patient-recipient, the result will be much better than if it is from a HLA nonsimilar donor. (This is true of all organs other than a cornea, where HLA typing seems to make little difference.)

2. Paternity testing: Since HLA is a much more specific genetic marker than blood group typing, it has become the best means of testing for parentage.

3. Diagnosis of various diseases: Studies now show that a variety of diseases correlate with certain HLA types. For example, HLA B27 is found in nearly everyone with ankylosing spondylitis (a form of arthritis). The list of diseases that correlates with certain HLA genes is growing each year, and HLA typing provides a powerful new tool (p. 355) for diagnosing these diseases.

COST: approximately $300.

HORMONES

Hormones are chemicals secreted by the body's glands. Once in the bloodstream, they circulate throughout the body and produce a variety of effects. Some typical hormones are insulin (secreted by the pancreas gland), cortisol (secreted by the adrenal gland), and renin (secreted by the kidney). Abnormal levels—both high and low—of hormones are associated with many diseases, so it is very important to be able to measure specifically the blood level of these critically important substances. Until recently, hormone blood levels could only be measured indirectly by studying the effects that the hormones produced. Within the past 20 years, however, a new way of doing these measurements was developed. This test—called a radioimmunoassay, or RIA—uses an antibody directed against the hormone to measure the actual hormone level in the blood. This procedure revolutionized the evaluation of hormonal diseases, and the developer of the RIA—Dr. Roslyn Yalow—received the Nobel Prize in Medicine for her work. Using the RIA methods, doctors can directly measure almost any hormone in the body. The most important ones include:

Cortisol: This hormone is produced by the adrenal gland, which, in turn, is under the control of the pituitary gland. Cortisol levels display a marked diurnal variation, meaning that they change with the time of day: the level is highest in the morning and lowest in the evening. Cortisol has a wide-ranging series of effects in the body. It plays a major role in regulating sugar, starch, protein, and fat metabolism; in producing insulin; and in acting as the body's "own" anti-inflammatory drug. Diseases of the adrenal or pituitary gland will cause the cortisol level to be abnormal. These diseases include:

Elevated level—Tumor (benign or malignant) of the adrenal or pituitary gland (a disease known as Cushing's syndrome resulting in obesity, hypertension, and diabetes).

Decreased level—Pituitary hypofunction and adrenal gland hypofunction (Addison's disease—causing fatigue or lethargy).

Cortisol levels are influenced greatly by steroid drugs as well as oral contraceptives or estrogen pills. There is no patient preparation necessary for the test, but the physician must be told if the patient is taking any of these medications. In addition, the time of day that the test is done is critical since the level varies significantly from morning to evening.

Cortisol levels are rarely performed as a simple one-time test. More often, they are measured both in the morning and in the evening to see if the normal diurnal variation is present. In addition, another variant of cortisol measurement that is frequently performed is the *dexamethasone-suppression test.* In this test the steroid drug dexamethasone is given to the patient, and then the levels of cortisol in the blood and cortisol breakdown products in the urine are measured. Normally, the dexamethasone suppresses the body's production of cortisol, but in patients with some diseases of the adrenal or pituitary glands the cortisol will still be made. This dexamethasone-suppression test is also useful in evaluating patients with severe depression. Certain patients with depression will have a normal suppression test, while others will have an abnormal result, and the difference seems to have important significance for therapy and prognosis.

NORMAL RANGE: morning cortisol—7–25 mcg / dl.
                evening cortisol—2–9 mcg / dl.
COST: approximately $45.

Thyroid hormones: The thyroid gland regulates the body's metabolic rate. A variety of blood tests are available to measure the function of the thyroid gland. These include measurement of T4 (thyroxine), T3 uptake (tri-iodothyronine resin uptake), and TSH (thyroid-stimulating hormone secreted by the pituitary gland). Abnormal thyroid function is very common. One or all of these tests will be done if abnormal function of the thyroid gland is suspected. Symptoms that suggest too much thyroid hormone (hyperthyroid) include increased heart rate, sweatiness, weight loss, tremor, nervousness, diarrhea, and sensation of always being hot. Conversely, symptoms that suggest too little thyroid hormone (hypothyroid) include sensation of always being cold, weight gain, fatigue, dry skin, constipation, and lethargy. Although there is no preparation necessary before the level is drawn, numerous drugs interfere with the test.

NORMAL RANGE: T4–4.5–12.5 mcg / dl.
                T3 uptake—23–34%.
                TSH–less than 11 micro IU / ml.
COST: T4–approximately $20.
        T3 uptake—approximately $10.
        TSH–approximately $55.

Testosterone: This hormone is the major male sex hormone and is produced by the adrenal gland and testes in males and, to a

VARIOUS PITUITARY HORMONES AND THEIR NORMAL RANGE

Hormone	Target Organ	Normal Range
Thyroid-stimulating hormone (TSH)	Thyroid	Less than 11 microIU/ml.
Adrenocorticotrophic hormone (ACTH)	Adrenal	Less than 94 pg/ml.
Follicle-stimulating hormone (FSH)	Ovary	Females: Premenopausal— 5–30 mIU/ml, but exact level will vary with phase of menstrual cycle. Postmenopausal— 40–200 mIU/ml. Males: 5–25 mIU/ml.
Luteinizing hormone (LH)	Ovary	Females: Premenopausal— 0–200 mIU/ml, but exact level will vary with phase of menstrual cycle. Postmenopausal— 35–120 mIU/ml. Males: 6–30 mIU/ml.
Prolactin		0–25 ng/ml.

lesser degree, by the adrenal gland and ovary in females. It is the major hormone responsible for male sex characteristics (libido, erection, deep voice, body hair, and muscle mass). Like cortisol, the highest level occurs in the morning and the lowest level occurs at night. The level is measured when symptoms suggest that the hormone is elevated (in females: increased body hair, menstrual irregularities, and large clitoris) or decreased (in males: impotency, small penis and testes, and decreased libido). If abnormal levels are found, it is usually indicative of abnormalities in the pituitary gland (which controls its secretion by the adrenal and testes) or in those glands themselves.

NORMAL RANGE: morning testosterone—(females) 25–100 ng / dl.
(males) 300–800 ng / dl.
COST: approximately $65.

Pituitary gland: The pituitary gland is often called the master gland of the body because it regulates the function of many other glands, including the thyroid, adrenals, ovaries, and testes. The pituitary gland regulates these other organs by secreting hormones that signal, in turn, the other target glands to release their own specific hormone. For example, the thyroid gland releases the various thyroid hormones in response to the pituitary gland releasing a thyroid-stimulating hormone. The various messenger hormones released by the pituitary gland and their normal ranges are listed in the table on p. 71.

These pituitary hormones will be measured whenever disease in the target gland, or pituitary itself, is suspected. These include pituitary tumors (visual disturbance, vomiting, headache, dizziness); hyperthyroid disease; hypothyroid disease; Addison's disease or an underactive adrenal gland (fatigue, sweatiness, vomiting, loss of appetite); Cushing's disease or an overactive adrenal gland (fullness in the face, neck, and back of the chest, muscle loss, weakness, and bruising); gynecologic dysfunction (infertility, menstrual irregularities) and hypopituitarism (infertility, menstrual disorders, decreased libido, and impotency). No patient preparation is necessary prior to these tests. Often, these tests will be done in conjunction with the measurement of these and related hormones in the urine.

COST: luteinizing hormone (LH)—$45.
follicle-stimulating hormone (FSH)—$45.
adrenocorticotrophic hormone (ACTH)—$110.
prolactin—$55.
thyroid-stimulating hormone (TSH)—$55.

IMMUNE SYSTEM TESTS

The immune system is a complex and multi-faceted part of the body whose overall job is to fight off infection and repel foreign substances. It is now possible to measure many different parts of the immune system. These tests include *immunoglobulin levels, complement levels,* and *lymphocyte analysis.* Immune system tests will be done in patients with a variety of symptoms (fever, swollen glands, rashes), recurrent infections, immunodeficiency diseases, and autoimmune diseases (rheumatoid arthritis and vasculitis). Some of the tests, especially the complement levels and lymphocyte analysis, may take as long as a week to perform.

Recently, it has become possible to analyze the white blood cells using powerful tools called monoclonal antibodies. These can identify the levels in the blood of certain white blood cells called T-lymphocytes that have specific functions in the immune system. Some of these lymphocytes (T4) help make antibodies, while others (T8) suppress the production of antibodies. It is now recognized that certain diseases may be associated with abnormalities in the number of these various T-cell populations, including multiple sclerosis (low T8), rheumatoid arthritis (low T8), and acquired immunodeficiency syndrome (AIDS), which appears to be associated with both decreased numbers of T4 helper cells and increased numbers of T8 suppressor cells.

COST: The cost for various tests that measure the immune system is highly variable.
Measurement of immunoglobulin levels—approximately $25.
Analysis with monoclonal antibodies of various T-lymphocyte groups—approximately $300.

INFECTIOUS-DISEASE ANTIBODY TITERS

Infection with almost any pathogen (viruses, bacteria, parasites) causes our immune system to produce antibodies against the foreign organism. Similarly, immunization will cause the patient to produce antibodies against the organism to which he is being immunized without having to actually have the real illness. Many of these specific antibodies can be measured and are useful in the diagnosis of the specific infection and as a monitor to ensure that a patient has been properly immunized and has sufficient antibodies present to protect against the disease. Antibody titers will often be repeated to see if the antibody level is rising or falling since this measurement indicates if the infection is worsening or improving, and if it is a recent infection or a past one. There is no such thing as a "normal value" with regard to antibody titers. Each result must be discussed with your physician. No patient preparation is necessary for these tests.

Rubella titer: This antibody is in response to a rubella (German measles) infection or immunization. Since a rubella infection during pregnancy can lead to birth defects, many states, prior to granting a marriage license, will require a woman to have this test performed. A woman with low titers of antibody—a sign that she is still susceptible to rubella infection—must have rubella immunization performed.

Antistreptolysin O (ASLO): This antibody is made in response to infection with the streptococcus bacteria. If infection with this bacteria is left untreated, serious complications can result, including rheumatic fever and kidney disease. When these illnesses are suspected (heart murmur, rash, swollen joints, fever), ASLO titers will be obtained.

Cold agglutinins: This term doesn't refer to antibodies made in response to a "head cold" but, instead, refers to those antibodies that are produced against a variety of organisms, most commonly mycoplasma, a frequent cause of pneumonia in young adults. The name, cold agglutinins, is derived from the fact that the antibodies are active only when the blood is cooled below the usual body temperature of 98.6°. This test is performed whenever a mycoplasma-caused pneumonia is suspected.

TORCH titers: This series of tests measures antibody levels against four organisms, all of which can cause birth defects if they occur in a pregnant mother: *t*oxoplasmosis, *r*ubella, *c*ytomegalovirus, and *h*erpes virus. Newborn babies with almost any kind of birth defect will have TORCH titers done to see if these infections were responsible.

Two other important infectious-disease antibody tests that are done are discussed separately: *hepatitis tests* (p. 65) and *mononucleosis tests* (p. 78).

COST: approximately $20 for each antibody measured.

IRON, TOTAL IRON BINDING CAPACITY (TIBC), AND FERRITIN

Iron, the element that is essential for the production of hemoglobin and red blood cells, is absorbed from the small intestines and coupled in the blood to a protein called transferrin. This protein carries iron to the bone marrow, where it will be used in producting hemoglobin and red blood cells. Iron that is not used immediately is stored in the bone marrow bound to another protein called ferritin. Iron-deficiency anemia results from (1) low levels of iron in the diet (common with young infants), (2) chronic blood loss from the gastrointestinal tract (people with bleeding disorders), (3) menstrual blood loss (common with many women).

Whenever iron-deficiency anemia is suspected, certain blood tests will be performed to evaluate the amount of iron present in the body. The most direct measurement is *serum iron,* but this result is not very reliable in determining the total amount of iron the body has stored away. The *total iron binding capacity* measures the various proteins—such as transferrin—to which iron can be bound. The combination of decreased serum iron and increased total iron binding capacity strongly suggests the presence of iron-deficiency anemia. Recently, another blood test has been developed that measures the amount of *ferritin,* the form in which iron is stored in the body. Decreased ferritin is associated with iron-deficiency anemia.

NORMAL RANGE: serum iron—45–200 mcg / dl.
             TIBC—250–350 mcg / dl.
             ferritin—20–330 ng / ml.
COST: serum iron and TIBC—approximately $25.
      ferritin—approximately $45.

KIDNEY TESTS (BUN, CREATININE, AND CREATININE CLEARANCE)

Urea is formed in the liver from the breakdown of protein and is found in the blood as *blood urea nitrogen* or BUN. Under normal conditions most of the BUN is excreted in the urine. Therefore, the BUN will be elevated if the kidneys are not working well or if a patient is dehydrated.

Creatinine is a by-product of muscle breakdown. All of the creatinine that is made is filtered out of the blood by the kidneys and excreted into the urine. This test is a more accurate measure of kidney function than the BUN test is.

The most accurate measurement of kidney function, however, is the *creatinine clearance.* This test is a combination blood and urine test that calculates the ability of the kidneys to filter the blood; it compares the amount of creatinine excreted into the urine over a 24-hour period with the level of creatinine present in the blood. A blood sample is collected and the patient then begins a 24-hour urine collection (p. 92). The blood and urine samples are sent to the laboratory and the amount of creatinine present in each is determined. Since all creatinine in the blood should be filtered into the urine, the test will determine just how well the kidneys are working.

These blood tests for kidney function are performed in people with known kidney disease to monitor the severity of the illness; in people with vomiting and diarrhea to measure the amount of dehydration; in people with decreased amounts of urine production; and in people with confusion, since kidney failure can cause this symptom.

NORMAL RANGE: BUN—10–20 mg / dl.

creatinine—0.5–1.5 mg / dl (varies with size of person being examined).

creatinine clearance—80–120 ml / min. (amount of blood the kidneys are filtering each minute).

COST: BUN—approximately $5.

creatinine—approximately $10.

creatinine clearance—approximately $20.

LEAD

Lead is an element with no known purpose in the body. Scientists believe that at one time, thousands of years ago, the human body had no lead in it at all. Today there is so much lead in our environment that everyone has minute quantities of this element in his body. When higher levels are present, the results can be serious. This problem is not limited to this century, however. Recent studies done on skeletons excavated from the time of ancient Rome, approximately two thousand years ago, revealed that many people living at that time had become dangerously poisoned with lead—probably from drinking wine that contained high levels of lead compounds.

Today the most common source of lead poisoning is lead-based paint. Years ago all paint contained lead. Although that is no longer the case today, walls, furniture, and old toys painted with lead-based paint are still found in many homes. Young children who eat loose chips of paint accumulate lead in their bones and other organs of the body. Symptoms associated with excessive lead levels in the body include abdominal pain, diarrhea, and changes in behavior. In communities where the problem of lead-based paints persists, a pediatrician frequently screens all young children for excessive lead levels even before symptoms develop.

NORMAL RANGE: 0–40 mcg / dl.
COST: approximately $30.

LIPIDS (CHOLESTEROL, TRIGLYCERIDES, HDL, AND LDL)

Heart disease is the major cause of death in the United States. Over the years information has accumulated that supports the relation between elevated cholesterol levels and increased risks of heart disease. Because of this association, we have become very sensitive to the amount of cholesterol in our diets. Although cholesterol, triglycerides, and HDL levels may be measured in people already known to have heart disease, they are also frequently measured in people without heart disease to determine the risk they have of developing it. And, finally, they are performed as well to monitor the effects of exercise and diet on altering the patient's blood levels.

Cholesterol is a compound found mostly in foods of animal origin and is necessary for the production of hormones and cell walls. Although everyone needs a certain amount of cholesterol, too much causes cholesterol plaques. These plaques can block vessel walls and are thought to cause heart attacks and strokes.

Triglycerides, which are fats, comprise the major portion of lipids in the body. The triglyceride level varies in relation to a meal: after a meal high in fats, the serum triglyceride level will be high. Since triglycerides cause serum to turn cloudy, a tube of blood placed in the refrigerator overnight that turns a whitish layer on top is a test for excessive amounts of triglycerides in the blood. Although the association of triglycerides and heart disease is unclear, triglycerides are elevated in people with diabetes, excessive alcohol intake, and pancreatitis. Before this test is performed, the patient must fast for 12 hours.

The triglycerides and cholesterol in the blood combine with other compounds to form lipoproteins. These lipoproteins are classified by their weight and density. *High density lipoproteins* (HDL) contain very little cholesterol; the *higher* the HDL, the *smaller* the chance of developing heart disease. The HDL is elevated by exercise, weight loss, and moderate alcohol intake. *Low density lipoproteins* (LDL) contain large amounts of cholesterol; the *higher* the LDL the *greater* the chance of having heart disease. The patient must fast for 12 hours before this test is performed.

NORMAL RANGE: cholesterol—depends on person's age and sex.
Under the age of 40—less than 190 mg / dl.
Over the age of 40—up to 250 mg / dl.
triglycerides—50–200 mg / dl.
HDL—36–59 mg / dl.
(Lower values are associated with an increased risk of heart disease, higher values with a decreased risk of heart disease.)
LDL—70–180 mg / dl.
COST: cholesterol—approximately $10.
triglycerides—approximately $15.
HDL—approximately $25.

LIVER FUNCTION TESTS

OTHER NAMES: LFTs, serum glutamic-oxaloacetic transaminase (SGOT), serum glutamic-pyruvic transaminase (SGPT), lactic dehydrogenase (LDH), alkaline phosphatase, bilirubin (see p. 45).

The liver is an amazing organ. Sitting in the upper right part of the abdomen, it is the largest of our internal organs. It plays a role in a great many bodily functions including the digestion and metabolism of our food, the breakdown and recycling of many proteins and chemicals in the body, the function of our immune system, and the secretion of many important hormones, to name but a few. Given the critical nature of the liver, it is not surprising that a series of blood tests has been developed to test for the health and functioning of the organ. These tests—which are really five separate blood tests—are usually performed at the same time and are called, as a group, *liver function tests* or LFTs. These blood tests will be obtained whenever liver disease is suspected, the common symptoms of which are jaundice or pain over the liver. In addition, LFTS will be done to diagnose hepatitis, cancer arising in the liver or spreading to that organ from other sites in the body, or gallstones blocking the ducts flowing out of the liver.

Four of the LFTS—SGOT, SGPT, LDH, and alkaline phosphatase—measure the level in the blood of enzymes that are normally present inside liver cells but leak out into the blood stream if liver damage or disease is present. These enzymes are found not only in liver cells but in other parts of the body as well. SGOT and LDH, for example, are found in red blood cells, while alkaline phosphatase is found in bone. Elevations in the levels of these enzymes can be caused by disease in those organs as well.

The fifth test in the LFTS measures the level of *bilirubin* (p. 45) in the blood. This chemical is a by-product of the breakdown of old red blood cells and is excreted by the liver through bile ducts and out into the intestines.

NORMAL RANGE: SGOT—1–70 IU / L.
                 SGPT—1–70 IU / L.
                 LDH—90–250 IU / l.
                 alkaline phosphatase—0–70 U / L.
                 total bilirubin—0.1–1.0 mg / dl.
COST: SGOT—approximately $10.
      SGPT—approximately $10.
      LDH—approximately $10.
      alkaline phosphatase—approximately $10.
      total bilirubin—approximately $10.

MONONUCLEOSIS TESTS

OTHER NAMES: monospot, heterophile test.

Mononucleosis is a viral infection caused by the Epstein-Barr virus. This infection—sometimes called the "kissing disease" because of the usual way it is spread between people (especially among high-school and college students)—causes symptoms similar to those caused by other viruses or bacteria: swollen glands, sore throat, and headache. In addition, mononucleosis can sometimes cause a swollen liver or spleen. The test is performed on patients with these symptoms to determine if mononucleosis is the cause. The test, which comes in two forms, measures the presence of certain antibodies in the blood.

There is a simple screening test, called a *monospot* test, that can be performed on a couple drops of blood in the doctor's office or hospital emergency room. If the monospot test is negative (the normal result), the patient probably does not have mononucleosis. If it is positive, the *heterophile* test is performed, since a positive monospot can occasionally be due to reasons other than mononucleosis. This test requires a laboratory to analyze the blood. The usual result for the heterophile in someone who does not have mononucleosis is zero or negative. These tests can be normal until several weeks after the mononucleosis infection has begun, so a negative result does not completely exclude the possibility of mononucleosis, and the test may be repeated if symptoms persist.

NORMAL RESULT: monospot test—negative.
          heterophile test—negative.
COST: monospot test—approximately $10.
    heterophile antibody test—approximately $20.

PROTEIN, ALBUMIN, GLOBULIN, AND SERUM PROTEIN ELECTROPHORESIS

Most proteins in the blood are either albumin or globulins. A variety of tests measures the levels of these proteins, including *total blood (or serum) protein, serum albumin, serum globulins,* and *protein electrophoresis.* The last of these measures the specific kinds of globulins present in the blood. Decreased serum albumin levels, in general, are signs of malnutrition, starvation, liver disease, or cancer. When the albumin is low, it is often due to kidney disease, the symptoms of which are fluid collecting in the ankles (edema) or lungs (congestive heart failure) and decreased urination. Increased serum protein levels, especially globulins, are found in patients with autoimmune disease, cirrhosis, cancer, and leukemia.

NORMAL RANGE: total blood protein—6.2–8.3 gm / dl.
          albumin—3.6–5.2 gm / dl.
          globulins—1.2–4.5 gm / dl.
COST: total blood protein—approximately $15.
    serum albumin—approximately $10.
    protein electrophoresis—approximately $25.

Prothrombin Time (pt), Partial Thromboplastin Time (ptt), and Bleeding Time

Clotting of the blood results from a complex series of interactions between various proteins in the blood (clotting factors) and platelets, a type of blood cell. The first two of these tests—PT and PTT—measure the clotting factors. The last—bleeding time—determines whether the platelets are working properly.

The PT and PTT tests are used only as screening tests; they do not determine which specific clotting factor is missing. If abnormalities are present, specific measurements of the different factors can be performed. Since many of the clotting factors are produced in the liver, the PT is a good measurement of liver function. Hemophilia, which results from Factor VIII deficiency, is best measured by the PTT. Vitamin K, which is absorbed from the intestines, is also necessary for many of these factors to be produced by the body, and problems with intestinal absorption (malabsorption) can be screened by this test. Not only are these tests done in people who have evidence of abnormal bleeding, but they are also done to monitor various medications, such as Coumadin and heparin, that are given to slow blood clotting in patients who have had excessive blood clots (as occurs in thrombophlebitis and pulmonary embolus) in the past. They will also be performed in some patients before major surgery to be sure that the blood will clot normally.

When the platelets are not working properly, the outcome of the bleeding time test will be abnormal. This can occur if the number of platelets in the body is decreased (thrombocytopenia) or if the platelets are present in normal numbers but are not working correctly. Although this latter condition can occur spontaneously, the more common cause of decreased platelet function in the presence of normal numbers of platelets is the drug aspirin. Even one 325 mg (5-grain) adult aspirin tablet can affect the bleeding time for a week. Therefore, it is critical that the physician know if the patient has taken aspirin or any of the hundreds of aspirin-containing compounds within the previous few days before the test is conducted.

The bleeding time test is performed as follows: a blood-pressure cuff is inflated around the upper arm and a small incision made with a metal lancet on the inner surface of the lower arm. Filter paper is used to blot the blood that seeps out, and a stop watch is used to time the number of minutes it takes until the bleeding ceases. A bleeding time will be obtained in patients with evidence of abnormal bleeding and sometimes prior to major surgery when the physician wants to be absolutely certain that a bleeding problem will not develop during the operation.

NORMAL RANGE: prothrombin time (PT)—10.5–12.5 sec.

partial thromboplastin time (PTT)—29–36 sec.

bleeding time—less than 5 min. (A greater time than 8 min. is abnormal; thus, a result between 5 and 8 min. is equivocal and the test will probably be repeated.)

COST: prothrombin time (PT)—approximately $10.

partial thromboplastin time (PTT)—approximately $15.

bleeding time—approximately $20.

RETICULOCYTE COUNT

Our bone marrow makes about 300 billion new red blood cells a day—more than 3 million every second. For about the first 24 hours after a red cell passes into the blood stream, it appears different when seen under a microscope. These new red blood cells— less than a day old—are called reticulocytes. After about a day the new red blood cell is fully mature and looks the same as all the others. There are many times when the doctor would like to know how many red blood cells the bone marrow is making. Although that information can be obtained from a biopsy of the bone marrow (p. 188), an easier way is simply to determine how many reticulocytes are circulating in the blood.

This *reticulocyte count* is reported as the percentage of total red blood cells that are reticulocytes. When the reticulocyte count is less than 0.5%, it is a good indication that the bone marrow's production of red blood cells is decreased, as will occur in iron-deficiency anemia as well as more serious diseases of the bone marrow, such as leukemia. An elevated reticulocyte count is found in patients with anemia caused by the body's destruction of too many red blood cells (hemolytic anemia, G6PD deficiency, sickle cell anemia) and in patients with blood loss due to bleeding. In these situations the bone marrow makes many more reticulocytes than normal in response to the red blood cells that are being destroyed or lost, and the test will be done whenever these conditions are suspected. An elevated reticulocyte count can also be found in patients with iron-deficiency anemia who are started on iron therapy. When these patients are iron deficient, they are unable to make new red blood cells. Once these patients begin iron therapy, however, the bone marrow will make increased numbers of red cells to compensate for the previous anemia. An important use of the reticulocyte count, therefore, is to monitor the effectiveness of iron therapy in these patients.

NORMAL RANGE: 0.5–1.5%.
COST: approximately $10.

SICKLE CELL ANEMIA TEST AND HEMOGLOBIN ELECTROPHORESIS

Red blood cells are little more than packages of hemoglobin that bind and deliver oxygen throughout the body. Hemoglobin is a large, complex molecule consisting of more than five hundred amino-acid building blocks. Depending upon the exact sequence of the amino acids that compose the molecule, a large number of different hemoglobins are found in nature. Only three of these are normal: hemoglobin F or fetal hemoglobin—present within the red cells of fetuses and infants until approximately the first few months of life; hemoglobin A or adult hemoglobin—found within the red blood cells of everyone, child or adult, after a few months of age; and hemoglobin A2—a close variant of hemoglobin A. If any of the amino acids that are usually present in these normal hemoglobin molecule are different, an abnormal hemoglobin molecule results.

More than 150 abnormal hemoglobin molecules have been discovered. The most common is hemoglobin S or sickle hemoglobin, the type of hemoglobin found within the red blood cells of patients (who are primarily black) with sickle cell anemia. The *sickle cell test* is a quick blood test that identifies those patients with sickle cell anemia and should be performed on all black babies within the first few months of life. In fact, many hospitals will perform this test before newborns go home from the nursery.

Hemoglobin electrophoresis is a more complicated biochemical test done on a patient's red cells. It answers two questions: (1) What types of hemoglobin are present? (2) How much hemoglobin is the body making? Abnormal hemoglobins cause the group of diseases called hemoglobinopathies of which sickle cell disease is an example. If the body makes insufficient amounts of hemoglobin, the patient has a disease called thalassemia.

NORMAL RESULT: sickle cell test for hemoglobin S—negative.
hemoglobin electrophoresis:
hemoglobin A—greater than 95%.
hemoglobin A2—2.0–3.5%.
hemoglobin F—0.5–2.0%.
COST: approximately $30.

SYPHILIS TESTS

OTHER NAMES: Wassermann test, Rapid Plasma Reagin (RPR), Venereal Disease Research Laboratory (VDRL), Fluorescent Treponemal Antibody Absorption (FTA-ABS).

Syphilis, a disease that is transmitted by sexual contact, is caused by Treponema pallidum—an unusual organism that is not visible with a normal microscope. The two tests used to screen for syphilis (RPR and VDRL), though inexpensive and easy to perform, are nonspecific. This means that a positive result can also be caused by other diseases unrelated to syphilis, such as lupus erythematosus, hepatitis, or mononucleosis. Consequently, if one of these tests is positive, a more specific test, the FTA-ABS, is performed. A positive FTA-ABS result indicates that the positive RPR or VDRL was due to infection with syphilis and not another disease.

A syphilis test is required in most states before marriage. Since syphilis can also be transmitted during pregnancy to the fetus, the test is also performed on all pregnant women so that the disease, if present, can be treated as soon as possible before it can do damage to the baby. This test is also done for people with unusual rashes on the penis or skin (symptoms of syphilis) or with other sexually transmitted diseases, such as gonorrhea. No preparation is necessary for this test.

NORMAL RESULT: negative.
COST: approximately $30.

URIC ACID

Gout is one of the oldest diseases known to man, having been described by Hippocrates in Ancient Greece nearly 2500 years ago.

This painful inflammation of one or more of the joints (often the big toe) has afflicted many notable people throughout history including Benjamin Franklin, who brought home with him colchicine (a drug used to treat gout) from France, where it had been in use for many years. Gout is due to an excessive level in the blood of *uric acid*, a by-product of our bodies' breakdown of deoxyribonucleic acid (DNA). Uric acid is excreted by the kidney into the urine. Elevation of the level of uric acid in the blood (hyperuricemia) also occurs in conditions other than gout, including kidney failure, leukemia, and cancer. This test will be performed in patients suspected of having any of these diseases. In addition, patients taking certain diuretics can have an elevated uric acid level and should also have the test done.

NORMAL RANGE: 2.5–8.5 mg / dl.
COST: approximately $5.

VITAMIN B12, FOLIC ACID, AND SCHILLING TEST

Vitamin B12 and folic acid (folate), another vitamin, are necessary for the proper maturation of red blood cells. These vitamins are found in a variety of foodstuffs, including green vegetables, liver, fruits, milk, and whole wheat bread. A lack of these foods in the diet is the main cause of vitamin B12 and folic-acid deficiency, conditions that result in anemia (p. 309). This is most commonly seen in children, older adults on poor diets, and alcoholics. Occasionally, pregnant women will develop folic acid deficiency, even though they are eating the "right" foods, because the fetus requires so much folic acid for proper development. Another common cause of these vitamin deficiencies is malabsorption; in this condition the vitamins are eaten in sufficient quantity but the intestine does not absorb them. Any patient with anemia or other signs of vitamin B12 or folic-acid deficiency (beefy, red tongue; diarrhea; tingling or numbness in the nerves) will have a *serum B12 and folic-acid level* drawn. This test requires no patient preparation. The results will indicate whether a deficiency of B12 or folic acid is present.

Patients in whom a deficiency of vitamin B12 is found usually have a *Schilling test* performed. Vitamin B12 is absorbed by the intestines only when combined with a substance produced in the stomach called the intrinsic factor. Lack of the intrinsic factor leads to a disease called pernicious anemia. The purpose of a Schilling test is to determine if the B12 deficiency is due to a deficit of the intrinsic factor (pernicious anemia), intestinal malabsorption, or dietary deficiency of the vitamin. The Schilling test is done in two phases. In the first phase the patient fasts for 8 to 12 hours and then swallows some vitamin B12 that has been made radioactive. One hour later an intramuscular injection of nonradioactive B12 is given. The urine is collected for 48 hours and the amount of radioactivity measured. If greater than 8% of the swallowed radioactive vitamin B12 is excreted in the urine, it is proof that the patient does not have pernicious anemia or malabsorption and the vitamin B12 deficiency is due to a lack in the diet of that essential nutrient. If less than 8% of the swallowed radioactive vitamin B12 is excreted in the urine, the second phase of the Schilling test will distinguish between malabsorption and pernicious anemia. This test is identical to phase one except that the patient is given radioactive B12 that is already attached to the intrinsic factor. If B12 is now excreted in the urine, it is evidence that the patient has pernicious anemia. Although the Schilling test uses radioactive compounds, there is no real risk since the compounds are of a potency and type that are nontoxic.

NORMAL RANGE: serum vitamin B12—200–900 pg / ml.
folic acid—3–16 ng / ml.
Schilling test—see explanation above.
COST: vitamin B12 and folic acid—approximately $65.
Schilling test—approximately $150.

VITAMINS

The good news about vitamins is that it is now possible to measure accurately the blood levels of many of them, including vitamins A, B1, B2, B6, B12, C, D, and E. Nevertheless, there are few times that these tests are of real value to your doctor. But to understand why this is so, it is necessary to review some information about vitamins. These chemicals—which are not manufactured within the body and thus must be supplied from the outside—are needed in only minute quantities. Because the minimum daily requirements (M.D.R.) for these vitamins—the amount that must be taken each day—will be supplied if you eat a well-balanced and nutritious diet, it is usually not necessary to take vitamin supplements. That practice is common, however, for two reasons. First, there are some people who don't trust their diet and want to be sure that they get sufficient vitamin intake. Second, other people, including some outstanding scientists and physicians, believe that vitamins should be taken in excess of the minimum daily requirement.

Many people who go to their doctor complaining of fatigue and a run-down, tired feeling think that they need vitamins. Rarely are those symptoms due to vitamin deficiency. Instead, those people who do not eat well and fail to maintain adequate vitamin levels will develop very specific symptoms, depending upon which vitamin is deficient. Some of the more common vitamin deficiencies include:

vitamin A: decreased nighttime vision, skin problems;
vitamin B_1 (thiamine): muscle weakness, heart failure;
vitamin B_2 (riboflavin): skin problems, light sensitivity;
vitamin B_3 (niacin): skin problems, diarrhea, irritability;
vitamin B_6 (pyridoxine): anemia, skin problems, nerve problems;
vitamin B_{12} (cyanocobalamin): anemia;
vitamin C: bleeding problems, gum disease;
vitamin D: rickets, weak bones;
vitamin E: anemia (infants only);
vitamin K: abnormal bleeding.

When a physician suspects that vitamin deficiency is present because of these symptoms, he may perform a vitamin level. More often, however, he will simply treat the patient with vitamin supplements. The bottom line is that although a physician can measure vitamin levels, there are not many reasons for him to want to do so.

Most vitamin tests require that the patient fast for eight hours prior to the test so that the recent ingestion of food that is rich in a particular vitamin will not influence the result. Vitamin supplements should not be taken for that period of time as well. Tests for vitamin B_{12} and folic acid are much more commonly performed and are discussed separately on p. 84.

COST: approximately $30.–$70., according to the individual vitamin.

5

Urine and Stool Tests

ROUTINE URINALYSIS

OTHER NAMES: UA, urine test.

PURPOSE OF THE TEST: to study and examine the urine.

BACKGROUND: Although the primary purpose of the kidneys is removal of waste materials from the body, their other functions are critically important as well. These include the regulation of minerals (potassium, sodium, calcium, magnesium, phosphorus), water balance, and the acid content in the body. The kidneys make approximately 1 quart of urine every day. In general, the content of the urine reflects the condition of both the kidneys and the body as a whole. A routine urinalysis consists of a series of tests aimed at studying the makeup of the urine; it is easy to perform, is of no risk to the patient, and can provide substantial information about many different organs in the body. Therefore, it is often performed on patients in apparently good health in an effort to detect any underlying illness or disease. Used in this way as a screening test, urinalysis is frequently done in the physician's office as part of the regular physical.

HOW THE TEST IS DONE AND WHAT THE RESULTS MEAN: The first urine that is passed upon awakening in the morning is the best specimen for routine urinalysis since it contains the highest concentration of the various chemicals and other components. Frequently, however, a routine urinalysis is also done on a sample obtained in the doctor's office. Regardless of which urine is used, the patient urinates into a clean, dry container, covers it, and returns it to the physician. If the specimen cannot be given to the doctor within one hour, it should be refrigerated; if it cannot be

87

returned within six to eight hours, a new urine should be collected.

Once the laboratory that will process the sample has the urine, it will conduct the following tests:

GENERAL APPEARANCE: The laboratory can evaluate a variety of characteristics simply by looking at the urine. These will include:

Color: The usual color of urine is yellow, although normal urines can range from clear (very light yellow) to dark amber. The differences in color among normal urines generally reflect the water balance in the patient. If the patient has recently ingested a lot of water and is making large quantities of urine, the specimen will be almost colorless. If, on the other hand, the patient has not drunk much that day, the urine will frequently be amber colored because it is very concentrated. In some diseases or conditions, the color of the urine is abnormal because of the presence of various pigments. Unusual colors of urine include:

colorless urine—reflects a very dilute urine that can be caused by excessive water intake, diabetes (p. 318), alcohol ingestion, or chronic kidney disease.

red or reddish-brown—usually derives from the presence of red blood cells (a condition called hematuria) or hemoglobin that has been released from destroyed red blood cells, various drugs, or various foods including beets and artificial food colorings.

orange—generally reflects a very concentrated urine that is due to insufficient water intake, excessive sweating, or high fever, although it can also be caused by various drugs or foods, including carrots, rhubarb, and artificial food colorings.

brownish-yellow—almost always due to the presence of bilirubin, as occurs in hepatitis or liver disease.

brownish-black—can be caused by red blood cells in the urine.

Clarity: Normal urine should be clear. Occasionally, however, even normal urine can be cloudy, especially if the urine sat in the refrigerator prior to urinalysis. Other causes of cloudy, milky, or hazy urine include pus or bacteria in the urine from a urinary tract infection (p. 326), a diet high in fat, or sperm (as is common if the urine specimen is obtained soon after ejaculation).

Odor: Normal urine has a characteristic odor due to the presence of its components. Unusual odors in the urine include:

very sweet or fruity—occurs in diabetes (p. 318) when the patient has excess sugar and ketones in the urine.

ammonia—common in urine that has stood for a long period of time (over eight hours) before analysis.

foul smell—frequently caused by urinary tract infections.

Foam: Normal urine always has a small amount of foam on its surface. Large amounts of foam are a sign of excessive bilirubin in the urine, usually found in conjunction with hepatitis or other liver disease.

DIPSTICK ANALYSIS: Urinalysis has been greatly helped by the development of dipsticks. These are strips of plastic, about 4 by ¼ inches, which are sold under a variety of names, including Multistix, Ketostix, Dextrostix, Acetest, and Clinistix. On the tip of the dipstick are small squares of paper that have been impregnated with chemicals designed to react with different components of urine. The person performing the dipstick analysis—laboratory technician, nurse, doctor, or patient—places the dipstick in the urine specimen, shakes it off, and then compares the color of the various squares with a color standard, usually found on the label of the bottle. Dipsticks can have only one square on their tip, to measure a single urine component, or multiple squares. Dipstick analysis is used to determine the possible presence in urine of blood, sugar (glucose), ketones, bilirubin, protein, urobilinogen, and acid. Since it is so easy to do, dipstick analysis is always performed as part of the routine urinalysis even if there are no symptoms present.

Let's discuss each of the different tests that can be done by dipstick analysis:

Blood: Normal urine should have no blood cells in it although a few red cells may be found after heavy exercise (jogging, football, wrestling). Other causes of blood in the urine include kidney injury, kidney inflammation, kidney or bladder stone, and a urinary tract infection. A woman's urine can sometimes be contaminated with menstrual blood.

Glucose: Sugar is normally not present in a urine sample. Diabetes (p. 318) is the most common cause of glucose in the urine. Urinalysis is done for two reasons with regard to diabetes: to screen for new patients with the disease and to monitor the success of therapy once the patient has begun treatment.

Ketones: Ketones are a by-product of the body's metabolism of fat. They are normally not found in the urine. Conditions in which they are present include high fever, malnutrition, starvation, dieting (especially when the diet is high in protein and low in carbohydrates), fasting, prolonged vomiting, and diabetes.

Bilirubin: Bilirubin (p. 45), which is usually not found in the urine, can be present in hepatitis or gallbladder disease or when there is increased destruction of red blood cells.

Protein: The healthy kidney does not normally allow passage of any protein from the blood into the urine. However, for reasons that are not clear, some patients will temporarily have protein in the urine because they have fever or because they have been on their feet for many hours. The persistent finding of protein in the urine (proteinuria) is one of the most reliable and sensitive indicators of kidney disease.

Urobilinogen: Besides bilirubin, another by-product of red cell destruction is urobilinogen. Normally, only a small amount is found in the urine. It is elevated, however, in liver or gallbladder disease or when there is increased destruction of red blood cells.

Acid: The acidity of urine is measured in units called pH. A pH value less than 7.0 is acidic, while a value greater than 7.0 is alkaline. Urine that is highly acidic is associated with uncontrolled diabetes, starvation, dehydration, or a diet high in meats.

Conversely, urine that is highly alkaline (very low in acid content) is associated with urinary tract infection, aspirin overdosage, kidney disease, diet high in citrus fruits and vegetables, and urine that has been left standing for more than one hour without refrigeration.

URINOMETER: An instrument called a urinometer is used to measure the specific gravity of the urine, a value that measures the concentration of the urine with comparison to plain water. The higher the specific gravity, the greater the amount of solids that are dissolved in the urine. Urine that is equal to water in concen-

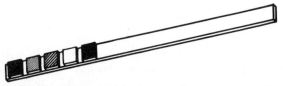

Dipstick used in urinalysis. This particular dipstick has five squares to detect blood, ketones, bilirubin, sugar, and protein in the urine.

tration would have a specific gravity of 1.000. The normal range for specific gravity is 1.006–1.030. Low specific gravity urine (very dilute) is found when there is excessive water drinking, kidney disease, and sickle cell anemia. Urine that is highly concentrated (increased specific gravity) is associated with dehydration, high fever, vomiting (p. 303), and diarrhea (p. 293).

MICROSCOPIC ANALYSIS: Once all the other lab tests have been completed, the technician will usually take a small portion of the urine and examine it under a microscope. Normally, blood cells are not seen in the urine. If red blood cells are present, they may be due to strenuous exercise, kidney injury, kidney or bladder stone, urinary tract infection, contamination of the sample with menstrual blood or cancer. White blood cells are usually found in association with a urinary tract infection.

COST: a full routine urinalysis, including a microscopic examination—approximately $20.

URINE CULTURE

Whenever we are concerned about the possible presence of a urinary tract infection in one of our patients, we will order a *urine culture*. The symptoms that will make us suspicious of an infection include abdominal pain, pain or burning on urination (dysuria), frequency of urination (polyuria), urgency with urination, foul smelling urine, the presence of white or red blood cells in the urine, and fever. If a urinary tract infection is diagnosed, the patient will be started on antibiotics; after approximately two weeks the urine culture will be repeated to be sure that the infection has cleared. For the specific description of how the urine is collected for a urine culture, as well as how the culture itself is performed, see urine culture (p. 175) and cultures in general (p. 167).

COST: approximately $25.

Twenty-Four-Hour Urine Collections

The concentration of many substances found in the urine will vary throughout the day, and so the amount of a substance excreted in the urine during an entire 24-hour period provides the most accurate and reliable indication of disease. Consequently, there are some substances for which measurements are made not on a single urine sample but on a 24-hour urine collection. Let's describe the way in which this is done:

At 8 A.M. on the day the collection starts, the patient urinates in the toilet and that sample is discarded. From then on, for the next 24 hours, all urine must be saved in the container given to the patient by the doctor or the hospital laboratory. This large container should be kept in the refrigerator, and the urine collected in smaller containers is then added to the larger one. At 8 A.M. the following morning the patient voids for the last time in the container and the collection is completed. Frequently, the container used to collect the 24-hour urine will have a small amount of liquid preservative in it.

Some of the most commonly measured substances in the urine include:

Calcium: Small amounts of this mineral are always excreted in the urine. Patients with increased urinary excretion of calcium will sometimes form kidney stones. Therefore, many patients who pass a kidney stone will have a 24-hour calcium collection done to determine if the stone was due to an abnormally high concentration of calcium in the urine.

NORMAL RANGE: 24-hour calcium—50–250 mg / 24 hours.
COST: approximately $10.

Protein: Persistent elevation of urinary protein is a sensitive indicator of kidney disease. Although routine urinalysis will provide some information concerning the presence of protein in the urine, a 24-hour urine collection will be a much more accurate indicator and is a useful way to distinguish patients with a small amount of protein on a routine urinalysis from those with significant levels of protein suggestive of serious kidney disease.

NORMAL RANGE: 24-hour protein—less than 50 mg / 24 hours.
COST: approximately $10.

Uric acid: Uric acid is a by-product of the body's metabolism of deoxyribonucleic acid (DNA). Elevated levels of uric acid in the urine may be found in patients with gout and leukemia. Sometimes, when excessive uric acid is present in the urine, kidney stones will form. Therefore, patients who pass a stone may have a 24-hour uric acid test performed on the urine.

NORMAL RANGE: 24-hour uric acid—250–750 mg / 24 hours.
COST: approximately $10.

Hormones: A variety of hormones secreted by the body can be measured in the urine. They reflect the function of the gland in which they are produced, and these tests—performed in order to determine their level in urine—are often done in combination with the measurement of the same or related hormones in the blood. The major hormones that are measured in this way include:

VMA and catecholamines—produced by the adrenal gland. They are most often measured in a patient with hypertension who also has heart palpitations, sweating, and headaches, symptoms that can sometimes be due to pheochromocytoma, a tumor of the adrenal gland. A major source of error in this test is that many foods contain high levels of VMA (vanillylmandelic acid) and consequently must be avoided by the patient for 72 hours before the test. These include coffee, tea, vanilla, chocolate, cheese, cocoa, and fruit. The complete list is very long and should be reviewed with the doctor or nurse before the test. In addition, many drugs can give false values to this test, such as aspirin and various cough medicines.

NORMAL RANGE: urine VMA—less than 1–8 mg in 24 hours.
COST: approximately $55.

Steroids and Estrogens: produced by the adrenal gland, ovaries, and testes. Their measurement will detect disease in these organs. Some symptoms for which these tests are performed include abnormal menses, abnormal genitalia, excessive body hair, and infertility. In addition, a specific type of estrogen—estriol—is measured frequently during pregnancy (p. 269).

NORMAL RANGE for some steroids found in the urine:
17-ketosteroids (17-KS):
    females—5–15 mg / 24 hours.
    males—5–23 mg / 24 hours.

17-ketogenic steroids (17-KGS):
    females—3–15 mg / 24 hours.
    males—5–23 mg / 24 hours.
total estrogens:
    females (during the menstruating years)—4–100 mcg / 24
        hours.
    males and postmenopausal females—4–25 mcg / 24 hours.

COST: approximately $30 for each of these tests.

5-hydroxyindoleacetic acid (5-HIAA)—produced by a tumor of the gastrointestinal tract called carcinoid. Doctors will order this test for patients who complain of excessive flushing and diarrhea, symptoms of carcinoid.

NORMAL RANGE: 5-HIAA—0–10 mg / 24 hours.
COST: approximately $35.

Urine Amino Acid Screening

Generally, only small amounts of amino acids (the building blocks of protein in the body) are found in the urine. Increased levels are due either to disturbances in protein metabolism or to kidney disease. An example of the former is a group of diseases known as aminoacidurias. These are usually present at birth and result from enzyme deficiencies that lead to excretion of amino acids in the urine. Afflicted children usually suffer from mental retardation or are delayed in their normal development. Children with such symptoms will often have a 24-hour urine collection done to screen for the presence of any amino acids.

NORMAL RANGE: 30–650 mg for 24 hours. If this level is elevated, the level of specific amino acids will be measured.
COST: approximately $50.

Routine Stool Examination

PURPOSE OF THE TEST: to examine and study the stool.

BACKGROUND: Stool is formed in a complex process that depends upon proper function of the small and large intestines as well as the liver. Normal stool is composed of a variety of substances including water, minerals (chiefly calcium and magnesium), bile, digested food, and bacteria. Abnormalities in the consistency, content, odor, and color of stool may reflect disease anywhere in the gastrointestinal tract or liver. Examination of stool is done when the patient has symptoms suggesting disease in these organs, including weight loss, anemia, and change in bowel habits. In this regard, examination of stool is different from a routine urinalysis, which is frequently done for patients who are apparently healthy.

HOW THE TEST IS DONE AND WHAT THE RESULTS MEAN: Stool for examination should be collected in a dry, clean container. It should not be scooped out of the toilet bowl or mixed with urine. The best specimen is a fresh one and only a small amount is generally needed. Stool collected from a patient who had an enema is not as useful. Much information can be gained by studying the overall appearance of the stool:

Consistency, shape, and form: Normal stool should be formed yet soft. Some common abnormalities and their interpretation are:

narrow ribbon-like stool: spastic or irritable bowel; partial bowel or rectal obstruction (sometimes tumors or polyps).

hard stool: constipation due to diet, certain medications, or sometimes cancer.

soft stool (diarrhea): spastic bowel or viral infection (stomach virus or flu, p. 293); when the stool is mixed with mucous and blood, it can indicate a more serious bacterial infection, such as shigella or salmonella; when mixed with blood or pus, it can indicate colitis.

Color: The usual color of stool is brown. Some differences in color are:

yellow or green—severe diarrhea.

black—gastrointestinal bleeding, taking iron pills, eating raw or rare meat.

tan or white—blockage of the liver or gallbladder ducts, as can occur in hepatitis and gallstones as well as cancer.

red—certain medications or bleeding in the colon or rectum.

Fat content: Most stool contains 10–20% fat. If the fatty content is higher than normal, the stool will appear pasty or greasy in appearance. The fat content can be determined in the laboratory.

Increased fat content is an important finding and may result from the intestine not absorbing food properly (malabsorption) or from disease in the pancreas.

Stool Culture

Normal stool contains large numbers of different kinds of bacteria; thus, a stool culture differs from cultures of most specimens (see cultures, p. 167) in that it is done to detect the presence of certain bacteria that cause disease and not bacteria in general. These disease-causing bacteria include salmonella, shigella, typhoid, and cholera. Symptoms that suggest a bacterial infection include diarrhea (especially when blood, mucus, or pus is present), fever, and dehydration. The details of collecting a stool specimen are described in Stool Culture (p. 173).

cost: approximately $25.

Stool for Ova and Parasites

Another test done on stool is a careful examination for the presence of parasites or their eggs (ova). The parasites that can be diagnosed in this manner include hookworm, whipworm, amoeba, tapeworm, and pinworm. Symptoms of these parasitic infections usually include weight loss, anemia, anal itching, and diarrhea. The examination for ova and parasites (sometimes called "stool for o and p" by the laboratory) is done carefully under a microscope by a skilled technician. It is important that the sample be as fresh as possible. In fact, sometimes when we are very worried about the presence of parasites, we will have the patient go to the hospital so that the laboratory can collect a warm, fresh specimen.

normal result: No ova or parasites seen.
cost: approximately $30.

Test for Blood in Stool

This is probably the most important test done on stool since the presence of blood is always a sign of gastrointestinal disease, including cancer, ulcerative colitis, polyps, hemorrhoids, and anal fissures. Sometimes the amount of blood in the stool is so great that its presence is obvious. Black stools imply bleeding from those portions of the gastrointestinal tract that are far away from the rectum (mouth, stomach, esophagus, small intestine), while bright red stool implies bleeding from the large bowel, rectum, or anus. Stool that is streaked with red blood is almost always due to hemorrhoids, an anal fissure, or rectal cancer. Often we will have the stool of our patients checked for blood even if it appears normal since bleeding into the stool can occur and yet not be visible to the naked eye. Symptoms that make us suspicious that this "occult" blood is present include anemia, abdominal pain, weight loss, and fatigue. The test for occult blood is conducted as follows: A small piece of stool is smeared on specially treated paper and a developing chemical is dripped on it. If the paper turns blue it is a positive test for blood in the stool. Eating a diet high in meat (especially when it is rare or raw) may give a positive result even though no gastrointestinal bleeding has occurred.

The test for occult blood in the stool is important to monitor in patients suspected of having gastrointestinal cancer or ulcerative colitis. This test can be done at home by the patient and is explained in greater detail elsewhere (Testing for Blood in the Stool, p. 340). Frequently, when the test is positive, a variety of other tests may then be ordered (p. 289).

COST: approximately $25.

6

X-Rays and Computerized Axial Tomography (CT Scans)

(SEE "X-rays" in "The Fifty Most Important
Questions about Medical Tests," p. 23.)

X-RAYS have become such a critical part of the practice of medicine that it is easy to forget that their discovery by Wilhelm Conrad Roentgen took place less than one hundred years ago. Working late one night in November 1895 at the University of Würzburg, Roentgen was doing some experiments with a cathode-ray tube, a sealed glass cylinder that emitted different kinds of radiation, when an electrical current was passed through it. Suddenly, quite to his surprise, he noticed that one form of radiation emanating from the tube had remarkable properties. It was capable of working on photographic film, but, most strikingly, it could pass through most objects. Only lead and other metals appeared to have the ability to stop this new kind of radiation.

As he studied this new phenomenon during the next several days he found its most unusual property. Once, while testing its effect, he held his hand between the cathode-ray tube and the photographic plate. When the plate was developed, he was amazed to find that he saw a clear and distinct outline of the bones in his hand. A few days later he presented his findings—including the term x-rays, the name he gave to his new form of radiation—to the monthly meeting of the Physico-Chemical Society of Würzburg. While initially his discovery, and especially the ability to "see inside the body," provoked some skepticism and cynicism (one French scientist proclaimed that with the new technique he could take photographs of the soul), few discoveries so completely and rapidly altered the world of science and medicine. Within weeks, serious physicists, scientists, and doctors had begun to explore the many uses of x-rays. In five years nearly every medical school or hospital had a machine capable of taking x-rays, and the importance of radiographic diagnosis has continued ever since.

Because x-rays have a shorter wave length than visible light, they are able to pass through material. Objects that are very dense, such as bone, permit very few x-rays to pass through, while gas, which is less dense, permits almost all x-rays to pass through. Bone will in turn produce a white shadow on the x-ray film, while gas will produce a dark shadow. X-rays take "pictures" of the body by making visible the contrast between tissues of different densities—bone, air, fat, and water. Tissues with a lot of contrast (as in the chest where bone and air are both present) enable the physician to see a great deal. The abdomen, on the other hand, which consists largely of tissues of the same density, permit little differentiation of structures.

In organs such as the intestines, brain, or kidney, where a contrast in densities does not occur naturally, it is possible to introduce a substance, either by mouth, through the rectum, or intravenously, that highlights these details. This substance is usually radiopaque (does not permit transmission of x-rays), such as a barium enema or intravenous pyelogram, but occasionally it may be radiolucent (permits passage of x-rays), such as air. Radiopaque contrast agents are generally safe but can sometimes cause damage to the kidneys or a serious, even life-threatening, allergic reaction. These risks are discussed separately in this part under the specific tests.

For *routine x-rays* the patient stands or lies in front of a photographic plate. The x-ray beam is directed towards the plate and through the part of the body to be examined. Examples of routine x-rays include x-rays of the bone that are taken to see if there is a fracture as well as x-rays of the chest and abdomen. Routine x-rays are simple to perform and require little patient preparation.

Fluoroscopy is an x-ray moving picture. It allows the movement of internal body organs to be seen on a television screen instead of as still pictures on photographic plates. It is very useful when the radiologist, the doctor whose speciality is the taking and inter-

X-ray of a fractured leg. The
larger bone in the leg (tibia)
has one break, while the
smaller bone (fibula) is
fractured in two locations.

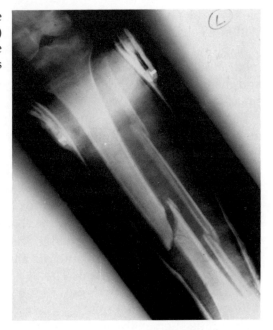

preting of x-rays, wants to see if the organ being investigated is
moving and functioning properly.

Another x-ray technique is *tomography* (also called *laminogra-
phy*), in which the x-ray beam is focused on only a small part of
the body while blurring out images in the surrounding tissues.
This is done by moving the x-ray machine in one direction while
simultaneously moving the film plate in the other direction. The
patient remains still throughout the test. Tomography permits small
abnormalities in an organ to be visualized. Organs that are commonly examined by this technique are the lungs, kidneys, and
gallbladder system. There is no special preparation required and
the test usually takes one hour to complete. A small tumor detected
on a chest x-ray can be visualized in much greater detail by this
technique because all of the tissues surrounding the tumor are
blurred, permitting a clear view of the area in question.

X-Rays: How to Evaluate and Lessen the Risk

Within a few years of Roentgen's discovery (for which he received
the first Nobel Prize in physics in 1901), scientists realized that x-
rays can be dangerous and could cause cancer. In fact, Roentgen
himself died from bone cancer, as did Marie Curie, the French

scientist who also did critical work in the development of x-rays. So there is little question that x-rays expose the patient to risk because of the radiation that is used. But just how dangerous are x-rays and what can be done to lessen the risk?

Radiation is generally measured in terms of a unit called the rad or, more commonly, the millirad (usually abbreviated as mrad). There are 1000 mrad to the rad, and the number of mrads that an x-ray exposes a patient to can be calculated. But first, let's get some ideas of how to judge that number.

Everyone living on earth is exposed to some radiation, even if he never has an x-ray taken. This radiation—called background radiation—results from natural sources (cosmic rays, for example) and amounts to an average of 100 mrad per year. The actual figure will vary from city to city, the change being mainly dependent upon the altitude (cities at higher altitudes have greater background radiation because there is less of the earth's atmosphere to protect them). Consequently, a person living in Denver with an elevation of over 5000 feet may have double the background radiation exposure that someone living in New York City at sea level has.

Now, in comparison to this average figure of 100 mrad of background radiation, how much radiation exposure is there in x-rays? A chest x-ray has only about 25 mrad, while an upper GI series may have 10 times as much—250 mrad—or more. The amount of radiation exposure to the entire body differs from the radiation exposure to parts of the body, such as the ovaries or testes. The table on page 102 gives both pieces of information.

We still haven't answered the basic question, however: how dangerous are x-rays? What does the danger of 200 mrad actually mean? One way that scientists evaluate the cancer danger of a factor is to compare it to some other factor in our society that has a cancer danger associated with it. With radiation exposure a comparison is often made to smoking. As everyone knows, cigarette smoking causes cancer. Since x-ray exposure also causes cancer, which is the more dangerous? The answer obviously depends upon how much smoking and how much radiation exposure are involved, but a rough guide has been established as follows: every 1000 mrad of radiation exposure a person receives from x-rays in a given year is equal in risk to smoking 20 cigarettes (one pack) every day during that year. A chest x-ray, for example, which exposes the patient to 25 mrad, would be approximately

Radiation Exposure from Various X-ray Procedures

	Average No. of Films per Exam (a)	Estimated Dose per Exam in Millirads (b)	Average Dose per Exam in Millirads to the Gonads (c)	
			Male (Testes)	Female (Ovaries)
Mammography	2/per breast	250–300	—	—
Upper GI	4.3	150–400	30	150
Barium Enema	2.9	150–400	200	800
Lumbosacral Spine	3.4	70–250	1000	400
Intravenous Pyelogram (IVP)	5.3	50–150	1300	800
Cholecystography (Gallbladder)	3.3	25–60	5	150
Abdomen (KUB)	1.6	10–60	500	500
Chest (Radiographic)	1.6	5–35	<10	<10
Extremities (Bone X-ray)	2.7	<5*	<10	<10

References:
(a) *Population Exposure to X-rays U.S., 1970* U.S. Department of Health, Education, and Welfare (FDA) Publication 73-8047, Appendix III. Rockville, Md.: Public Health Service, Nov. 1973.
(b) Laws, P.W., and M. Rosenstein, "A Somatic Dose Index for Diagnostic Radiology," *Health Physics*, 35:629-642, Nov. 1978.
(c) *Gonad Doses and Genetically Significant Dose from Diagnostic Radiology*, 1964 and 1970, U.S. Department of Health, Education, and Welfare (FDA) Publication 76-8034, Public Health Service, Apr. 1976.

This table adapted from *The X-ray Information Book* by Priscilla W. Laws and the Health Research Group. Copyright © 1983 by Priscilla W. Laws and the Health Research Group. Reprinted by permission of Farrar, Straus and Giroux, Inc.

equal to smoking half a cigarette every day for one year.

How does a patient decide if the x-ray risk from any proposed study is too great? If an x-ray study is medically appropriate, it should be done, regardless of how much radiation it involves. So the real question is: how do you know if an x-ray study is really needed? The best way is to discuss it with your doctor, using the guidelines we outlined in Chapter 3. The key question to ask your doctor is: what difference in my medical care will this x-ray make? If the x-ray result will not influence the treatment, then it is probably an unnecessary x-ray and should not be done. If the doctor indicates to you how the x-ray result will alter the medical care that you receive, then the study is probably appropriate—regardless of the radiation exposure. Obviously, this means that x-rays should not automatically be done on a routine screening basis, for example, in preemployment physicals or as part of every visit to your doctor or dentist.

Even if an x-ray study is necessary, you can lessen the radiation exposure by following these six guidelines:

1. Ask if the results from previous recent x-rays will suffice so that new films do not need to be taken. Many times x-rays taken within the last few months are good enough so that new films are not necessary. We remember one patient who had a complicated knee problem and eventually went to see four different orthopedists. Each of them requested that x-rays of the knee be taken. Obviously, only one set of x-rays was necessary and the films from the first doctor were sufficient for the others, but it is the responsibility of the patient to bring his previous x-rays to the attention of his doctor.

2. Ask if fewer x-ray pictures can be taken. Most x-ray studies consist of more than one x-ray picture. A standard chest x-ray, for example, consists of two pictures: one taken from the patient's side, the other from his back. A complete series of x-rays of the skull consists of six films. Often, however, not all of these pictures are required. Again, x-rays should be taken only when there is a specific purpose, and, frequently, the particular question being answered by the x-ray study can be achieved with fewer films. Here are some examples: A patient with a possible diagnosis of appendicitis will usually have an x-ray of the abdomen taken (p. 105). Routinely, an abdominal x-ray will consist of two films: one with the patient lying flat, the other with him standing up. Often, only one of these is necessary to provide the surgeon with all the information he requires. So remember the basic rule: even if x-rays are necessary, fewer pictures are better.

3. Ask that only the area of concern be x-rayed. Often, the x-ray beam can be made very narrow so that only the small area that is of interest to the doctor will be exposed. For example, if a patient falls and the doctor is worried that the leg may be broken, the x-ray picture should be limited to that area in the leg that is of concern and not the entire limb. Always request that the technician use the smallest beam possible.

4. Always cooperate during the x-ray study so that repeat films

are not necessary because you failed to sit still or hold your breath.

5. Insist on lead shields to protect the reproductive organs (ovaries in female, testes in male) as well as other parts of the body not being x-rayed. These shields will include aprons or small pieces of lead that can be placed over your body. Always ask that they be used.

6. Have x-rays taken only by skilled technicians using modern equipment in an up-to-date office or hospital. How do you know if the x-ray facility meets these criteria? One way of judging can be its response to the other five guidelines listed here. A quality x-ray facility will honor your request to use previous films or to restrict the number of x-rays. Its equipment will expose you to the fewest number of mrads possible and the technicians will give you, without being asked, the lead shields that are appropriate. If the x-ray facility resents your concern with safety and limited x-ray exposure, you should have your x-rays done elsewhere. The basic rule is: a good x-ray facility will be as concerned with your safety as you are.

X-ray use during pregnancy involves another whole set of issues. Generally, the reasons for doing x-rays during pregnancy must be even more convincing than usual. And if x-rays are being considered for whatever reason, be sure that the radiologist and your doctor know that you are pregnant.

Dental x-rays are sometimes considered to be inconsequential, but that is not the case. Just like all x-rays, dental x-rays should be done only when there is a specific reason. It is probably inappropriate to have a full set of dental x-rays done each year when you go to the dentist for a cleaning and checkup. As with your physician, you should ask the dentist the reason for the x-ray being taken.

Finally, x-rays on children are thought to be even riskier than those on adults, since their tissues are growing more quickly and have a greater chance of suffering damage from the radiation exposure. Safe x-rays in children require special equipment and expertise and should, therefore, be done only at x-ray facilities that are experienced in the examination of children. If this is not the case, then take your child to a facility that has the special expertise required.

In summary, x-rays are an invaluable aid for the physician, but they can be dangerous for the patient. As an informed patient, you should work with your physician whenever x-rays are being considered. Discuss these guidelines with him and make it a team effort to use x-rays as safely as possible.

ABDOMINAL X-RAY

OTHER NAMES: KUB (kidney-ureter-bladder x-ray), abdominal plain film, flat plate of the abdomen.

PURPOSE OF THE TEST: to diagnose tumors, kidney stones, abnormal collections of gas, and other abnormalities in the abdomen.

BACKGROUND: Although our abdomen contains many organs, most of these are not seen on a routine x-ray. When blockage of the intestines occurs, however, large amounts of fluids and air will remain trapped inside these organs. The contrast between this air and fluid is easily detected on an abdominal x-ray. When the wall of the intestines is torn, air that has leaked out of the intestines will be seen in the abdomen. Likewise, calcium deposits that can occur in the kidney and pancreas are easily seen because the high density of the calcium contrasts with the surrounding air. Although this x-ray is frequently used as an initial screening test for abdominal complaints, many diseases such as ulcer or colon tumor will not be seen by this technique and will need other x-ray contrast studies. This test is performed routinely before all IVPS (p. 121) and barium enemas (p. 109) are done.

HOW THE TEST IS DONE: The patient undresses and puts on a hospital gown. While he lies on his back on the x-ray table, a single x-ray is taken. A second x-ray is obtained with the patient standing (upright film). The x-rays take only several minutes to perform.

HOW THE RESULTS ARE GIVEN: The x-rays are immediately developed and interpreted by the radiologist. A written report is sent to the patient's physician. In an emergency, an oral report can be given immediately.

PATIENT PREPARATION: None.

RISKS AND DISCOMFORTS: Other than the minimal radiation exposure, there are no risks.

SYMPTOMS FOR WHICH THIS TEST IS COMMONLY OBTAINED:
Abdominal pain (p. 285).
Fever (p. 296).
Weight loss (p. 306).
Vomiting (p. 303)
Diarrhea (p. 293).

DISEASES FOR WHICH THIS TEST IS COMMONLY OBTAINED:
Kidney stones—Because most kidney stones contain calcium, they
will be easily seen on this x-ray.
Cancer (p. 313)—Tumors in the wall of the large intestines will
tines are not actually seen on KUB, they will cause changes in the
abdomen that can be seen on an x-ray. When a tumor obstructs
the intestines, excessive air and fluid will be seen on the x-ray.
Appendicitis.

COST: approximately $80.

ANGIOGRAPHY

OTHER NAMES: arteriogram, angiogram.

PURPOSE OF THE TEST: to detect abnormalities in the arteries of the
brain, lung, heart, kidneys, and abdomen as well as the organs
supplied by these vessels.

BACKGROUND: Arteries, the blood vessels that carry blood from the
heart to the organs of the body, are not visualized on normal x-
rays. But when a contrast dye is injected into these vessels, they
become outlined on x-rays. The physician can then easily identify
abnormalities in the lining of the artery, blood clots within the
vessel, and irregularities in the path of the vessels indicating injury
or a tumor.

HOW THE TEST IS DONE: The patient fasts for eight hours prior to
the test. He must remove any dentures and metal objects such as
hair pins and jewelry before he is placed on his back on an examining table. The skin over the groin or elbow region where the
plastic tube (catheter) is to be inserted is then shaved and cleaned.
Sedatives are given to reduce the patient's discomfort, and an
anesthetic is injected into the skin of the groin or elbow. The catheter is inserted through the skin into the artery to be examined,
contrast dye is injected, and x-ray pictures are taken. During the

entire study the patient must remain still. The catheter is then removed from the artery. This entire exam takes up to three hours; afterwards, the patient stays in bed for 24 hours with dressing packs over the site of the injection.

HOW THE RESULTS ARE GIVEN: The radiologist reviews the x-ray pictures taken of the arteries that were examined. A report describing blood clots and other vessel abnormalities is given the patient's physician.

PATIENT PREPARATION: The patient must restrict his eating and drinking for eight hours before the procedure; no additional preparation is necessary.

RISKS AND DISCOMFORTS: The patient will feel a stinging sensation when the anesthetic is injected into the skin. A burning sensation and flushing can occur when the contrast dye is injected through the catheter, and allergic reactions to the contrast dye, sometimes serious ones, can also occur. Occasionally, bleeding will develop at the site where the catheter is placed. The most dangerous complication involves the dislodging of deposits present on the artery wall, which might then clog the arteries leading to the brain and heart causing a stroke or heart attack. In addition, patients with diabetes can suffer kidney damage from the dye. Finally, it is uncomfortable to lie very still for up to three hours while the procedure is being done.

SYMPTOMS FOR WHICH THIS TEST IS COMMONLY OBTAINED:
Chest pain (p. 291).
Fever (p. 296).
Bleeding (p. 288).
Shortness of breath (p. 290).
Slurred speech.

DISEASES FOR WHICH THIS TEST IS COMMONLY OBTAINED:
Heart attack (p. 319)—See "cardiac catheterization" (p. 111).
Pulmonary embolus (blood clot in the lung)—The angiogram will detect where the blood clot is in the lung.
Cancer (p. 313)—Tumors frequently have more arteries surrounding them than would ordinarily be the case. The tumor also causes normal arteries to bend from their usual course.
Stroke (p. 324)—Narrowing and blockage of the arteries feeding the brain will be identified.

Transient ischemic attack (TIA)—This is a temporary blockage of the blood flow to the brain; it will cause symptoms similar to those of a stroke but lasts for a few minutes.
Ulcer (p. 325)—If the ulcer is bleeding, the angiogram will tell the source of the bleeding. Occasionally, drugs can be introduced through the catheter to help stop the bleeding.

COST: approximately $400.

ARTHROGRAM

OTHER NAMES: arthrography.

PUSPOSE OF THE TEST: to evaluate the tissues and structures of joints, especially the knee.

BACKGROUND: Joints are the junction of two or more bones and contain ligaments (which bind bones to each other), tendons (which bind muscle to bone), cartilage (which protects bones that rub against each other), and membranes that line the entire structure (synovium). The joints in the body are prone to numerous problems, including injury and arthritis. When the joint is thought to be damaged by injury or disease, routine x-rays do not often reveal much information since most of these structures are of the same density and do not appear as distinct images on the x-ray. Furthermore, the surrounding bones that are more dense than these tissues will often overlay the joint tissue and mask any findings that would otherwise appear on the x-ray.

Arthrography consists of x-rays that are taken of the joint cavity after a radiopaque contrast dye or air is injected into it. It is used to evaluate the status of the joint and the tissues within it. Both arthroscopy (p. 154) and arthrogram can be used to evaluate the tissues within the joint. The decision as to which test to use is not always clear and it is often a matter of style. Some orthopedists prefer using arthroscopy, which does have the added advantage of enabling minor surgery to be performed at the same time. In other hospitals, where the radiologists are skilled at arthrography, that procedure may be recommended.

HOW THE TEST IS DONE: The joint to be examined—most often the knee—is cleaned with an antiseptic, and sterile drapes are applied. A local anesthetic is injected into the skin and a needle is inserted into the joint. Then contrast dye or air is placed in the joint and fluoroscopic pictures are obtained. For further study some permanent x-ray pictures are taken as well. The patient may be asked to move the joint during the study so that the physician can see the interaction of the various joint tissues.

HOW THE RESULTS ARE GIVEN: The radiologist reviews the films and sends a report to the patient's doctor.

PATIENT PREPARATION: None.

RISKS AND DISCOMFORTS: Pain may occur when the local anesthetic is given and when the joint is moved during the study. There is a very slight chance of infection within the joint from the procedure as well.

SYMPTOMS FOR WHICH THIS TEST IS COMMONLY OBTAINED:
Knee or other joint pain—especially if it is persistent, severe, or otherwise suggestive of joint injury.
Joint swelling.
Pain with joint movement.

DISEASES FOR WHICH THIS TEST IS COMMONLY OBTAINED:
Joint injury.
Arthritis (p. 310).

COST: approximately $300.

BARIUM ENEMA

OTHER NAMES: air contrast study, double contrast study.

PURPOSE OF THE TEST: to visualize the large intestines (colon).

BACKGROUND: The large intestines are ordinarily not seen clearly on a routine x-ray of the abdomen. In order for the physician to evaluate the inner lining of the colon, a radiopaque contrast material—barium—is used. This permits x-ray visualization of tumors in the wall of the colon. Occasionally, air is used in addition to the barium (double contrast) to increase the ability to visualize small abnormalities, such as polyps, on an x-ray.

HOW THE TEST IS DONE: First, a flat plate of the abdomen (p. 105) is taken. While the patient is lying on his side, barium is introduced by enema into the rectum. As the patient is moved into different positions, barium is passed throughout the colon. The radiologist does fluoroscopy of the colon and takes x-rays of any suspicious areas. Afterwards, the patient goes to the bathroom and has a bowel movement to remove the barium. Additional x-rays are taken at this time. If polyps are suspected, air is introduced into the rectum to create further contrast within the colon. The examination takes approximately one hour.

IVP, ultrasound, and nuclear medicine studies must be done before, and not after, a barium enema since the barium will make it difficult to interpret these other tests.

HOW THE RESULTS ARE GIVEN: Many x-rays are taken of the large intestines during the barium enema. After the study a radiologist reviews the x-rays and prepares a written report that is sent to the patient's physician.

PATIENT PREPARATION: Although the specific preparation will vary with each hospital, laxatives and enemas are given the day before and the morning of the x-ray. On the night before the x-ray, no food may be eaten after dinner and no liquids after midnight. After the x-ray is completed, another enema is given to remove as much of the remaining barium as possible.

RISKS AND DISCOMFORTS: The laxative that the patient takes before the study can dehydrate him and cause fatigue. He may develop cramps and a sense of fullness while the barium is being administered as well as an urge to defecate. Cramps will occur while the air is being introduced as well. Occasionally, constipation from the barium remaining in the colon can occur.

SYMPTOMS FOR WHICH THIS TEST IS COMMONLY OBTAINED: All of these symptoms may be due to cancer, polyps, ulcerative colitis, or diverticulitis. A barium enema is performed to see if any of these conditions is present.
Abdominal pain (p. 285).
Blood in bowel movements or bleeding from the rectum (p. 289).
Weight loss (p. 306).
Diarrhea (p. 293).
Constipation.

DISEASES FOR WHICH THIS TEST IS COMMONLY OBTAINED:
Cancer (p. 313)—Tumors in the wall of the large intestines will appear as irregularities on the barium enema x-ray since the barium does not fill that area of intestines completely.

Ulcerative colitis—A unique x-ray pattern showing small ulcers and polyps is seen with the barium enema. The extent and severity of the disease can also be determined.

Polyps—Air contrast studies are necessary to visualize small polyps.

Diverticulitis—Small sacs filled with barium will protrude from the intestinal wall.

COST: approximately $130.

CARDIAC CATHETERIZATION

OTHER NAMES: cardiac cath, coronary angiography, cardiac arteriography.

PURPOSE OF THE TEST: to visualize and evaluate the function of the heart as well as the veins and arteries leading to and from the heart.

BACKGROUND: Heart disease is one of the most common causes of disability in our society, but it is not one specific disease. Rather, the term encompasses all the various diseases and abnormalities that can occur in the heart. In the past it was not always possible to pinpoint accurately what the particular problem was and where in the heart it was located. However, cardiac catheterization now allows for the accurate diagnosis of those parts of the heart that cause the patient's problems. Once the location and nature of the problem are pinpointed, cardiac surgery can often correct conditions that previously might have been fatal. All patients for whom cardiac bypass surgery is being considered must have this procedure performed. With cardiac catheterization the severity of narrowed heart valves can be determined, the ability of the heart to pump blood to the rest of the body can be measured, and the location of blocked arteries feeding the heart can be detected. None of these can be determined by simple blood tests or routine x-rays.

The history of cardiac catheterization is a fascinating one. In 1929 a young German doctor, Werner Forssmann, requested permission from the medical staff at his hospital to perform cardiac catheterization on patients with suspected heart disease. The medical staff refused, claiming that it was too dangerous. Forssmann, still convinced that it was a reasonable experiment, had no choice but to perform it on himself. He threaded the catheter (long, thin tube) up the vein in his arm and into his heart. Walking through the hospital corridors with the catheter in place, he made his way to the x-ray department so that x-rays could be taken to prove that the catheter was in place. Over the next few months he performed cardiac catheterization on himself numerous times and eventually won the Nobel Prize in medicine for his efforts in this field.

As medical tests go, cardiac catheterization is both costly and relatively risky. It should be performed only after extensive discussion between the patient and physician, and, in this regard, a second opinion may be helpful. Once the decision has been reached to go ahead with the test, it should be done only in a medical center where the test is performed several times a week and not in a facility where, for example, one catheterization is done every few weeks.

HOW THE TEST IS DONE: The patient undresses and puts on a hospital gown. He then lies on a special table that can move back and forth and tilt to each side. It is necessary to strap the patient to the table to prevent unwanted movement. While the patient is being monitored by EKG (p. 193), catheters are inserted through the skin into the artery and vein in the elbow or groin region. The catheters are guided with the aid of fluoroscopy into the vessels around the heart and into the chambers of the heart. Blood samples and pressure measurements are obtained from these sites. A contrast dye is injected through the catheter into the small arteries feeding the heart, and moving x-ray pictures are taken. This permits the doctor to see how well the heart pumps as well as whether any of these arteries are blocked. The test lasts approximately two to three hours. Afterwards, the patient remains in bed for 24 hours. EKGS are obtained immediately after the test and one day later.

HOW THE RESULTS ARE GIVEN: With the information obtained from the blood samples and pressure measurements, the quality of heart function is determined as well as whether any of the heart valves are narrowed. Analysis of the moving pictures will detect if there is blockage of the arteries feeding the heart. The cardiologist who performs this test will prepare a written report for the patient's doctor.

PATIENT PREPARATION: The patient fasts for eight hours before the test and is given a sedative. To minimize pain, a local anesthetic is then placed on the skin before the catheter is inserted.

RISKS AND DISCOMFORTS: It is uncomfortable for the patient to lie in one position during the test. He will feel a stinging sensation when the anesthetic is injected into the skin. A burning sensation and occasional flushing occurs when the contrast dye is injected through the catheters. Allergic reactions to the dye, even life-threatening ones, can also occur. Although dangers to the patient have been reduced in recent years, there are still serious risks associated with this test. Irregular heart beats and even a heart attack can occur. Occasionally, the contrast dye, which is excreted from the body in the urine, causes kidney damage.

SYMPTOMS FOR WHICH THIS TEST IS COMMONLY OBTAINED:
Chest pain (p. 291).
Shortness of breath (p. 290).

DISEASES FOR WHICH THIS TEST IS COMMONLY OBTAINED:
Angina pectoris—If chest pain continues even though the patient takes medications to control the symptoms, catheterization will be helpful in determining which heart blood vessels are blocked and whether heart surgery is necessary.
Heart attack (p. 319)—Pictures obtained of the vessels feeding the heart will tell if one or more of them are blocked. Blockage of these vessels can cause angina pectoris or a heart attack. The ability of the heart to pump blood throughout the body after a heart attack is also measured.
Congestive heart failure—Decreased pumping ability by the heart causes fluids to back up from the heart into the lungs. The heart's pumping ability will be measured during catheterization, and the cause of this problem may be determined.
Aortic stenosis, mitral stenosis (heart valve narrowing)—Pressure measurements on both sides of a heart valve can determine whether a narrowing of the valve has occurred.

COST: approximately $1200.

CHEST X-RAY

OTHER NAMES: chest radiograph, lung film, chest film, PA (posterior-anterior) and lateral of the chest.

PURPOSE OF THE TEST: to detect abnormalities and diseases of organs found within the chest, including the lungs, heart, rib, and thorax.

BACKGROUND: The principle behind all x-rays is that organs and tissues in the body will show up differently on x-ray pictures because of their different densities. The chest contains many critical organs of different densities, including the air-filled lungs, the blood-filled heart, and the solid, bony ribs. A chest x-ray provides the physician with much information about these vital tissues, and for this reason it is the most commonly performed x-ray. In fact, more than half of all x-rays that are done are of the chest.

HOW THE TEST IS DONE: The patient undresses to the waist and stands with his chest against the x-ray film. Usually two x-rays are taken. The first is a view from the back to front (posterior-anterior film), and the other is a view from the side (lateral film). The patient is generally asked to take a deep breath and hold it while the x-ray is taken. Thus, his lungs are filled up with air, producing a better picture. Once the x-ray is taken, the film is developed (this procedure takes only a few minutes) and is ready for interpretation.

HOW THE RESULTS ARE GIVEN: A physician skilled in reading and interpreting x-rays (radiologist) will examine the film and report any abnormalities that are found. Although the patient's physician may have to wait a few days to receive the written report, he can immediately obtain an oral report from the radiologist if necessary, or he may read and interpret the film himself.

PATIENT PREPARATION: During the x-ray a lead shield should be placed over the genital area in males and lower abdomen in females to protect the reproductive organs.

RISKS AND DISCOMFORTS: As with all x-rays, there is a slight risk from the radiation.

SYMPTOMS FOR WHICH THIS TEST IS COMMONLY OBTAINED:
Cough (p. 292).
Shortness of breath (p. 290).
Chest pain (p. 291).
Wheezing.
Production of phlegm or sputum.

DISEASES FOR WHICH THIS TEST IS COMMONLY OBTAINED:
Congestive heart failure (fluid in the lungs)—to judge the size of the heart and determine if fluid has filled the lungs because the heart is not functioning properly.

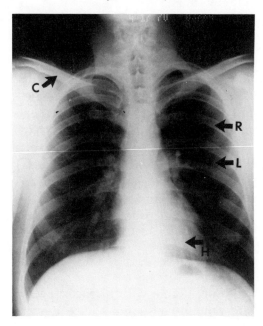

This is a normal chest x-ray. The arrows and letters identify normal structures within the chest: heart (H), lungs (L), and bones: rib (R) and clavicle (C). The bones are white because of their high density, while the lungs are black because of their low density, essentially filled with nothing but air.

Pneumonia (p. 321)—to detect the extent and location of the disease.

Asthma (p. 312)—to detect any pneumonia accompanying the asthma.

Pulmonary embolus (blood clot in the lung)—to detect the location and extent of lung tissue that has been damaged by the blood clot.

Bronchitis and emphysema (p. 315)—to detect the extent of the disease and possible presence of any accompanying pneumonia.

Cancer (p. 313)—to detect any cancer growing in the lung (that either arose in the lung or has spread there from another part of the body).

COST: approximately $70.

CT SCANS

OTHER NAMES: CAT scan, computerized transaxial tomography, computerized tomography, computerized axial tomography, brain CT scan, body CT scan.

PURPOSE OF THE TEST: to detect and evaluate diseases and abnormalities in the brain, lungs, abdomen, and spine.

BACKGROUND: Although the CT scan has been in use for only 10 years, it has had a great impact on the way doctors diagnose diseases. Before, painful and dangerous tests such as pneumoencephalography and angiography (p. 106) were needed to evaluate people with persistent headaches, strokes, and brain tumors. Now they are rarely done, as the CT scan of the head is easier and safer to do and provides as much, if not more, information. The CT scan examines body sections from many different angles. A detector records the many x-rays that are taken and sends the impulses to a computer, which analyzes them and produces a composite picture of the scan.

HOW THE TEST IS DONE:

Brain CT scan: The patient lies on a table with his head placed in a circular box (scanner) and remains motionless as x-rays are taken from many different angles. The x-ray procedure takes one hour to perform. Occasionally, iodinated contrast material is injected to increase the scan's ability to diagnose small abnormalities. If the patient is known to be allergic to the iodine, medicines are given beforehand to reduce the risk of complications.

Body CT scan: The patient undresses and puts on a hospital gown. All jewelry is removed. He lies on a table and his body is placed in the circular opening of a scanner, which revolves around parts of the body that are to be examined. X-rays will be taken from many different angles. Frequently, contrast dyes are used to enable better differentiation of the body's tissues. The scan takes one hour.

HOW THE RESULTS ARE GIVEN: The computer's analysis of the many impulses are seen on a television screen and pictures are taken. A radiologist reviews these pictures and prepares a written report.

PATIENT PREPARATION: For a body CT scan, enemas are frequently given beforehand. In addition, the patient is told not to eat for three to four hours before the exam. A sedative is sometimes given to ensure that he is relaxed and does not move during the study.

RISKS AND DISCOMFORTS: If a contrast agent is used, the patient may develop an allergic reaction to the dye. But medicines can be given beforehand to reduce this risk. A warm sensation through-out the body may be experienced by the patient when the contrast substance is injected. In addition, the patient may experience a claustrophobic sensation while lying inside the scanner.

SYMPTOMS FOR WHICH THIS TEST IS COMMONLY OBTAINED:
Brain CT scan:
Headache (p. 297).
Dizziness (p. 293).
Seizures.
Head trauma.
Fever (p. 296).
Body CT scan:
Fever (p. 296).
Weight loss (p. 306).
Abdominal pain (p. 285).

DISEASES FOR WHICH THIS TEST IS COMMONLY OBTAINED:
Brain CT scan:
Cancer (p. 313)—Tumors of the brain will appear as abnormal areas on the scan.
Stroke (p. 324)—Areas of the brain affected by the stroke will appear darker than normal.
Dementia (p. 316).
Body CT scan:
Cancer (p. 313)—Cancers in the lung, liver, kidney, and pancreas

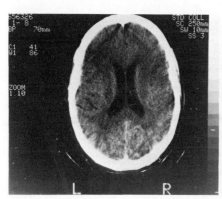 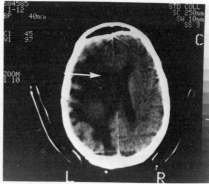

CT scan of the brain in a 23-year-old man with a brain tumor who had been having severe headaches for three weeks. The scan on the left is normal, while the arrow points to the tumor in the abnormal scan on the right.

can be detected by this technique. Enlarged lymph nodes that suggest a cancer or infection can also be detected.
Abscess (collection of pus from an infection).
Aortic aneurysm (enlargement of the aorta).
Pleural effusion (fluid around the lung).

COST: approximately $500.

DIGITAL SUBTRACTION ANGIOGRAPHY (DSA)

PURPOSE OF THE TEST: to evaluate the status of arteries or veins in the body.

BACKGROUND: Currently, there are a number of procedures available to evaluate blood vessels in the body. These include angiography (p. 106), venography (p. 130), and CT scanning (p. 115). Digital subtraction angiography, or DSA, represents a new method for radiographic evaluation of blood vessels. It is easier to perform than other techniques yet is safer while providing detailed information. Simply, before a contrast dye is injected, a fluoroscopic image of the area to be studied is made. The computer converts the information from the fluoroscopic image into digital information. After the contrast dye is injected, additional fluoroscopic pictures are taken. In the subsequent computer analysis, anything that was found in both the pictures taken before and after injection of the dye is "subtracted" from the resultant radiographic picture. This leaves behind a detailed picture of the blood vessels through which the contrast dye flowed.

HOW THE TEST IS DONE: The patient lies on a table in the x-ray suite or radiologist's office. A fluoroscopic picture of the area to be studied is taken, and the computer records with that picture all the images that are there prior to the injection of the contrast dye. A needle is used to inject the contrast dye into the patient's vein. After a few minutes new fluoroscopic pictures are taken. The computer performs the subtraction analysis, leaving behind a detailed picture of only the contrast dye flowing through the blood vessels.

HOW THE RESULTS ARE GIVEN: The radiologist will interpret the film and send the report to the patient's own doctor within a few days.

PATIENT PREPARATION: None.

RISKS AND DISCOMFORTS: The patient may experience slight pain from the needle that is used to inject the dye. Rarely, an allergic reaction to the dye may occur. There may also be some discomfort because the patient must lie still on the x-ray table for an extended period of time while the test is being done.

SYMPTOMS FOR WHICH THIS TEST IS COMMONLY OBTAINED: DSA is used in the same kind of situations as angiography (p.106). These include patients with:
Bleeding (p. 288).
Shortness of breath (p. 290).
Weight loss.
Slurred speech.

DISEASES FOR WHICH THIS TEST IS COMMONLY OBTAINED:
Pulmonary embolus—to see if a clot is present in the lungs.
Brain tumor—to see where the tumor is.
Cancer (p. 313)—to diagnose tumors, which frequently have an unusual number of arteries within them.
Stroke(p. 324)—to detect abnormalities in the arteries of the brain.
Transient ischemic attack (TIA)—to see if there is a temporary blocking of blood flow to the brain, which will cause transient symptoms similar to those of a stroke.
Aneurysm—to detect a weakening in the wall of an artery.

COST: approximately $400.

GALLBLADDER X-RAYS

OTHER NAMES: oral cholecystogram,
OCG, intravenous cholangiogram.

PURPOSE OF THE TEST: to evaluate the function of the gallbladder and to see if gallstones are present.

BACKGROUND: Ordinarily, gallstones or other gallbladder disease cannot be seen on a routine x-ray of the abdomen. A variety of techniques is available to visualize the gallbladder and the ducts connecting it to the liver and small intestine. In the most common of these—an oral cholecystogram—an iodine contrast substance, telepaque, is taken orally and concentrates in the gallbladder, allowing visualization of gallstones. If the gallbladder is still not seen on the x-ray, despite using this contrast material, there is a good chance that there is inflammation in the organ. An intravenous contrast material may then be given to see if the ducts leading from the gallbladder are blocked by stones.

HOW THE TEST IS DONE: The telepaque tablets are taken orally 12 hours before the x-ray. Three x-rays of the abdomen are taken while the patient lies on his stomach, followed by fluoroscopy of the gallbladder while the patient stands. If an intravenous contrast substance is used, the person lies on the table as the x-rays are being taken. This study takes two hours.

Abdominal ultrasound is presently used more frequently to detect gallstones than these x-rays. If a barium enema or a thyroid scan is to be performed in addition to the gallbladder x-rays, the thyroid scan must be done before the gallbladder x-rays and the barium enema must be done after.

HOW THE RESULTS ARE GIVEN: The x-rays are reviewed by a radiologist who determines whether gallstones are present and whether the gallbladder is functioning properly. A written report is sent to the patient's physician.

PATIENT PREPARATION: The night before the x-ray, a fat-free meal is eaten. This meal prevents the gallbladder from emptying and enables the contrast dye to be stored in the gallbladder. As mentioned above, the telepaque tablets are taken 12 hours before the planned study. The patient fasts for 10 hours before the x-ray is done. Before the intravenous contrast study, a laxative is given to eliminate gas from the intestines, which could interfere with the x-ray.

RISKS AND DISCOMFORTS: The oral contrast agent can cause nausea or vomiting. The intravenous contrast agent can cause allergic reactions, including skin rashes or, very rarely, severe life-threatening complications such as loss of blood pressure. The patient must remain still during the entire study.

SYMPTOMS FOR WHICH THIS TEST IS COMMONLY OBTAINED:
Abdominal pain (p. 285).
Jaundice (p. 300).

DISEASES FOR WHICH THIS TEST IS COMMONLY OBTAINED:
Gallstones.
Cholecystitis (inflamed gallbladder).

COST: approximately $80.

HYSTEROSALPINGOGRAM

PURPOSE OF THE TEST: to visualize the uterus and fallopian tubes.

BACKGROUND: A common cause of infertility is blockage of the fallopian tubes, where the egg and sperm usually meet and conception occurs. This blockage prevents the egg from coming in contact with the sperm. Normally, when a contrast material is placed into the uterus, it will flow freely through the fallopian tubes and can be seen on an x-ray. When there is a blockage in the tubes, flow of the contrast material will be stopped.

HOW THE TEST IS DONE: The woman undresses from the waist down and lies in the usual position for a gynecological exam with her legs up in stirrups. The vagina is cleansed and a speculum is placed into the vagina. A tube is passed into the cervix and the contrast material is injected. X-rays are then taken for about two to three minutes. Usually the test is done seven days after the menstrual cycle begins.

HOW THE RESULTS ARE GIVEN: The radiologist reviews the x-rays to see if there is blockage of the fallopian tubes. A report is sent to the patient's doctor.

PATIENT PREPARATION: Occasionally, a sedative is given before the test is done.

RISKS AND DISCOMFORTS: The patient may experience dizziness or abdominal cramping and pain during and after the test. She will also have a discharge from the vagina for several days afterwards.

SYMPTOMS FOR WHICH THIS TEST IS COMMONLY OBTAINED:
Infertility (p. 299).

DISEASES FOR WHICH THIS TEST IS COMMONLY OBTAINED:
Fibroid uterus—Irregularities or tumors in the wall of the uterus will be seen.

COST: approximately $120.

INTRAVENOUS PYELOGRAM

OTHER NAMES: pyelogram, IVP.

PURPOSE OF THE TEST: to evaluate the size, shape, and function of the kidneys.

BACKGROUND: The kidneys are not ordinarily seen on a routine abdominal x-ray because of the lack of contrast with surrounding tissues. When a radiopaque contrast substance, such as Hypaque or renografin, is injected intravenously, it travels through the blood stream to the kidneys. There it is filtered into the urine and excreted via the tube (ureter) connecting the kidneys with the bladder. X-ray pictures are taken as the contrast material makes its way out of the kidneys, thus enabling the doctor to visualize the kidney, ureter, and bladder as well as any stones, tumors, or cysts that are present. Kidney function can also be evaluated by measuring the time it takes for the contrast dye to concentrate in the urine. This test is not as effective in people with impaired kidney function since the dye will not be concentrated or excreted.

HOW THE TEST IS DONE: The contrast material is injected intravenously while the person lies on his back. Several x-rays are taken during the next half hour. The person then goes into the bathroom to urinate, and afterwards another x-ray is taken.

HOW THE RESULTS ARE GIVEN: A radiologist reviews the x-rays that have been taken and prepares a written report for the patient's physician.

PATIENT PREPARATION: Since stool in the large intestines can prevent interpretation of the x-rays, a laxative and enemas are given the evening before as well as the day of the x-ray. Usually, the person does not eat or drink for 12 hours before the study.

RISKS AND DISCOMFORTS: The patient may experience a warm sensation throughout his body when the contrast material is injected. Occasionally nausea or headache may occur. Some people develop an allergic reaction to the iodine in the contrast material; the allergic reaction may be as mild as a rash, but in rare instances severe life-threatening reactions occur. In diabetics, or patients who are dehydrated, as can occur in the elderly, the dye may cause kidney damage. This problem can be minimized by ensuring that the person is given enough fluids intravenously before the x-rays are done.

SYMPTOMS FOR WHICH THIS TEST IS COMMONLY OBTAINED:
Abdominal pain (p. 285).
Burning or difficulty on urination.
Blood in the urine.
Protein in the urine.

DISEASES FOR WHICH THIS TEST IS COMMONLY OBTAINED:
Cancer (p. 313)—Cancer in the kidney itself can be seen. In addition, other cancers in the abdomen may displace the ureters from their normal position, indicating the presence of a tumor.
Urinary tract infections (p. 326)—Anatomic abnormalities in the kidney, which predispose the patient to urinary tract infections, may be seen.
Kidney stones—Stones, if present, will be seen in the kidney or ureter.
Hypertension (p. 320)—Some forms of hypertension are caused by abnormalities in the kidney or its blood vessels. If patients with hypertension do not respond to simple medications, an IVP might be done to see if kidney abnormalities are the cause of the elevated blood pressure.
Kidney disease—When patients have blood tests obtained that suggest poor kidney function, an IVP will help in determining the cause. The size of the kidneys will also be measured. Small kidney size will indicate that the kidney disease has been present for a long time.

COST: approximately $60.

LYMPHANGIOGRAM

PURPOSE OF THE TEST: to visualize the lymph glands and lymph nodes.

BACKGROUND: The lymph glands are located throughout the body. These glands may become enlarged when infection, cancer, or leukemia is present. Normal x-rays, however, do not permit visualization of these tissues. The lymphangiogram will detect these glands and aid in diagnosing and monitoring the treatment of cancers.

HOW THE TEST IS DONE: The patient lies on an examining table. After a local anesthetic is injected, the radiologist doing the test makes a small incision in the skin, usually in the foot, and with the help of a blue dye finds a lymph vessel. A catheter (plastic tube) is inserted into the lymph vessel; then more dye is injected and it diffuses throughout all the lymph tissue of the body. This process takes several hours. X-rays will be taken at that time and again after 24 hours when the lymph nodes become filled with the dye. The dye remains in the glands for six months and x-rays can be taken during that time to recheck the status of the lymph tissue.

HOW THE RESULTS ARE GIVEN: The radiologist reviews the x-rays to determine if lymph glands are enlarged or if they have changed in size during the past several months. A report will be sent to the patient's physician.

PATIENT PREPARATION: No special preparation is necessary.

RISKS AND DISCOMFORTS: The major complaint patients have with this test is that they have to lie perfectly still for several hours while it is performed. This is especially true during the initial phases of the test when the radiologist is trying to locate the small lymph vessel. The injection of the local anesthetic causes a stinging sensation. A bluish discoloration in the urine and stool, as well as on the toes, occurs for one to two days after the test is performed. The oil-based contrast dye can occasionally cause blood clots in the vessels of the lungs, causing shortness of breath and pulmonary embolus. For this reason this test should not be done in patients with prior history of heart or lung disease.

SYMPTOMS FOR WHICH THIS TEST IS COMMONLY OBTAINED:
Weight loss (p. 306).
Fever (p. 296).
Abdominal pain (p. 285).
Swollen lymph nodes (p. 305).

DISEASES FOR WHICH THIS TEST IS COMMONLY OBTAINED:
Cancer (p. 313)—The presence of lymph nodes in the abdomen suggests cancer. A biopsy can be performed on the lymph nodes to make a specific diagnosis. In a patient who is being treated for cancer, changes in the size of the lymph nodes can be monitored to help the doctor follow the course of the disease.

COST: approximately $400.

MAMMOGRAPHY AND XEROGRAPHY

PURPOSE OF THE TEST: to detect breast cysts or tumors.

BACKGROUND: Mammography and xerography are special x-rays done on breasts to locate the presence of abnormal tissue, such as tumors and cysts.

HOW THE TEST IS DONE: The patient undresses and puts on a hospital gown that opens in the front. While sitting, she places each breast, in turn, on an x-ray table. In mammography two x-rays are generally made of each breast; in xerography the x-ray picture is developed in conjunction with photocopier paper, but the actual procedure for taking the picture is the same as in mammography. The entire procedure takes about 15 minutes.

HOW THE RESULTS ARE GIVEN: The radiologist will interpret the x-ray and send a report to the patient's doctor. The x-ray cannot tell with certainty that an abnormality is cancer. If the mammography result is suspicious, a final diagnosis can be made only by biopsy (p. 187). The mammography must be considered in light of the physical examination of the breasts as well as the patient's age and other medical problems.

PATIENT PREPARATION: None

RISKS AND DISCOMFORTS: The test is not uncomfortable. In recent years, significant improvements have been made in the safety of

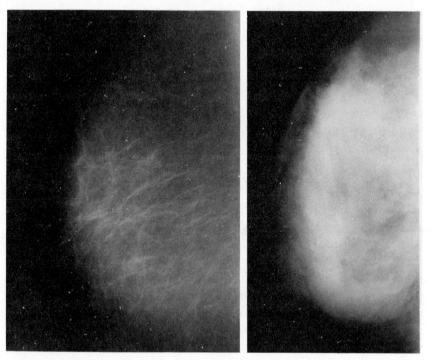

Normal mammogram (left side) and one from a patient with a breast cancer (right side).

this test because newer technology allows for the use of much lower radiation dosages. Even still there has been much publicity concerning the risk that mammography poses to women. The indiscriminate use of mammography is dangerous because it exposes breast tissue to x-rays that can themselves cause cancer. The way to evaluate the risk is straightforward: if the test is indicated because of the presence of a breast mass, or a family history that is strong for breast cancer, the risk is acceptable. If the test is being done without good reason or in women without symptoms under the age of 40, then the risk from the radiation is too high, and the procedure should not be performed. See p. 244 for a more detailed discussion.

SYMPTOMS FOR WHICH THIS TEST IS COMMONLY OBTAINED: These symptoms are suggestive of breast cancer, and the test is therefore done to search for tumors when these symptoms are present:
Breast lump or swelling (p. 302).
Nipple discharge.

The use of mammography and xerography in screening healthy women for breast cancer is discussed on p. 244.

COST: approximately $90.

MYELOGRAM

PURPOSE OF THE TEST: to evaluate the spinal cord and nerves that flow from it, the membranes lining it, and the vertebrae that surround it.

BACKGROUND: In order to understand myelography, it is necessary to explore the anatomy of the area involved. The spinal cord begins at the base of the brain in the neck and runs to the lower back. Throughout its length, nerves flow from it to control the many parts of the body. This critical organ is protected by a series of membranes, called meninges, which form a protective lining for it, as well as by the vertebrae that encircle it and offer a bony "suit of armor." The nerves that extend from the spinal cord run between the vertebrae before entering the body. Between each of these vertebrae are pads that cushion the bones from each other. These pads—discs—are formed from cartilage.
    Numerous diseases can affect any of these tissues and organs,

including tumors of the spinal cord itself, degeneration or rupture of the discs, abscesses of the spinal cord or meninges and arthritis of the vertebrae. Routine x-rays of the vertebrae will demonstrate any abnormality within the vertebral bone. The anatomy of the spinal cord and discs is not well seen, however. In myelography, a contrast dye is injected into the cerebrospinal fluid, which flows within the meninges and bathes the spinal cord. This will outline the tissues and make x-ray analysis possible.

HOW THE TEST IS DONE: The test is usually done in the x-ray department of the hospital. In addition to the radiologist, a neurologist or neurosurgeon may be present. The patient lies on the table and is prepared in the exact same way as for a lumbar puncture (p. 210). The lower back is washed well with a disinfectant, and sterile drapes are applied, exposing only a small area of skin. A local anesthetic is given and a needle is then placed through the skin between the vertebrae and into the cerebrospinal fluid. The contrast dye—about one to three teaspoonfuls—is then injected through the needle into the cerebrospinal fluid. The dye used is different from other contrast dyes in that it is very oily and much denser than the cerebrospinal fluid. This is important because it enables the radiologist to tilt the table in different directions while the oily, thick contrast dye flows up and down the spinal cord. As the radiologist does this, the patient is fluoroscoped and x-ray pictures are taken of any abnormalities. The needle is kept in the patient's back during the procedure, and at the end of the study the table is tilted so that the dye flows towards the needle and is removed as much as possible. The test takes approximately one hour. Following the removal of the dye, the needle is taken out, and the patient lies flat for several hours. In this way the procedure is similar to that done after a lumbar puncture.

HOW THE RESULTS ARE GIVEN: The radiologist, neurologist, or neurosurgeon will be able to tell from the fluoroscopy if any abnormalities are present. This may be told to the patient immediately after the procedure, or, more commonly, a report will be sent to his doctor after the x-rays have been carefully examined.

PATIENT PREPARATION: Occasionally, a sedative is given to relax the patient. If the test is done in the morning, he should avoid eating breakfast until after the procedure. If scheduled in the afternoon, a light breakfast is permitted.

RISKS AND DISCOMFORTS: A myelogram is an uncomfortable procedure. The lumbar puncture may be painful and may result in a headache—sometimes severe—following the test. The presence of the dye can cause a chemical inflammation throughout the spinal cord that can result in fever, stiff neck, headache, or vomiting. More rarely, the patient may suffer an allergic reaction to the dye. In addition, it is never possible to completely remove all the dye following the procedure. During the test itself the patient may be uncomfortable as the table is tilted back and forth. Although he is strapped securely to the table, he may feel as if he is about to "fall off."

SYMPTOMS FOR WHICH THIS TEST IS COMMONLY OBTAINED: All these symptoms can be due to disease within the area, including ruptured disc, arthritis, tumors of the spinal cord, compression of the spinal cord, abscesses, and injury:
Back pain (p. 287)—This test is performed for back pain only if the patient has not responded to medical treatment or if neurological symptoms are present.
Weakness or paralysis.
Incontinence.
Pain along nerves.

DISEASES FOR WHICH THIS TEST IS COMMONLY OBTAINED:
This test is done to confirm the presence of these diseases when surgery is being considered:
Ruptured (slipped) disc.
Tumor (benign or malignant) of the spinal cord, meninges, vertebrae, or nerves.
Spinal cord abscess.
Vertebrae arthritis.

COST: approximately $200.

UPPER GI SERIES

OTHER NAMES: upper GI, barium
swallow, small bowel series, UGI.

PURPOSE OF THE TEST: to visualize the esophagus, stomach, duodenum, and small intestines.

BACKGROUND: Ordinarily, the esophagus, stomach, duodenum, and small intestines are not seen clearly on a routine x-ray. When barium (a radiopaque contrast agent) is ingested, it coats the lining of these organs as it is swallowed and permits visualization by x-ray. Ulcers, tumors, and inflammation can be diagnosed by this procedure.

HOW THE TEST IS DONE: The patient stands against an x-ray table and drinks a barium "milkshake," which has a chalky taste. As the barium passes through the esophagus and into the stomach, the table is tilted in different directions in order to spread the contrast material throughout the organs to be examined. Occasionally, pressure is applied to the outside of the patient's abdomen to allow better distribution of the barium and better visualization of the organs. X-rays are taken at various points during the study. The x-ray of the esophagus, stomach, and duodenum takes about half an hour. If the entire small intestine is to be examined, an additional four hours may be necessary.

HOW THE RESULTS ARE GIVEN: The many x-rays taken are reviewed by a radiologist. He prepares a written report which is sent to the patient's physician.

PATIENT PREPARATION: The patient must not eat or drink for eight hours before the study. A laxative is given afterwards to help remove the barium from the body.

RISKS AND DISCOMFORTS: The barium has an unpleasant taste but is often flavored with chocolate or strawberry. Slight abdominal discomfort may occur during the study.

SYMPTOMS FOR WHICH THIS TEST IS COMMONLY OBTAINED:
Trouble swallowing—As the barium flows from the mouth through the esophagus and into the stomach, abnormalities in the swallowing mechanism can be detected.
Indigestion (p. 298).
Abdominal pain (p. 285).
Blood in stool (p. 289).
Vomiting (p. 303).

DISEASES FOR WHICH THIS TEST IS COMMONLY OBTAINED:
Ulcer (p. 325)—Irregularities will be seen in the wall of the stomach or duodenum.
Cancer (p. 313)—Tumors in the wall of the esophagus or stomach,

or obstruction to the free flow of barium in those organs will suggest cancer.

Reflux esophagitis—This occurs when part of the stomach slides into the esophagus (hiatal hernia) and stomach contents are forced up into the lower portion of the esophagus causing inflammation. An upper GI series will detect this abnormal movement.

COST: approximately $70.

VENOGRAPHY

OTHER NAMES: venogram.

PURPOSE OF THE TEST: to visualize the veins in the legs.

BACKGROUND: Blood clots in the veins of the legs (thrombophlebitis) occur commonly. The clots, if not treated, can lead to blockage of the veins higher up in the legs and abdomen. Parts of these clots can dislodge and cause a pulmonary embolus (blood clot in the lung). Early diagnosis allows for treatment and prevention of this dangerous problem. The venogram is used to detect abnormal flow in the veins and to diagnose thrombophlebitis.

HOW THE TEST IS DONE: There are two slightly different ways for venography to be conducted. In both, the patient cannot eat for four hours before the test and must lie on a table that is capable of being tilted in different directions. The skin over a vein in the leg is cleaned. A needle is placed into the vein and radiopaque contrast material is injected. In one method of venography tourniquets are applied around the leg to exert pressure on the vein and enable the dye to circulate throughout the various veins in the leg. In the other method the table is tilted up so that the patient is nearly standing upright. The patient stands on one leg, and because of gravity the dye will flow throughout all the veins. In either method fluoroscopy and x-ray pictures are taken of the veins, which are now filled with radiopaque material. A salt solution is injected into the vein after the study to wash out the contrast agent. Only one leg can be studied at a time. The test takes one hour to perform.

HOW THE RESULTS ARE GIVEN: A radiologist reviews the x-rays of the vein patterns and determines if a blood clot is present. A written report is sent to the patient's physician.

PATIENT PREPARATION: A sedative is occasionally given before-hand to decrease the patient's apprehension.

RISKS AND DISCOMFORTS: The major risk in venography is that the procedure itself—especially the use of tourniquets—can actually cause blood clots to develop where none existed previously. In addition, the placing of the needle in the vein can be slightly pain-ful.

SYMPTOMS FOR WHICH THIS TEST IS COMMONLY OBTAINED:
Leg pain and swelling.
Shortness of breath (p. 290).
Chest pain (p. 291).

DISEASES FOR WHICH THIS TEST IS COMMONLY OBTAINED:
Thrombophlebitis—Demonstration of blockage of the normal blood flow in the veins will help in the diagnosis of this disease.
Pulmonary embolus—The most common cause of this disease is thrombophlebitis of the legs, which then releases blood clots that lodge in the lungs. A venogram cannot detect if this has happened but will often be done to see if thrombophlebitis is present in suspected cases of pulmonary embolus.

COST: approximately $250.

7

Nuclear Medicine

NUCLEAR medicine (sometimes called nuclear scanning or radionuclide organ imaging) is a series of tests that are used to evaluate the anatomy and function of internal organs and tissues. Nuclear medicine centers around the use of radioisotopes, materials that emit radiation. These substances, when injected into the body, concentrate differently in abnormal tissue than in healthy tissue. This allows for clear visualization of diseased tissue within an organ.

There are many different radioisotopes. Each one, when administered to a patient, concentrates in a specific organ, so different radioisotopes are used for scanning different organs. When the isotopes are administered to a patient, the radiation that is released is detected by scanning devices—similar to Geiger counters—called rectilinear or gamma cameras. These cameras measure the intensity of the isotope and allow visualization of parts of organs that are not usually seen by normal x-rays. A permanent record is made on a photographic plate.

Although the details of the technique will vary with the individual scanning test, the basic procedure is the same. The radioactive isotope is either taken orally or injected into the patient's vein. The isotope is allowed to concentrate over time in the organ that is to be evaluated, and a scanner is placed over the tissue to be examined. Measurements of the amount of radiation released by the organ are then recorded. The scanning machine converts this measurement of the radioactivity into a picture of the tissue to be examined. This picture will then be interpreted by a doctor, usually a radiologist who is a specialist in the field of nuclear medicine. A written report is sent to the referring physician within several days.

Not surprisingly, when patients first hear about nuclear medicine tests they become apprehensive about the risk from radioactivity. Therefore, when we describe these tests to our own patients, we take special care to explain that as far as we now know, there is very little or no risk to the use of these radioisotopes. The amount of radioactivity they emit is very small, and the radioisotopes themselves are excreted from the body (either in urine or stool) within a few days. Nevertheless, we recommend that these tests not be performed in pregnant women or mothers who are breast feeding (since the radioisotope may be excreted in the milk) and that alternative diagnostic procedures be used for them instead.

Although we do not believe that the radioactivity is dangerous, there are some discomforts associated with these tests. The patient must lie very still during the scan, and this can be mildly uncomfortable. When the isotope is injected into the vein, slight pain may result. In addition, the isotopes may cause an allergic reaction in some people, although this is rare.

Generally, little patient preparation is required for these tests. The patient must tell the doctor if she is pregnant or is breast feeding so the test can be postponed or canceled. Also, it is important to tell the radiologist if any nuclear medicine scans have been done in the recent past since the radioisotopes often interfere with each other and the test will be impossible to interpret correctly.

BONE SCAN

PURPOSE OF THE TEST: to detect areas of abnormal bone that cannot be seen on x-ray.

BACKGROUND: Even though bones stop growing when a person becomes an adult, bone remains a living tissue that continuously requires minerals and nutrients like any other organ in the body. A bone scan is based on the principle that the mineral phosphate is absorbed by the bone from the blood. If this mineral is made radioactive, a scanner can be used to determine the amount of the phosphate that has been absorbed into the bone. Diseased bone will absorb the radioactive phosphate at a different rate than normal bone and consequently show up differently in the bone scan picture. Both x-rays and bone scans are used to detect diseased bone. Generally speaking, a bone scan is better than an x-ray in detecting abnormal bone but gives less specific information than an x-ray concerning the exact nature of the abnormality that is found. Therefore, depending upon the history in any given patient, the physician may decide to get one or both tests.

HOW THE TEST IS DONE: Radioactive technetium-99m diphosphonate is injected intravenously into the patient. A two-hour waiting period is necessary for the radioactive phosphate to be absorbed by the bone. Before the actual scan begins, the patient is asked to urinate because a full bladder will hide many of the pelvic bones. Following this the patient lies still on a table while the scanner moves slowly around the body. The scan takes about 30 to 60 minutes to complete.

HOW THE RESULTS ARE GIVEN: The scanning machine converts this measurement of the radioactivity into a picture of all the bones in the body. This picture looks like a drawing of the skeleton. Normally, in adults all the bones will absorb the same amount of phosphate and give off equal amounts of radioactivity. Diseased bone will absorb the phosphate abnormally and give off either more or less radioactivity. Physicians refer to these abnormal areas on the bone scan as "hot spots" or "cold spots." Bone scans done on children are more difficult to interpret because the bones of children are still growing. Therefore "hot spots" or "cold spots" might be related to the growing pattern of normal bone and may not indicate a disease process.

PATIENT PREPARATION: Although all the bones of the body are seen on a bone scan, laxatives are given the night before the scan if the bones near the abdomen are of special interest to the physician.

RISKS AND DISCOMFORTS: See "Nuclear Medicine," p. 132.

SYMPTOMS FOR WHICH THIS TEST IS COMMONLY OBTAINED:
Bone pain.
Weight loss (p. 306).
Fever (p. 296).

DISEASES FOR WHICH THIS TEST IS COMMONLY OBTAINED:
Cancer (p. 313)—to look for its spread into the bone.
Osteomyelitis (infection within the bone)—to locate the site of the infection.

COST: approximately $270.

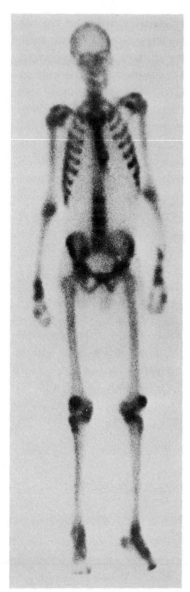

Normal bone scan. The bones of the body are visible as darkened areas, giving this bone scan the appearance of a "miniature skeleton."

BRAIN SCAN

PURPOSE OF THE TEST: To evaluate possible strokes or brain tumors.

BACKGROUND: Normally, substances do not cross over from the blood vessels in the brain into the brain tissue itself. This so-called blood-brain barrier serves to protect the brain. When lesions occur in the brain, however, this barrier breaks down and high concentrations of substances can leak from the blood vessels into brain tissue. The isotope technetium-99m pertechnetate, which is injected in this test, is found only in low concentrations in the normal brain but will be present in higher amounts when a stroke, tumor, or hematoma (collection of blood) is present. Because the findings from the brain scan are nonspecific, the brain CT scan (p. 115) has all but replaced the brain scan in evaluating brain tumors and strokes. If your physician recommends a brain scan, you should ask why this test—which is now slightly outmoded—and not a CT scan is being ordered.

HOW THE TEST IS DONE: The person lies on his back with his hands at his sides. At least one hour before the isotope is to be injected intravenously in the arm, a solution is taken by mouth to prevent the uptake of the isotope by the thyroid or salivary glands (where this particular isotope also tends to collect). The examining time is about one hour.

HOW THE RESULTS ARE GIVEN: Abnormalities in the brain are visualized by increased uptake of the isotope. Unfortunately, strokes, tumors, and hematomas will all have a similar appearance when this technique is used and cannot be differentiated. When a stroke has occurred, the brain scan does not become abnormal until after a few days. Hematomas and tumors in the brain, however, can be visualized and localized earlier.

PATIENT PREPARATION: None.

RISKS AND DISCOMFORTS: See "Nuclear Medicine," p. 132.

SYMPTOMS FOR WHICH THIS TEST IS COMMONLY OBTAINED:
Headache (p. 297).
Dizziness (p. 293).
Fainting (p. 294).

DISEASES FOR WHICH THIS TEST IS COMMONLY OBTAINED:
Stroke (p. 324)—Increased uptake of the isotope occurs after a stroke.
Cancer (p. 313)—Primary brain tumors or tumors from other parts of the body that have spread to the brain can be detected.
Aneurysm.
Brain hematoma.

COST: approximately $240.

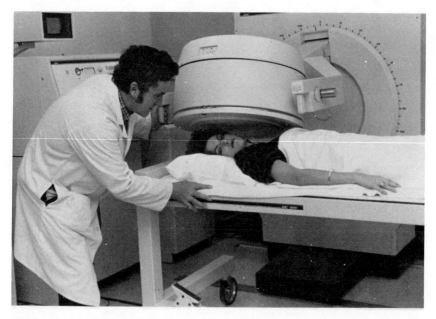

Patient having a brain scan. She is lying still while the scanning machine moves slowly over her head.

GALLIUM SCAN

PURPOSE OF THE TEST: to detect tumors and inflammation within the body tissues.

BACKGROUND: The radioisotope gallium citrate is picked up by abnormal tissue—such as a tumor or infection—that may be present in many different tissues (i.e., liver, bone, brain, and lymph nodes). Although increased uptake on the scan usually implies an abnormal condition, a normal scan does not rule out cancer or infection.

HOW THE TEST IS DONE: A laxative is taken the night before and enemas are given on the morning of the test. Gallium is injected intravenously and scans are obtained of the body 48 and 72 hours later. The patient must lie still while the scan is performed.

HOW THE RESULTS ARE GIVEN: Areas of increased radioisotope uptake indicate possible infection or cancer. Unfortunately, the gallium isotope collects in the stool making it difficult to interpret abnormalities in the intestines. Enemas done after the radioisotope is injected will lessen this problem. A picture of the body is taken from the scan which is then interpreted by a radiologist.

PATIENT PREPARATION: None.

RISKS AND DISCOMFORTS: See "Nuclear Medicine," page 132.

SYMPTOMS FOR WHICH THIS TEST IS COMMONLY OBTAINED:
Fever (p. 296).
Weight loss (p. 306).
Abdominal pain (p. 285).

DISEASES FOR WHICH THIS TEST IS COMMONLY OBTAINED:
Cancer (p. 313)—Tumors can be diagnosed by this technique. Response to cancer therapy can be measured by a decreased amount of isotope uptake as compared to a previous scan.
Abscess—An infection in the abdomen or elsewhere will demonstrate increased uptake of the isotope.

COST: approximately $330.

HEART SCANS

OTHER NAMES: gated blood pool scan,
thallium scan, stress-thallium scan, technetium scan.

PURPOSE OF THE TEST: to evaluate whether damage to heart muscle has occurred as well as to estimate how well the heart is functioning.

BACKGROUND: Heart disease continues to be one of the leading health problems today. Accurate detection of heart disease is an important task for the physician. The use of the heart scans described in this part has revolutionized the way in which a doctor can evaluate patients with proven or potential heart disease. These tests allow for a more accurate diagnosis in patients with angina or heart attack. Three different radioisotopes can be used for these heart scans:

1. Technetium-99m pyrophosphate—helps to determine whether actual death of heart tissue (myocardial infarction, or heart attack) has occurred; it can be done as early as 12 hours after the suspected heart attack.

2. Thallium-201 scan—used in association with an exercise tolerance test (p. 202) to determine whether any areas of the heart are not receiving sufficient amounts of oxygen (ischemia) during exercise.

3. Red cells labeled with technetium-99m (blood pool scan)—allows measurement of how well the heart is actually able to pump blood throughout the body. Since some of these labeled red cells enter the heart, actual changes in the heart's shape during a contraction are displayed by the scan as well.

The information obtained from heart scans will be used by the doctor in deciding whether additional testing (such as cardiac catheterization) is necessary. Since the scans involve little risk and often provide all the information necessary, they will always be performed before more dangerous procedures such as cardiac catheterization. If heart surgery is being considered, however, the surgeon will want the more detailed information obtained by catheterization, even if the heart tests have already been done.

HOW THE TEST IS DONE: Technetium pyrophosphate scan—While the patient is resting comfortably, the isotope is injected intravenously. After 30 minutes the scan is performed.

Thallium scan—The patient exercises to a maximum heart rate on an exercise treadmill. Immediately afterwards, the thallium is injected intravenously and the person lies down. After several minutes, scanning of the heart is performed.

Blood pool scan—While the patient is resting, the isotope is injected intravenously and the scan is performed.

HOW THE RESULTS ARE GIVEN: Areas of abnormal uptake of the isotope in the heart indicate either heart tissue death or insufficient oxygen to the heart muscle, depending on whether the isotope technetium or thallium is used. Measurements are made with the blood pool scan to determine how forceful each heart contraction is.

PATIENT PREPARATION: The patient should not eat or drink after midnight prior to a thallium or blood pool scan.

RISKS AND DISCOMFORTS: See "Nuclear Medicine," p. 132.

SYMPTOMS FOR WHICH THIS TEST IS COMMONLY OBTAINED:
Chest pain (p. 291)—thallium or technetium pyrophosphate scan.
Shortness of breath (p. 290)—blood pool scan.

DISEASES FOR WHICH THIS TEST IS COMMONLY OBTAINED:
Heart attack (p. 319)—The technetium-99m pyrophosphate scan will determine if a heart attack has occurred and what part of the heart was involved. The blood pool scan will evaluate how well the heart is functioning after a heart attack.
Congestive heart failure—A blood pool scan will document impairment in the heart's ability to transport blood throughout the body.
Angina pectoris—The thallium scan will determine which portions of the heart are receiving insufficient oxygen during chest pain.

COST: approximately $200.

KIDNEY SCAN

OTHER NAMES: renal scan, renogram.

PURPOSE OF THE TEST: to evaluate blood flow to the kidneys as well as the location and structure of the kidneys.

BACKGROUND: One of two isotopes—^{131}I hippuran or technetium-99m glucoheptanate—is used in a kidney scan. Both isotopes concentrate in the kidney and can be used to outline the size and shape of this organ as well as the blood vessels that supply it.

HOW THE TEST IS DONE: The patient will be asked to drink several glasses of water before the radioisotope is injected. If ^{131}I hippuran is used, it is injected intravenously and scanning is performed immediately. The patient must lie quietly for one hour during the scan. When technetium-99 glucoheptanate is used, the patient must be still for 30 minutes after the isotope is injected to allow for a complete picture of the kidney to be outlined. This study should be delayed for at least 24 hours after an IVP (p. 121) has been performed in order to insure that no residual dye remains.

HOW THE RESULTS ARE GIVEN: With ^{131}I hippuran, both the uptake and excretion from the kidney are measured and are compared for the right and left kidneys. The technetium-99m glucoheptanate scan creates a picture of the kidney. Areas of decreased uptake suggest tumors, cysts, or a nonfunctioning kidney. These measurements are analyzed by a radiologist.

PATIENT PREPARATION: None.

RISKS AND DISCOMFORTS: See "Nuclear Medicine," p. 132.

SYMPTOMS FOR WHICH THIS TEST IS COMMONLY OBTAINED:
Hematuria (blood in the urine).

DISEASES FOR WHICH THIS TEST IS COMMONLY OBTAINED:
Hypertension (p. 320)—A difference between the blood flow to the two kidneys may cause high blood pressure.
Kidney failure—Decreased uptake by the kidney will indicate abnormal kidney function.
Cancer (p. 313)—Decreased uptake by part of the kidney can occur with cancer.

COST: approximately $200.

Liver Scan

OTHER NAMES: liver-spleen scan.

PURPOSE OF THE TEST: to evaluate the size, shape, and function of the liver and spleen.

BACKGROUND: One of the liver's primary functions is to filter out foreign particles from the blood. If such particles are coated with radioactive technetium-99m pertechnetate and injected into the vein, they are rapidly trapped by the liver and spleen cells.

HOW THE TEST IS DONE: Thirty minutes before the scan is performed, technetium-99m pertechnetate is injected intravenously. At various times the person lies on his back, halfway on his left side, and on his abdomen, while the scanning is done. This allows visualization of the entire liver. The entire procedure takes approximately one hour.

HOW THE RESULTS ARE GIVEN: The scanner creates a picture of the liver. Cysts, tumors, and abscesses will show up on the scan as an irregular uptake of the radioisotope.

SYMPTOMS FOR WHICH THIS TEST IS COMMONLY OBTAINED:
Jaundice (p. 300).
Itching.
Fever (p. 296).
Weight loss (p. 306).

DISEASE FOR WHICH THIS TEST IS COMMONLY OBTAINED:
Hepatitis—Irregular uptake of the isotope by the liver will occur.
Cancer (p. 313)—The liver scan will detect liver cancer as well as
cancer from other parts of the body that has spread to the liver.
Repeat scans are helpful to determine if treatment of the cancer
has been effective.
Cirrhosis—Irregular uptake of the isotope by the liver will be
detected.

COST: approximately $220.

LUNG SCANS

PURPOSE OF THE TEST: to evaluate lung function and detect blood
clots in the lung.

BACKGROUND: Two different radioisotopes are used to evaluate the
lung. Radioactive serum albumin is used to evaluate blood flow,
and xenon-81m is used to evaluate how well the lung exchanges
oxygen for carbon dioxide. When injected, radioactive albumin
enters the blood stream and is trapped by the small vessels of the
lung. If a blood clot is present, the albumin cannot enter the small
vessels and decreased radioactivity will be measured by the scanner. Inhaled xenon demonstrates which parts of the lung are
effectively exchanging air.

HOW THE TEST IS DONE: The radioactive serum albumin is injected
intravenously and scanning of the lungs begins immediately. The
patient must remain still throughout the study. When xenon is
used, the patient inhales the isotope and then holds his breath to
allow the radioactive gas to be distributed throughout the lungs.
A chest x-ray is obtained for comparison with the nuclear medicine study.

HOW THE RESULTS ARE GIVEN: A film showing the distribution of
the isotope throughout the lungs is made. When the xenon study
and comparison chest x-ray are entirely normal, decreasd uptake
of radioactive albumin is suggestive of a pulmonary embolus. With
pneumonia the uptake of both albumin and xenon is decreased.

PATIENT PREPARATION: None.

RISKS AND DISCOMFORTS: See "Nuclear Medicine," p. 132.

SYMPTOMS FOR WHICH THIS TEST IS COMMONLY OBTAINED:
Shortness of breath (p. 290).
Chest pain (p. 291).
Hemoptysis (coughing up blood).

DISEASES FOR WHICH THIS TEST IS COMMONLY OBTAINED:
Pulmonary embolus—The radioactive albumin will be decreased in the involved area, while the xenon study will be normal.
Emphysema (p. 315)—The lung scan indicates which part of the lung is functioning abnormally.

COST: approximately $190

THYROID SCAN

PURPOSE OF THE TEST: to evaluate the size and functioning of the thyroid gland.

BACKGROUND: Iodine is actively taken up by the thyroid gland and utilized in the formation of the thyroid hormone. For this reason radioactive iodine, ^{131}I or ^{123}I, is used to measure the gland's function.

HOW THE TEST IS DONE: The patient swallows a capsule of radioactive iodine. He returns after six hours and again after 24 hours to have the actual scans performed. Each time the test takes 30 minutes. The dyes used in other X-ray studies will interfere with the uptake by the thyroid of the radioisotope. Consequently, a thyroid scan cannot be performed for at least six weeks after an IVP (p. 121) or six months after an oral cholecystogram (p. 119).

HOW THE RESULTS ARE GIVEN: The information obtained from the scanner is plotted on film, outlining the thyroid gland. Normally the iodine uptake is equal throughout the gland. Areas of increased iodine uptake indicate overactive thyroid function, while areas of decreased iodine uptake indicate underactive thyroid function or possibly cancer.

PATIENT PREPARATION: Care must be taken not to eat items that contain iodine for at least one week before the scan because this will interfere with the gland's uptake of the radioisotope. Iodine-containing compounds include thyroid drugs, oral contraceptives, cough medicines, and iodized salt.

RISKS AND DISCOMFORTS: See "Nuclear Medicine," p. 132.

SYMPTOMS FOR WHICH THIS TEST IS COMMONLY OBTAINED:
Diarrhea (p. 293).
Constipation.
Weight loss or gain (p. 306).
Hair loss.
Cold or heat intolerance.

DISEASES FOR WHICH THIS TEST IS COMMONLY OBTAINED:
Thyroid nodule—A thyroid scan may be ordered when a physician feels a nodule on the thyroid during a physical exam. Decreased uptake of the radioisotope iodine by the nodule—"cold" nodule—raises the possibility that the nodule may be cancerous. Hyperthyroidism and hypothyroidism—Activity of the thyroid gland is measured by the concentration of iodine uptake by the gland.

COST: approximately $190.

8

Ultrasound

AT FIRST glance one would not think that there is much in common between porpoises, burglar alarms, submarines, and the modern hospital. But, in fact, all rely heavily on the principles of ultrasonic waves. Sound travels through air or water by waves, and humans can generally hear sound when the waves range between 100 and 16,000 times per second. When the sound waves are at a very high speed—greater than 20,000 times per second—they are called ultrasonic, and the sound they produce is not heard by the human ear. These ultrasonic waves have one property that makes them very useful: they will reflect or bounce back when they hit solid objects.

Porpoises transmit ultrasonic waves and use the resultant reflection of the waves from solid objects as a navigation system, alerting them to the presence of obstacles in the water and allowing them to swim safely at high speeds. In the 1930s, the principles behind this sytem were adapted to use by boats. Called SONAR for SOund Navigation And Ranging, this system transmits ultrasonic pulses towards a target and then listens for the reflected sound waves with a sensitive microphone. SONAR was critical to the navy during World War II and is still used on most ships to detect the depth of the ocean floor and warn of approaching rocks and other underwater obstacles.

About 30 years ago a similar system of ultrasonic transmission and detection was adapted for use in the area of medical testing to provide information about internal organs, including the heart and blood vessels. All ultrasound devices used since that time have depended on the same principles. Ultrasonic waves are transmitted from the tip of a device called a transducer; also in the tip is a sensitive microphone. The transducer is pointed at the desired area of the body. Since the different parts of the body will have differing densities, the sound waves are reflected differently from the many structures that are present. These reflected waves are processed and either displayed on an oscilloscope—an instrument that resembles a television screen—or recorded permanently on special paper. Abnormal structures are easily detected when their densities are different from the normal surrounding tissue. Because ultrasonic waves are completely reflected by air-containing organs, such as the lungs and the gas-filled intestines, the test is not useful in diagnosing abnormalities in these organs.

There are many advantages to ultrasound. Since this technique does not use radiation, it is safe to the patient and technician performing the test. It takes only a short time to perform and requires little patient preparation. For these reasons it is being used with increasing frequency and may be performed safely more than once on the same patient within a short interval. On the other hand, ultrasound is difficult to perform in patients with abdominal bandages or scars, as these cause erratic deflections of the ultrasonic waves. Barium remaining in the abdomen from a previous barium enema may also affect the quality of the ultrasound study. In addition, because the patient must remain still for the test, it is often difficult to perform on young children.

Since the equipment is expensive, this test is most often performed in a hospital on an out-patient basis. Occasionally, however, individual physicians may have the necessary equipment in their office. To prepare the patient a lubricant is applied to the skin of the area to be studied. This acts as a conductor for the sound waves. The transducer is held by a technician and moved back and forth over the lubricated skin surface. The height of the sound waves as well as the time required for the sound waves to be reflected from the body are displayed on the oscilloscope screen. Permanent records are made from the pictures obtained from the oscilloscope.

A specialist trained in the interpretation of ultrasound will study the test and report the results. This specialist might be a radiologist, or, in the case of certain ultrasound examinations, a cardiologist (for ultrasound of the heart), or an obstetrician (when the uterus of a pregnant mother is being studied). Although the ultrasound pictures can be interpreted immediately, and an oral report given if necessary, it generally takes several days for your own physician to receive a written report. At the present time, there are no known risks to ultrasound. There is no radiation involved in an ultrasound and, consequently, no radiation-associated risk exists from the test. Nevertheless, numerous research studies are underway to determine if the technique is safe as it is presently used.

Ultrasound is most effective when a particular organ is being studied or a specific disease is being considered. It is not useful as a screening test, and your physician should be able to give you a precise reason for doing the study and not simply "to see if everything is all right."

The particular details of the various kinds of ultrasound examination are discussed on the following pages.

ABDOMINAL ULTRASOUND

OTHER NAMES: abdominal sonogram.

PURPOSE OF THE TEST: to evaluate the organs located in the abdomen.

BACKGROUND: Many of the structures located in the abdomen can be analyzed by ultrasound. These include the gallbladder, liver, spleen, kidney, lymph nodes, pancreas, and abdominal aorta as well as the uterus and ovaries. Gas-filled structures, such as the small and large intestines, cannot be seen by this technique. The ultrasound is most helpful when it is directed specifically at one of these organs instead of attempting to evaluate several structures at once.

HOW THE TEST IS DONE: The patient undresses to the waist. Lubricant and the transducer are applied to the portion of the abdomen that is to be examined.

HOW THE RESULTS ARE GIVEN: A radiologist will interpret the pictures obtained from the oscilloscope and report if any abnormalities are present. A written report will be sent to the patient's physician.

PATIENT PREPARATION: If the pelvic area is to be evaluated, the patient will be asked to drink three or four glasses of water and not urinate until after the ultrasound is obtained. When the gallbladder is evaluated, the patient should not eat solid food for 12 hours beforehand to permit the gallbladder to enlarge. Likewise, the patient will fast for eight hours prior to an ultrasound of the pancreas, liver, and spleen. In addition, any wound dressings should be removed from the abdomen before the test is performed. Care should be taken to ensure that a barium enema (p. 109) or upper GI series (p. 128) is not performed before an abdominal ultrasound because the sound waves cannot penetrate the barium used in these studies.

RISKS AND DISCOMFORTS: See "Ultrasound," page 145.

SYMPTOMS FOR WHICH THIS TEST IS COMMONLY OBTAINED:
Fever (p. 296).
Weight loss (p. 306).
Abdominal pain (p. 285).
Back pain (p. 287).
Jaundice (p. 300).

DISEASES FOR WHICH THIS TEST IS COMMONLY OBTAINED:
Gallbladder—Stones in the gallbladder or the ducts that drain from the gallbladder are frequently seen by ultrasound. Inflammation of the gallbladder (cholecystitis) can also be diagnosed with this technique.
Pancreas—Inflammation of the pancreas (pancreatitis) and cancer of the pancreas are detected.
Liver—Fluid-filled cysts, solid tumors, and areas of infection (abscesses) are distinguished by differing intensities of the ultrasonic waves that are reflected.
Abdominal aorta—Abnormal dilation of the aorta (aneurysm) can be measured. This technique will also indicate when surgery is necessary to repair the aneurysm.
Lymph nodes—Enlarged lymph nodes are present with cancer or infection. Repeated ultrasounds are performed after treatment to evaluate the success of the treatment.
Kidney—Urinary tract infection (p. 175), obstructions to the passage of urine, and congenital abnormalities can be diagnosed by this test.
Uterus and ovaries—Proper position of intrauterine devices IUDs can be checked. Ultrasound can also detect fibroid tumors of the uterus, masses in the ovaries, and inflammation in the fallopian tubes.

COST: approximately $100.

DOPPLER ULTRASOUND

OTHER NAMES: carotid flow study.

PURPOSE OF THE TEST: to detect blood flow in the veins and arteries in the body.

BACKGROUND: Since ultrasound can detect motion, this technique is used to differentiate between normal and abnormal blood flow in the arteries and veins as well as to record blood flow in the fetus and placenta.

HOW THE TEST IS DONE: With the patient lying on his back, the lubricant and transducer are placed over the blood vessels to be examined. Frequently, the blood vessels that supply the brain and the legs are examined. When the legs are examined, blood pressure cuffs are placed along the limbs to determine exactly where changes in the blood flow occur. When the test is done to detect blood flow in the fetus and placenta, the lubricant and transducer are placed on the woman's abdomen over the uterus.

HOW THE RESULTS ARE GIVEN: Differences in blood flow to the parts of the leg will be interpreted as obstruction of the blood vessels. The obstruction is classified as mild, moderate, or severe. A radiologist analyzes the Doppler flow readings and sends a written report to the referring physician. When used in a pregnant woman, the Doppler records the heart rate of the fetus.

PATIENT PREPARATION: None.

RISKS AND DISCOMFORTS: See "Ultrasound," page 145.

SYMPTOMS FOR WHICH THIS TEST IS COMMONLY OBTAINED:
Leg pain or swelling.
Dizziness (p. 293).
Shortness of breath (p. 290).

DISEASES FOR WHICH THIS TEST IS COMMONLY OBTAINED:
Stroke (p. 324)—This technique will detect obstruction in the arteries that supply the brain.
Pulmonary embolus—Ultrasound can look for blood clots in the legs that might break off and lodge in the lung.
Thrombophlebitis—Blockage and inflammation of the veins in the legs can be detected.

COST: approximately $100.

Echocardiogram

OTHER NAMES: heart echogram, echo.

PURPOSE OF THE TEST: to detect abnormalities in the heart.

BACKGROUND: This use of ultrasound has revolutionized our ability to evaluate the internal structures of the heart in a safe and easy way. Because the heart is filled with blood, sound waves are transmitted easily through the heart to its walls. The size, shape, and position of the heart as well as the movement of the heart valves and chambers can then be recorded.

HOW THE TEST IS DONE: The patient undresses to the waist and lies on his back with the lubricant and transducer placed over the chest wall. The transducer is directed in towards the chambers of the heart and the valves separating the chambers.

HOW THE RESULTS ARE GIVEN: Specific measurements of the size of the heart chambers are made and compared with normal values. Function of the mitral and aortic valves as well as the pumping ability of the heart are also determined. These measurements are interpreted by either a radiologist or a cardiologist. A written report is made and sent to the referring physician.

PATIENT PREPARATION: None.

RISKS AND DISCOMFORTS: See "Ultrasound," page 145.

SYMPTOMS FOR WHICH THIS TEST IS COMMONLY OBTAINED:
Chest pain (p. 291)—to detect whether pericardial effusion—fluid around the heart sac—or abnormalities of the heart valves are causing the pain.
Palpitations.
Shortness of breath (p. 290).

DISEASES FOR WHICH THIS TEST IS COMMONLY OBTAINED:
Stroke (p. 324)—to determine whether blood clots from the heart caused the stroke.
Heart attack (p. 319)—to detect whether the heart's ability to pump blood has been impaired by the heart attack.
Heart valve abnormality (mitral stenosis, aortic stenosis, and mitral valve prolapse)—to detect whether the heart valves are functioning properly.

Pericardial effusion.
Rheumatic fever.

COST: approximately $100.

OBSTETRIC ULTRASOUND

OTHER NAMES: fetal ultrasound.

PURPOSE OF THE TEST: to evaluate the fetus during pregnancy.

BACKGROUND: Because no radiation is involved, this test is used extensively in evaluating the fetus during pregnancy. The amniotic fluid-filled uterus provides strong transmission of ultrasonic waves, which permits easy distinction between the fluid, placenta, and fetus. This test can detect a pregnancy as early as five weeks after a missed menstrual period and can be used to evaluate the fetus throughout the pregnancy.

HOW THE TEST IS DONE: The patient lies on a table with her abdominal area uncovered. Lubricant is spread over the lower abdomen and the transducer is placed on the lubricated skin. The ultrasound waves are recorded on an oscilloscope.

HOW THE RESULTS ARE GIVEN: Pictures are taken from the oscilloscope and analyzed by the obstetrician or radiologist. A written report is sent to the patient's physician.

PATIENT PREPARATION: The patient drinks three to four glasses of water and should not urinate until after the test is done. This fluid distends the bladder and makes it easier to visualize the fetus.

RISKS AND DISCOMFORTS: At this time there is no known risk to a pregnant woman or to the fetus from ultrasound. There is much research currently being done on the subject, however, and the final verdict on potential risks is still pending.

ALTHOUGH NOT USED AS A ROUTINE PREGNANCY TEST, THE OBSTETRIC ULTRASOUND CAN DO THE FOLLOWING:
Diagnose pregnancy.
Determine fetal age—This can be done by measuring the size of the fetus's head.
Determine fetal position—This is important in determining whether

there is a breech presentation and in deciding whether a vaginal delivery is possible.

Identify placenta—Abnormal location or separation of the placenta can be identified.

Determine number of fetuses—Twins and other multiple pregnancies can be determined as early as the second month of pregnancy.

Determine fetal death—The absence of fetal growth over a period of several weeks, as determined by repeated ultrasounds, suggests fetal death.

COST: approximately $100.

9

Endoscopy

For many years physicians have inserted tubes attached to a light source into various orifices of the body in order to see directly the internal structures and organs. Until a few years ago these tubes were rigid and hard and had to pass as a straight line between the light and the organ to be examined. But in the last few years these procedures, called endoscopy, have been altered dramatically by the development of fiberoptic instruments. These tubes, which can bend easily, come in various lengths and widths, ranging from one-eighth to one-half inch in diameter.

The tube is inserted into the body and the doctor looks through a lens attached to the opposite end. In this way he can visualize the organs and surrounding structures. In addition, small tweezers (forceps) can be attached to the end of the tube, enabling the doctor to use the endoscopy procedure as a means of obtaining biopsy specimens of any questionable tissue. Although the general name for these procedures is endoscopy, the specific tests are more commonly referred to by their own names, such as gastroscopy or sigmoidoscopy. These tests frequently provide information that could previously be obtained only by surgery. Most of them require special training and experience and are done by specialists, not family practitioners, general internists, or pediatricians. For example, bronchoscopy is done by lung specialists (pulmonologists) or thoracic (chest) surgeons, and colposcopy is done by gynecologists. If you have symptoms or diseases that require these procedures, your own doctor will refer you to one of these specialists.

How does the patient get the results from an endoscopy? Since the specialist actually sees the part of the body being examined during the test, he should be able to tell the patient the results at that time—and this is often the case. Sometimes, however, a biopsy may be required, the results of which will take several days to process. Also, since the patient is frequently sedated for these tests, it might be difficult for the doctor doing the procedure to discuss the findings with him. What's more, if the physician doing the test is not the patient's own doctor but a specialist to whom the patient has been referred, the results may be sent directly to the patient's own doctor, who will then meet with the patient to discuss them in detail.

Arthroscopy

PURPOSE OF THE TEST: The purpose of arthroscopy is to see directly the inside of the joint as well as the cartilage and ligaments that support it. The joint most commonly studied by arthroscopy is the knee, but other joints, such as the shoulder and ankle, can be studied as well. In addition, arthroscopy can be used to perform minor joint surgery, usually the removal of injured cartilage.

BACKGROUND: Injuries to the knee and other joints are not unique to star quarterbacks or basketball players, although they receive the most publicity when it happens. In fact, injuries to the knee are relatively common. This is not surprising considering the heavy use that our exercise- and fitness-oriented society gives to the knee, a rather delicate structure. Until recently, the doctor caring for a patient with a persistent knee problem would have to make a difficult decision: should he place the patient under general anesthesia and surgically explore the joint? Although this might enable the doctor to know for certain what is going on, it exposes the patient to the risk of anesthesia and infection to the joint and requires many days of hospitalization and recuperation time. Today, however, the doctor has another option—arthroscopy. This test will provide nearly all the information obtained by surgery with greater convenience and much less risk to the patient.

HOW THE TEST IS DONE: This test is done by orthopedists and is performed either in the doctor's office or in the operating room at the hospital. In either case sterile conditions are strictly maintained. A local anesthetic is injected into the skin and a small incision is made through which the arthroscope is passed into the joint. The orthopedist will first look to see if the cartilage, ligaments, and other joint tissues are normal. If he finds that the cartilage has become torn or injured, he may remove it at that time with forceps attached to the arthroscope. The test takes less than an hour and shortly thereafter the patient can return home. The knee will be bandaged or splinted, and usually the patient will need to walk with the aid of crutches and rest the leg for several days. Occasionally, if the patient is very uncomfortable, the procedure may be done under general anesthesia. If this is the case, the test must be done in the hospital and the patient will have to spend a few hours in the recovery room before being discharged.

HOW THE RESULTS ARE GIVEN: See "Endoscopy," page 153.

PATIENT PREPARATION: Frequently, the patient will be given a sedative before the test. If general anesthesia is used, eating and drinking are prohibited for at least six hours prior to the test.

RISKS AND DISCOMFORTS: The local anesthetic, given by injection, will be slightly painful. Although the entire procedure is done under sterile conditions, infection in the joint—a potentially serious problem—may occur as a result of arthroscopy, although this is rare. For several days after the test, the patient will be uncomfortable, especially if minor joint surgery was performed during the arthroscopy.

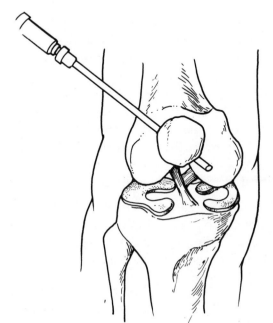

Location of the arthroscope in the knee joint.

SYMPTOMS FOR WHICH THIS TEST IS COMMONLY OBTAINED: The doctor may perform arthroscopy if the following symptoms are present in the knee (or occasionally in other joints as well). This test is usually not done when these symptoms first appear but only if conservative medical management (rest and possibly an exercise program, splinting, ice, or heat) does not result in improvement.
Joint pain.
Joint swelling.
Joint weakness or instability.

DISEASES FOR WHICH THIS TEST IS COMMONLY OBTAINED:
Joint injury.
Arthritis (p. 310)—to see how severely the joint is affected.

COST: approximately $400.

BRONCHOSCOPY

PURPOSE OF THE TEST: Bronchoscopy allows the doctor to see the airways—trachea and bronchi—when tumors and other diseases of these organs are suspected. In addition, bronchoscopy will be done in patients to remove an object that has lodged in their airway or windpipe.

BACKGROUND: Lung cancer, tuberculosis, and other serious chest diseases are difficult to diagnose by x-ray alone. When the chest x-ray is abnormal, it rarely provides a specific diagnosis but only indicates that some disease is present. What's more, even though the x-ray is perfectly normal, a disease may be present. Bronchoscopy allows the doctor to see directly the site of disease and to take a biopsy of tissue in order to make the specific diagnosis. This test will be done only when these diseases are suspected and other simpler tests such as sputum culture (p. 173) and cytology (p. 192) have not been helpful.

HOW THE TEST IS DONE: Bronchoscopy can be performed as an outpatient procedure in the hospital clinic. Prior to the test the patient receives a sedative as well as atropine, a medicine that decreases secretion in the airways. A local anesthetic is sprayed on the mouth, tongue, and throat to decrease the gag reflex—the uncontrollable reflex that causes gagging when something touches the throat. The patient's head is tilted as far back as possible and the bronchoscope inserted through the mouth or nose and down into the windpipe and airways. The doctor will first look around the area and then take a biopsy of any suspicious tissue or remove the object that is lodged. Bronchoscopy takes approximately one hour to perform. Occasionally, if a patient is unable to tolerate the procedure while awake, the test is done under general anesthesia. In that case the patient will have to spend a few hours in the recovery room before being discharged.

HOW THE RESULTS ARE GIVEN: See "Endoscopy," page 153.

PATIENT PREPARATION: The patient must not eat or drink for a minimum of six hours before the test so that if he gags during the insertion of the bronchoscope, there will be no food in the stomach to vomit and choke on. The sedative and atropine are administered prior to the procedure, and dentures must be removed from the mouth. A good exercise to do before the test is to practice breathing through the nose with the mouth open—the process that will be required when the bronchoscopy is being done. If the patient can be taught to do this before the procedure is performed, the suffocating feeling will be substantially diminished.

RISKS AND DISCOMFORTS: This test is an uncomfortable one. The presence of the bronchoscope may cause patients to have a choking sensation or feel that they cannot breathe. The medications given will make the patient feel drowsy and will cause a dry mouth. Following the procedure the patient will usually have a sore throat and often be hoarse. Bleeding from the lung may occur following the procedure, especially if a biopsy was performed. There is a very slight chance that the bronchoscope will injure the airway or windpipe, sometimes requiring surgery. Finally, if the procedure is done under general anesthesia there is the additional risk that always comes from the use of anesthesia.

SYMPTOMS FOR WHICH THIS TEST IS COMMONLY OBTAINED:
For all three symptoms, the purpose of the bronchoscopy is to see if cancer, tuberculosis, or pneumonia is present.
Cough (p. 292).
Spitting up blood.

DISEASES FOR WHICH THIS TEST IS COMMONLY OBTAINED:
Cancer (p. 313).
Tuberculosis.
Foreign object in the windpipe or airway.

Lung abscess.
Pneumonia.
Abnormalities seen on chest x-ray.

COST: approximately $250.

COLONOSCOPY

PURPOSE OF THE TEST: To visualize directly the interior surface of the large intestine (colon) and permit biopsy of suspicious areas.

BACKGROUND: A variety of diseases that afflict the large intestine can cause similar symptoms: blood in the stool, altered bowel habits, and abdominal pain. X-ray examination is sometimes insufficient to make the specific diagnosis. Colonoscopy is done to allow a direct examination of the entire colon, while sigmoidoscopy (p. 165) permits examination of only the 10 inches closest to the rectum.

HOW THE TEST IS DONE: The test is done in the doctor's office and does not require hospitalization. The patient is heavily sedated and lies on his left side. The colonoscope is inserted through the rectum and the physician doing the test—usually a gastroenterologist—passes the instrument through the twists and turns of the colon, looking at the inner surface as he goes along. Biopsies are taken of suspicious sites. The procedure takes from one to two hours.

HOW THE RESULTS ARE GIVEN: See "Endoscopy," page 153.

PATIENT PREPARATION: It is critical that the bowel be clean and without stool so that the colon can be seen. In order to do this, the patient must drink only clear liquids (juices, broths, soda) for 72 hours before the test. Laxatives will be given, usually for one to three days before the procedure. The night prior to the test, as well as the day of the test, an enema may be given. The patient should fast for eight hours before the test. The sedatives must be given immediately prior to the test.

RISKS AND DISCOMFORTS: During the test the patient will feel pressure in the rectum and colon but usually not sharp pain. Bleeding may occur from the colon, especially if a biopsy has been performed or a polyp removed. There is a slight chance that the colonoscope may perforate the colon, a very serious complication that may possibly require surgery.

SYMPTOMS FOR WHICH THIS TEST IS COMMONLY OBTAINED:
This test will be done whenever the patient has any of these symptoms to see if cancer, diverticulitis, polyps, or ulcerative colitis is present:
Abdominal pain (p. 285).
Gastrointestinal bleeding or blood in the stool (p. 289).
Diarrhea (p. 293).
Contipation.
Weight loss (p. 306)

DISEASES FOR WHICH THIS TEST IS COMMONLY OBTAINED:
Cancer (p. 313)—used to diagnose the presence of cancer, and once it has been removed to make sure it has not returned.
Colon polyps—used to see if polyps are present; can also be used to remove the polyps with the aid of the tweezers on the end of the instrument.
Ulcerative colitis and regional enteritis (Crohn's disease)—can often be used in several ways in these patients. When symptoms first occur, the test can be an aid in diagnosis. A biopsy can be obtained during the procedure as well. Once the patient is on medication, the test is valuable as a means of following and monitoring the disease. Finally, since patients with these diseases have an increased risk of cancer in the colon and rectum, the test is used to check periodically to be sure that they have not developed a malignancy.
Anemia (p. 309)—used especially in iron-deficiency anemia. Patients with bleeding from the gastrointestinal tract due to a variety of causes, including cancer, polyps, and ulcerative colitis, will often develop iron-deficiency anemia because of the chronic blood loss that they suffer.

COST: approximately $400.

COLPOSCOPY

PURPOSE OF THE TEST: To examine the vagina and cervix.

BACKGROUND: Cancer of the cervix is an important problem, and it is clear that early detection greatly increases the possibility of cure. Pap smears (p. 212) are now done routinely on most women to aid in the diagnosis of that disease. In the past, if abnormal cells were seen, the woman would have been admitted to the hospital to have cervical conization performed. This is minor surgery that involves taking a biopsy of the cervix and examining it. Today, however, a colposcopy enables the gynecologist to examine the cervix directly and determine whether further therapy is required. Besides those with abnormal Pap smears, another group of patients who have colposcopy are those whose mothers received the chemical DES (diethylstilbestrol) during their pregnancy. Use of this drug has been associated with cancer of the vagina and cervix, and female children of these women should be screened periodically for this problem.

HOW THE TEST IS DONE: The patient prepares for a pelvic examination in the usual manner. She is placed in stirrups and a speculum is inserted into the vagina (exactly as is done during a routine internal). No part of the colposcope is actually inserted into the vagina. Instead, the instrument—which looks like a microscope—is placed at the vaginal opening and the gynecologist looks through the eyepieces and examines the vagina and cervix. Small tweezers may be used to take a biopsy of abnormal tissue. Cotton swabs will dry any vaginal secretions or "paint" the area with a chemical that allows for better visualization of any abnormal tissue.

HOW THE RESULTS ARE GIVEN: See "Endoscopy," page 153.

PATIENT PREPARATION: None.

RISKS AND DISCOMFORTS: There might be some slight vaginal bleeding, especially if a biopsy was obtained.

SYMPTOMS FOR WHICH THIS TEST IS COMMONLY OBTAINED:
Vaginal bleeding.
Maternal exposure to DES (even without any symptoms).

DISEASES FOR WHICH THIS TEST IS COMMONLY OBTAINED:
Cancer (p. 313).
Abnormal Pap smear.

COST: approximately $200.

CYSTOSCOPY

PURPOSE OF THE TEST: In both men and women the purpose of a cystoscopy is to examine the bladder, the ureters (tubes connecting the kidney to the bladder), and the urethra (tube connecting the bladder to the outside). In addition, in males, this test allows the urologist to see the prostate gland. The procedure can also be used therapeutically to remove stones and small tumors from the bladder and kidney.

BACKGROUND: Cystoscopy enables the urologist to visualize directly a variety of tissues that cannot be seen on any x-ray study. In this manner specific diagnoses can be made.

HOW THE TEST IS DONE: The patient is sedated and placed on his back with legs in stirrups. The genitalia are swabbed with an antiseptic and a local anesthetic is applied to the urethra. At that time the cystoscope is inserted into the urethra and the bladder and adjacent tissues are examined. The procedure takes about 15 minutes. Occasionally, if the patient is uncomfortable or if the cystoscopy is being used to remove substantial amounts of tissue from the bladder or prostate gland, the test will be done under general anesthesia. Sometimes, the cystoscope is used to inject a contrast dye (which shows up on x-rays) into the bladder and ureters, and x-rays are then taken. This procedure is called *retrograde ureteropyelogram* and allows for more detailed examination of these tissues.

HOW THE RESULTS ARE GIVEN: See "Endoscopy", page 153.

PATIENT PREPARATION: On the morning of the test the patient can eat only liquid foods. A sedative must be administered prior to the procedure.

RISKS AND DISCOMFORTS: The procedure is uncomfortable and may cause a urinary tract infection or bleeding from the bladder. If the blood clots that results from such bleeding are large or if swelling of the urethra occurs, the patient may be unable to urinate and a catheter would have to be placed to release the urine. In rare instances perforation of the bladder may occur.

SYMPTOMS FOR WHICH THIS TEST IS COMMONLY OBTAINED:
Cystoscopy might be performed whenever a patient has the following symptoms, which suggest disease in the bladder, ureters, or kidneys:
Hematuria (blood in the urine).
Dysuria (pain with urination).
Inability to initiate urination (hesitancy) or other urinary symptoms, such as frequent urination or straining at urination.

DISEASES FOR WHICH THIS TEST IS COMMONLY OBTAINED:
Cancer (p. 313).
Enlarged prostate.
Narrowing of the urethra (urethral stricture).
Urinary tract infection.
Kidney or bladder stones.
Kidney obstruction.

COST: approximately $300.

GASTROSCOPY

OTHER NAMES: endoscopy, esophagoscopy,
duodenoscopy, esophagogastroduodenoscopy.

PURPOSE OF THE TEST: To allow the physician to view the tissues and organs of the upper gastrointestinal tract—esophagus, stomach, duodenum (first part of the small intestine).

BACKGROUND: A large number of diseases can affect the upper gastrointestinal tract causing symptoms of gastrointestinal bleeding, indigestion, vomiting, and abdominal pain. X-ray studies are sometimes not enough to determine the specific diagnosis. In these instances direct visualization of the organs is helpful.

HOW THE TEST IS DONE: The procedure is usually done by a gastroenterologist in the outpatient clinic of the hospital. The patient is asked to gargle with a topical anesthetic and is sedated with Valium or a similar drug. The endoscope is inserted slowly into the throat, down the esophagus, into the stomach, and then into the duodenum. Pictures can be taken through the endoscope, and biopsies of suspicious tissue will be obtained. In addition, forceps on the tip of the endoscope can remove any foreign objects that may have been swallowed (coin or pin).

HOW THE RESULTS ARE GIVEN: See "Endoscopy," page 153.

PATIENT PREPARATION: Patients must fast for four to six hours prior to the test. Dentures must be removed from the patient's mouth. The sedative and local anesthetic must be administered.

RISKS AND DISCOMFORTS: Placing of the tube into the stomach produces an uncomfortable feeling and may cause a gagging sensation or stomach cramps. Occasionally, the endoscope can perforate the gastrointestinal tract, a complication that sometimes requires surgery. Hemorrhage, which might be severe, can also result from the procedure.

SYMPTOMS FOR WHICH THIS TEST IS COMMONLY OBTAINED:
Gastrointestinal bleeding—to look for ulcers, gastritis, esophagitis, and cancer.
Indigestion (p. 298).
Weight loss (p. 306).
Abdominal pain (p. 285).
Difficulty swallowing (dysphagia).

DISEASES FOR WHICH THIS TEST IS COMMONLY OBTAINED:
Ulcer (p. 325).
Cancer (p. 313).
Anemia (p. 309)—especially iron-deficiency anemia, since that disease can result from excessive blood loss from bleeding in the gastrointestinal tract.
Gastritis.
Esophagitis.

COST: approximately $250.

LAPAROSCOPY

PURPOSE OF THE TEST: to evaluate the abdominal and pelvic organs.

BACKGROUND: Although there are many techniques available to evaluate the internal abdominal or pelvic organs, including x-ray, ultrasound, and nuclear medicine scans, sometimes it is best simply to see them directly. Some endoscopic tests, like gastroscopy or sigmoidoscopy, allow the doctor to visualize directly the interior surface of abdominal organs; laparoscopy allows him to see directly the outer surface of abdominal organs.

HOW THE TEST IS DONE: Laparoscopy in many ways resembles minor surgery. The procedure is done in a small operating room, where the patient wears a hospital gown and lies on the table. His lower abdomen is cleaned well with an antiseptic, and a local anesthetic is applied to the skin and underlying muscle. A small ($1/2$ inch) incision is made in the skin and the laparoscope—a short tube with a rotating tip—is placed through the skin and into the abdominal cavity. By rotating the tip, the physician (either a surgeon or gynecologist) is able to see the abdominal and pelvic organs. Biopsies can be obtained using tweezers on the end of the laparoscope. The entire procedure takes less than one hour.

HOW THE RESULTS ARE GIVEN: See "Endoscopy," page 153.

PATIENT PREPARATION: Patients are not allowed to eat or drink for eight hours prior to the test. A sedative may be given to the patient if he appears very anxious.

RISKS AND DISCOMFORTS: Although in some ways this test resembles minor surgery, there are very few risks associated with it. Rarely, the laparoscope may cause internal bleeding, or the incision site may become infected. After the procedure, the skin over the incision may be tender for a few days.

SYMPTOMS FOR WHICH THIS TEST IS COMMONLY OBTAINED:
Laparoscopy is most commonly done by gynecologists to evaluate the female reproductive organs. Symptoms that would prompt such an examination include:
Infertility (p. 299).
Abnormal menses.
Tumor or mass on any of the reproductive organs.
In addition, the procedure may be done in men and women when diseases of the abdomen are suspected and direct visualization will be helpful to make a diagnosis. Symptoms suggestive of these diseases include:
Weight loss (p. 306).
Weakness.
Blood in stool (p. 289).
Abdominal pain (p. 285).
Abdominal mass or tumor.
Diarrhea (p. 293).

DISEASES FOR WHICH THIS TEST IS COMMONLY OBTAINED:
Cancer (p. 313).
Endometriosis.
Ovarian cyst.
Liver disease.

COST: approximately $550.

Proctosigmoidoscopy

OTHER NAMES: proctoscopy, sigmoidoscopy, anoscopy.

PURPOSE OF THE TEST: To see directly the 10 inches of the gastrointestinal tract closest to the rectum.

BACKGROUND: These last few inches of gastrointestinal tract are the site of many diseases that can cause similar symptoms: bleeding, a change in bowel habits, and pain. A barium enema does not work well for the area closest to the rectum and therefore cannot be used to evaluate these symptoms. Instead, a proctosigmoidoscopy will be performed in which the endoscope will be inserted and the area seen directly.

HOW THE TEST IS DONE: The patient is given an enema just prior to the test. He lies on a table with his chest and knees drawn together. The instrument is slowly and carefully inserted through the rectum and the physician—usually a gastroenterologist or internist—examines the area. Biopsies are taken from suspicious tissue. The test takes approximately 15 minutes.

HOW THE RESULTS ARE GIVEN: See "Endoscopy," p. 153.

PATIENT PREPARATION: The night before the test the patient should have only a light meal.

RISKS AND DISCOMFORTS: The test will cause the patient to have a strong urge to defecate. He may also feel pressure during the exam but usually no pain. Bleeding can result, especially if a biopsy was performed during the procedure.

SYMPTOMS FOR WHICH THIS TEST IS COMMONLY OBTAINED:
For all four of these symptoms, the test is performed to see if cancer, polyps, or hemorrhoids are the cause:
Rectal pain.
Blood in stool (p. 289).
Change in bowel habits.
Diarrhea (p. 293).
Constipation.

DISEASES FOR WHICH THIS TEST IS COMMONLY OBTAINED:
Cancer (p. 313).
Rectal polyps—used not only to find the polyps but to remove them as well.

Ulcerative colitis—to diagnose the disease initially and to monitor therapy.
Hemorrhoids.
Anemia (p. 309)—especially iron-deficiency anemia, since that disease can result from excessive blood loss caused from bleeding in the gastrointestinal tract.

COST: approximately $60.

10

Microbiology

The purpose of all cultures is to identify those microscopic organisms or microbes that are causing an infection in the patient. Microbiology is the study of these microbes. At one time microbiology was called bacteriology, but the name was changed when it was recognized that many different organisms besides bacteria—including viruses, fungi, rickettsia, and parasites—can cause disease. In many hospitals, however, the laboratory that is involved in culture work is still called the bacteriology lab. The reason is this: while it is possible to do special cultures to detect these other organisms, when a doctor or nurse uses the term culture, unless otherwise specified, he is talking about a culture to detect bacteria.

A culture, therefore, is performed on a patient with symptoms that suggest an infection to determine: (1) Is the infection caused by bacteria? (2) If so, which bacteria? While it is possible to do special cultures to detect viruses and organisms other than bacteria that are causing an infection, these are less commonly done and are discussed under "Cultures for Viruses and Other Nonbacterial Organisms", p. 177.

When a culture is positive and bacteria are detected, antibiotic sensitivity testing is almost always conducted. This test will determine which of the many available antibiotics is effective against this particular strain of bacteria. Another test called Gram staining will often be done to the specimen itself. In this test, named after a famous 19th-Century Danish microbiologist, a small piece of the specimen is stained with special chemicals. Examination of the stained specimen under a microscope may reveal the presence of bacteria and give the doctor strong clues as to their identity.

To understand well the concepts behind cultures, it is important to remember that we are all living in a sea of bacteria. Within 24 hours of our birth, our skin as well as the inside lining of our large intestines are covered with bacteria, a condition that will persist for the duration of our lives. Bacteria are found on almost every object that we touch, on our food, in our drinking water, in the air we breathe. Generally, these bacteria cause no problem, but occasionally we will be exposed to bacteria that cause disease. Infection with these disease-causing bacteria can occur anywhere in the body. It can be localized—the infection is limited to one site only (such as throat, skin, or lung)—or systemic—bacteria are found in the bloodstream and the entire body is involved.

Until the discovery of antibiotics in this century, the detection and identification of the specific bacteria causing an infection were of value only because of scientific curiosity. But now as a result of these drugs, it is possible to treat almost all bacterial infections effectively. The prompt use of the right antibiotic will eradicate the infection as well as eliminate potential complications, such as rheumatic fever resulting from a strep throat, or mental retardation from meningitis. Consequently, culture and antibiotic sensitivity testing are among the most important and useful medical tests that can be done.

All cultures are done in essentially the same manner regardless of the site of the infection. A specimen is collected from the infected site. The specific technique for this will be discussed under the individual cultures, but examples are: blood from someone suspected of having a systemic blood infection, or cerebrospinal fluid from someone who might have meningitis. Once the specimen is collected, it is placed in a culture medium in the laboratory that is either a broth-like liquid contained in bottles or a jelly-like substance placed in petri dishes. All kinds of media contain the nutrients that bacteria need to grow. The cultures are kept at 98.6° so that the bacteria can grow at body temperature. If many bacteria are present, they can be detected as early as 24 hours after the culture is started. Most often, however, it takes from 36 to 48 hours for the culture to reveal the presence of bacteria; if after 72 hours they are not evident, it is assumed that they are not present, and the culture is discarded.

If bacteria are detected, the laboratory technician will take them from the culture medium and attempt to grow them in the presence of different antibiotics. Those antibiotics that have the ability to kill or slow the growth of the bacteria as well as those that have no effect will be noted. This antibiotic sensitivity testing takes an additional 24 to 48 hours after the bacteria have been detected. Therefore, it takes from two to five days for the final results of culture and sensitivity testing to be available.

Culture results have two parts. Those in which no abnormal bacteria are detected are termed "negative," while cultures that grow harmful bacteria are called "positive." In addition, positive cultures will identify, by name, the specific bacteria that are found. For example, a doctor may say that the blood culture was "positive for pneumococcus bacteria." Antibiotic sensitivity testing reports will inform him which antibiotics were tested and whether they are effective in treating this particular bacteria. If a certain antibiotic prevented the growth of the bacteria, the bacteria is then reported as being "sensitive" to that drug. If the antibiotic had no effect on the growth of the bacteria, the bacteria are termed "resistant" to that particular drug.

Once a specimen is collected from a specific part of the patient's body, the remainder of the test is conducted in the microbiology or bacteriology laboratory. There are no risks associated with the actual culture, but the collection of the specimens, such as a throat culture, spinal tap to collect cerebrospinal fluid, or venipuncture to obtain a blood culture, may be uncomfortable.

SYMPTOMS FOR WHICH CULTURES ARE COMMONLY OBTAINED:
Abdominal pain (p. 285)—Urine cultures are done to check for bladder or kidney infection.
Breathing difficulty (p. 290) and cough (p. 292)—Sputum cultures are done to detect pneumonia.
Diarrhea (p. 293)—Stool cultures are done to look for shigella or salmonella bacteria as the cause of the diarrhea.
Fever (p. 296)—If no cause for the fever can be established, cultures from many different sites (blood, urine, sputum) will be obtained in an effort to see whether infection may be causing the fever.
Headache (p. 297)—Cerebrospinal fluid cultures might be done in a patient with headache, especially if he has fever, to see if meningitis is present.
Sore throat (p. 304)—Throat culture will be done to see if the infection is caused by streptococcus bacteria (strep throat).

Swollen glands (p. 305)—Cultures from many different sites, including blood, may be done if no specific cause for the swollen glands is found.

DISEASES FOR WHICH CULTURES ARE COMMONLY OBTAINED:
This test is done whenever any bacterial infection is suspected, including the specific kinds of infection listed below. Cultures will sometimes be repeated after antibiotics have been used to see if the treatment was successful.
Urinary tract infection (p. 326).
Pneumonia (p. 321).
Meningitis.
Strep throat.
Endocarditis (infection of the heart valves).
Gastroenteritis with diarrhea.
Sexually transmitted diseases (p. 323).

BLOOD CULTURE

BACKGROUND: The finding of disease-causing bacteria in the blood, a condition called bacteremia or septicemia, is always a serious matter because it indicates that the infection is not localized but is systemic and throughout the entire body. Bacteremia can result from the spread into the blood stream of a localized infection that has not been adequately controlled or originate in the blood stream itself. For example, if a patient has pneumonia and does not receive appropriate antibiotic therapy, the bacteria causing the pneumonia can spread throughout the blood stream. In other instances, especially in patients who are particularly susceptible to infections, the bacteria can overwhelm the body's defenses and begin growing in the blood without first causing a localized infection. The most important symptom of a blood infection is fever, and patients who have fever without an identifiable cause will always have blood cultures done. This is especially true in those patients who are especially susceptible to blood infections, including those who are malnourished, debilitated, or undergoing chemotherapy for cancer, as well as infants or the elderly.

HOW THE SPECIMEN IS COLLECTED: The specimen for a blood culture is collected from a vein, most commonly from the vein in the interior surface of the elbow. The skin over the vein is thoroughly cleansed with an antiseptic, such as Betadine. This is done so that the culture does not pick up any of the bacteria that are on the skin. The doctor, nurse, or technician will collect the blood in the same way as he does for blood tests (p. 43). Frequently, patients suspected of having a blood infection will have numerous blood cultures done over a couple of days, thereby increasing the chances that one of them will be positive.

COST: approximately $35.

CEREBROSPINAL FLUID (CSF) CULTURE

BACKGROUND: Infection of the tissue that lines the brain and spinal cord (meningitis) remains a very serious disease. Meningitis can be caused by numerous organisms, including viruses, bacteria, and fungi. A culture of the cerebrospinal fluid is essential to the diagnosis of bacterial meningitis. Symptoms that make the doctor suspect meningitis include headache and stiff neck, especially when accompanied by fever. In children and infants meningitis usually causes irritability as well. Because it is critical to begin treatment of bacterial meningitis as early as possible, most patients having a cerebrospinal fluid culture will be started on antibiotics before the culture report is available. If the report is negative, and no bacteria are detected, the antibiotics can be stopped and no harm has been done. If the culture result is positive, the doctor will have saved a critical 48 to 72 hours by starting the antibiotics at the time the culture was obtained instead of waiting for the result.

HOW THE SPECIMEN IS COLLECTED: Cerebrospinal fluid is obtained from the patient during a spinal tap or lumbar puncture (p. 210). For this procedure the patient is placed in a position that spreads open the spaces found between the vertebrae of the lower back, the usual puncture site. This is done in two ways: either the patient sits and bends forward, placing his head on his knees, or he lies on his side and draws the head and knees together in what is called the "fetal position." Once he is in position, the skin over the puncture site is cleaned and scrubbed with soap and an antiseptic, such as Betadine. The doctor will inject a local anesthetic into the skin using a very small needle and then carefully place the spinal tap needle through the skin and into the space between the two vertebrae he has selected. If successful, the needle will then enter directly into the space surrounding the spinal cord that contains cerebrospinal fluid. Occasionally, the doctor will have to try two or three times for this to be successful.

After the spinal tap is completed, the patient should lie flat on his back with his head level to decrease the chance of a "post-spinal tap headache." Other tests are done on the spinal fluid besides culture. These are described under lumbar puncture (p. 210). Since early diagnosis of meningitis is so important, the cerebrospinal fluid will also be Gram stained (p. 167) in addition to being cultured, and, occasionally, the bacteria can be identified by this procedure so that the doctor doesn't have to wait for culture results.

COST: approximately $25.

CULTURES FOR GONORRHEA

OTHER NAMES: Thayer-Martin culture of
the cervix, urethra, throat, or rectum.

BACKGROUND: Cultures are done to detect gonorrhea in persons who have symptoms of that disease. In males such symptoms include penile discharge or pain on urination, while females might have lower abdominal pain or vaginal discharge. Cultures must also be done on anyone who has had sexual relations with someone who has gonorrhea. In female patients the best site for a specimen is the cervix, while in males it is the urethra. Depending on the symptoms and the patient's sexual activity, cultures of the throat or rectum may be done as well. The standard culture medium does not allow for the growth of the gonorrhea bacteria, and, therefore, a specially prepared medium, called Thayer-Martin medium or chocolate agar, must be used whenever gonorrhea is suspected.

At one time antibiotic sensitivity testing was not done on patients with cultures positive for gonorrhea because all strains of that bacteria could be effectively treated with penicillin. Today this is no longer the case, and increasingly we find strains of gonorrhea that are resistant to penicillin. Although most patients with gonorrhea will be treated with penicillin, sensitivity testing is sometimes done to determine if the particular bacteria being treated is penicillin sensitive or resistant.

HOW THE SPECIMEN IS COLLECTED:

Urethra—A sterile swab is inserted into the penile opening (urethral opening) approximately 1 inch and rotated. This is slightly uncomfortable. Occasionally, if gonorrhea is suspected but has not been cultured on previous tries, the physician may do a rectal exam with his finger at the same time as he does the urethral culture and express pus by massaging the prostate gland.

Cervix—The woman is placed on the table with her legs in stir-rups in the same manner as for a routine pelvic examination. A speculum is used to hold open the vaginal opening, then a swab is placed within the cervix, rotated, and removed.

Throat—A swab is used to collect the specimen.

Rectum—A swab is used to collect the specimen.

COST: approximately $15.

SPUTUM CULTURE

BACKGROUND: Numerous infections can occur within the airways (bronchitis) and lungs (pneumonia); a sputum culture is useful to determine the bacteria that are causing these infections. Sputum is not saliva but consists of secretions from deep within the air-ways and lungs. In addition, sputum culture is the most impor-tant way to detect active tuberculosis.

HOW THE SPECIMEN IS COLLECTED: A patient can bring up sputum by deep coughing. The sputum is collected in a sterile cup and brought to the laboratory for culturing. Sometimes, if the patient is unable to bring up the sputum, the nurse, doctor, or physical therapist will help by pounding on the chest to loosen the spu-tum. Occasionally, it is necessary for the patient to breathe a warm aerosol mist to further loosen the sputum. Finally, if all else fails, and especially in patients who are very weak, paralyzed, or have their breathing assisted by a respirator, the nurse may insert a small plastic tube down the windpipe to collect the specimen. It is always useful to obtain a Gram stain (p. 167) of the sputum so that an early diagnosis of a bacterial infection can be made.

COST: approximately $25.

STOOL AND RECTAL CULTURES

BACKGROUND: Diarrhea can be due to a variety of causes, usually viruses. Occasionally, however, diarrhea is caused by bacteria, especially shigella, salmonella, Escherichia coli, or staphylococcus. Patients with persistent diarrhea or diarrhea that is bloody and accompanied by high fever will have a stool culture done to see if one of these bacteria is the cause. The most reliable results are obtained from a fresh stool specimen, but sometimes a physician will use a rectal swab instead.

HOW THE SPECIMEN IS COLLECTED: Cultures from stool are best done on a fresh stool specimen. It should be collected in a clean, dry container and brought to the physician. The specimen should not contain urine or toilet paper, as these might interfere with the culture. A rectal swab is performed by inserting a swab (a Q-tip on a longer than usual stick) through the anus and into the rectum. For the best results the swab must be placed at least 2 to 3 inches inside the rectal opening since this is where the bacteria are found.

COST: approximately $25.

THROAT CULTURE

BACKGROUND: Sore throats (pharyngitis) can be caused by many different organisms, including viruses and bacteria. The most dangerous form of sore throat is that caused by infection with Group A beta-hemolytic streptococcus—a condition called a strep throat. Infection with this particular bacteria can result in rheumatic fever as well as inflammation of the kidneys (glomerulonephritis). All throat cultures will reveal the presence of some bacteria (since many different kinds of bacteria are found in a throat that is not infected), but only if the disease-causing strep bacteria are found will the physician treat with antibiotics. Antibiotic sensitivity testing is not done for positive throat cultures since penicillin is always effective in treating strep.

Individual physicians have different policies in deciding which patients get a throat culture. Although some physicians will do a throat culture on all patients with a sore throat to determine if strep is the cause, most physicians, including ourselves, will do a throat culture only when the patient has other symptoms that suggest strep, and not a virus, is the cause. These symptoms include fever (p. 296), pus on the tonsils or in the throat, and swollen lymph node (glands) (p. 305). Other factors to consider are the age of the patient and his exposure to others with strep throat.

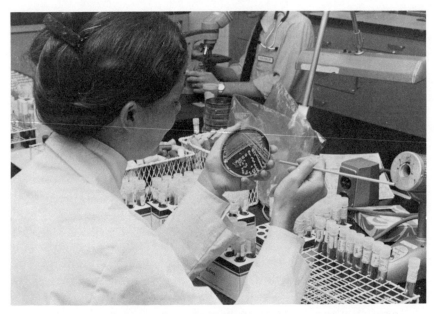

Technician in a hospital microbiology laboratory smearing a swab used in a throat culture on the appropriate culture medium.

HOW THE SPECIMEN IS COLLECTED: The person doing the throat culture (usually a doctor or nurse) takes a sterile swab (essentially a Q-tip on a longer-than-usual stick) and rubs it over the back of the throat and tonsils. This frequently produces a momentary gagging sensation.

COST: approximately $5.

URINE CULTURE

BACKGROUND: Urine cultures are used to detect bacterial infections of the kidneys or bladder. Urinary tract infections are found in patients of all ages and both sexes, but they are most common in females because of anatomic differences between the sexes. The female urethra (the tube that runs from the bladder to the outside) is shorter than the one for the males, allowing for bacteria to enter the bladder more easily and cause infection. In addition, in comparison to males, the urethral orifice in females is closer to the anus, a site from which bacteria can come, especially in young girls with less than optimal toilet hygiene. A urine culture is usually done in conjunction with a urinalysis (p. 87). Symptoms that will make the doctor suspicious of a urinary tract infection and prompt him to do a urine culture include dysuria (pain or burning on urination), hematuria (blood in the urine), polyuria (increased frequency of urination), urgency before urination, and foul-smelling urine.

HOW THE SPECIMEN IS COLLECTED: The patient cleans the genital area well using swabs and an antiseptic. Since the first drops of urine may contain bacteria that were not cleaned away, the patient begins urinating into the toilet, then stops the urine stream midway, positions the sterile container appropriately and starts to urinate again, this time into the container. After a sufficient quantity has been collected (about 1 ounce), the patient stops urinating again, removes the container, and then finishes voiding. This method of urine collection, termed a mid-stream specimen, is the best to use for a urine culture. In patients who have a bladder catheter, the urine can be collected directly from the tubing. In very small infants the urine is collected by placing a needle directly into the bladder. This is very safe, the only complication being slight bleeding from the bladder. Gram staining (p. 167) of the urine specimen is frequently done as well to identify the bacteria immediately.

COST: approximately $25.

WOUND CULTURES

BACKGROUND: Any open wound in the body, whether resulting from an accident, illness, or surgery, provides a perfect site for bacterial infection. When this happens, the wound will become swollen, tender, red, and usually have pus. It is important to identify a wound infection early for two reasons. First, infected wounds do not heal well, and if they do, they will heal with much more scarring. Second, an infection in a wound can easily and quickly spread throughout the body, a life-threatening complication. Whenever infection of a wound is suspected, the doctor will order a culture. If patients have large areas of open wounds, as might happen in a burn patient, the wound will routinely be cultured periodically, so that if an infection develops, it will be detected as early as possible.

HOW THE SPECIMEN IS COLLECTED: A swab is used to collect any pus or drainage from the wound. Often, a wound must be debrided, meaning that dead tissue and skin are removed. If this is done, the dead tissue and skin are often sent to the laboratory and used directly as a specimen. Gram stain of the pus from a wound will almost always reveal the nature of the bacteria that are causing the problem and is very important in the diagnosis of these infections.

COST: approximately $25.

CULTURES FOR VIRUSES AND OTHER NONBACTERIAL ORGANISMS

BACKGROUND: The routine cultures described earlier in this chapter are designed to detect bacterial infection. Sometimes, it is important to know if an infection or illness is caused by organisms that are not bacteria. This includes viruses, rickettsia, fungi, and parasites. Cultures can be done to detect these organisms as well. The methods are much more sophisticated and complex than those used for bacterial culture and, consequently, are not done in most hospitals. Often, the state or county health department runs a special laboratory that is used to culture these organisms.

The cultures for nonbacterial organisms grow much more slowly than those for bacteria; thus it may take weeks, and occasionally months, until the lab has an answer. Therefore, the results of these cultures rarely affect the actual medical treatment given to a patient since the doctor will have to make decisions without the results being available. The cultures are done for public health purposes, for it is important that officials know if certain dangerous viruses or other organisms are causing disease in a given locale. In addition, although treatment may have to be initiated before the results are available, it is important for the patient's medical record to list accurately the microbes causing a particular illness.

COST: This will vary widely depending upon the type and number of cultures that are done.

11

Miscellaneous Tests

ALLERGY TESTS

OTHER NAMES: skin tests, scratch tests, patch tests, RAST test (Radio-Allergo-Sorbent-Test)

PURPOSE OF THE TEST: to determine if the patient is allergic to various substances.

BACKGROUND: When a patient comes in contact with a substance (allergen) to which he is allergic, a reaction will occur. These allergic reactions can be mild, such as hives, or life-threatening. The most important medical treatment for allergies is avoidance of the specific allergens—the substances that cause the allergic reaction. This requires identifying the patient's particular allergens. There are three general ways by which the doctor determines what substances the patient is allergic to: by history (every time the patient is exposed to or eats a certain substance the allergic reaction occurs), by skin testing, and by blood testing (also called RAST test).

This part will describe the skin tests and blood tests used to identify specific allergens in a patient suspected of having allergies. The choice between skin tests and RAST tests is controversial. Skin tests are generally considered to provide more accurate information than RAST tests but are slightly more painful and risky. Also, they are unreliable for children under three years of age since their immune system is not yet mature enough to provide reliable evidence of the allergy in the blood. A good compromise is to do the initial screening (for everyone over three years of age) with skin tests and monitor any therapy used to treat the allergy with RAST tests.

Skin Tests

HOW THE TEST IS DONE: A few drops of several liquid extracts, derived from substances to which patients are commonly allergic (foods, molds, grasses, weeds, trees, insects), are placed on the skin of the arm or back, approximately 1 inch apart. A small needle is used to prick the skin beneath the drop of extract. The skin is observed for 30 minutes for the formation of a red, raised swelling around the extract, similar in appearance to an insect bite. As many as 15 to 25 extracts can be tested at one time. The entire test takes about 45 minutes.

HOW THE RESULTS ARE GIVEN: The presence of a red, raised circular lesion, at least ¼ inch in diameter, around the prick in the skin, is interpreted as proof that the patient is allergic to that particular substance. Redness without the raised swelling is less important and is not considered conclusive evidence of allergy.

PATIENT PREPARATION: The patient should not take any antihistamines for at least 72 hours prior to the test. But if he has to take them during that time, he should inform the physician, who then may decide to postpone the test.

RISKS AND DISCOMFORTS: The pricking is slightly painful but lasts only a moment. There is a very slight risk that a patient will have a serious allergic reaction during the actual skin test to a substance to which he is allergic. Medicine is always nearby to treat such a reaction if it develops. This risk is highest when testing for allergies to insect bites.

RAST Test (Radio-Allergo-Sorbent-Test)

HOW THE TEST IS DONE: Blood is obtained from the patient's vein by routine venipuncture and sent to the lab where it is analyzed for the presence of antibodies (IgE—Immunoglobulin E) directed against particular allergens. If such antibodies exist, it is strong evidence that the patient has an allergy to that material. The same allergens tested for by skin test can be tested for by the RAST test: weeds, trees, molds, dust, animals, insects.

HOW THE RESULTS ARE GIVEN: The physician receives a report from the laboratory in two to three days detailing the list of allergens against which the patient had IgE (antibodies) present in the blood.

PATIENT PREPARATION: None.

RISKS AND DISCOMFORTS: The only risk to this test is the slight pain and possible bruising that accompanies a venipuncture.

For Both Tests (Skin and RAST)
SYMPTOMS FOR WHICH THESE TESTS ARE COMMONLY OBTAINED:
In these cases the tests are done in an effort to find out the particular substances to which the patient is allergic:
Hives.
Runny Eyes.
Rash.
Wheezing.
Sneezing.

DISEASES FOR WHICH THIS TEST IS COMMONLY OBTAINED:
Allergies (p. 308)—The tests are done for two reasons: first, to detect the substances to which the patient is allergic; and, second, once those allergens have been identified, if the patient is receiving desensitization shots (allergy shots), the test will be repeated to see if the treatment is working.

COST: approximately $30 for each test.

AMNIOCENTESIS

(In addition to reading this part, please read the other part on amniocentesis in this book, p. 271.)

PURPOSE OF THE TEST: To study the amniotic fluid and the fetal cells that are found within it.

BACKGROUND: The fetus is surrounded in the uterus by amniotic fluid. Cells from the fetus are shed continuously into the fluid. Collection of the fluid, its subsequent examination, as well as evaluation of the fetal cells, can tell the doctor much about the fetus, including its sex, the presence of certain chromosomal diseases and other inherited illnesses, the gestational age, and overall fetal condition. Amniocentesis is performed on a pregnant woman in whom there is sufficient reason to worry about these abnormalities that it warrants the risk that amniocentesis entails.

The decision to perform amniocentesis is not always a simple one. As explained below, there are real risks to the procedure. The question that must be asked to help in the evaluation of possible amniocentesis is: What difference would the result make? If a woman will not have an abortion, regardless of the result of the test, then amniocentesis is probably inappropriate. If, on the other hand, a woman would decide to have an abortion if the test disclosed that the fetus has Down's syndrome, and the woman is at high risk for that particular disorder, then the test is likely to be warranted. It is important that these issues be discussed with the obstetrician or gynecologist before amniocentesis is performed so that an appropriate decision is reached.

HOW THE TEST IS DONE: Amniocentesis is usually performed in the hospital between the 14th and 18th week of pregnancy. Before that time there is not enough amniotic fluid to safely perform the procedure, and inserting the needle will have an unacceptably high risk of hurting the fetus. Beyond the 18th week it is no longer simple or safe (and in many states not legal) to perform an abortion—a likely consequence if the results indicate a serious birth defect is present. Sometimes, the purpose of amniocentesis is not to screen for birth defects. Rather, it is done to evaluate how well the fetus is maturing or to see if a disease is present that affects the fetus, such as Rh incompatability (p. 46). In these instances when abortion is not an issue, amniocentesis may be done very late in the pregnancy, right up till the time of delivery.

Regardless of when amniocentesis is done, the procedure remains the same. The woman voids before the procedure in order to empty her bladder and prevent the accidental puncture of that organ. She lies on a table and the location of the fetus is determined by ultrasound of the abdomen (p. 151). The fetus is manually pushed up (towards the woman's head). The suprapubic area, usually just above the pubic hair, is cleansed well with soap and an antiseptic applied. Sterile drapes are placed so that only a small area of skin is visible and a local anesthetic is injected. The amniocentesis needle—approximately 4 inches long—is inserted through the skin and into the uterus. A small amount of amniotic fluid—usually half an ounce—is withdrawn. The needle is then removed and a tight bandage applied to the skin.

HOW THE RESULTS ARE GIVEN: The following items can be measured on the amniotic fluid specimen:

L / S ratio—This is a measurement of two chemicals—lecithin and sphingomyelin—and is a useful indicator of fetal age and maturity. When the doctor is considering an induction of labor or a Caesarean section, this test may be done late in pregnancy to determine if the fetus is ready for birth.

Bilirubin (p. 45)—If present, it is a sign of a blood incompatibility between the pregnant mother and the fetus (see blood typing, p. 46).

Cells—The fetal cells can be examined and the following ascertained:

Sex of the fetus.

Chromosomal analysis (p. 208).

In addition, the cells from the fetus can be grown in the laboratory, and after a few weeks the following items ascertained:

Presence or absence of certain critical enzymes (p. 61).

Presence or absence of sickle cell anemia (p. 82).

RISKS AND DISCOMFORTS: The injection of the local anesthetic is slightly painful and may cause a burning sensation. The insertion of the amniotic needle will cause pressure but not sharp pain. The risks to the fetus must also be considered. Approximately 1 in 300 amniocenteses will cause a miscarriage or premature delivery. In comparison, this risk—1 in 300—is approximately equal to that of a woman over 35 giving birth to a baby with Down's syndrome.

PATIENT PREPARATION: None, other than voiding before the procedure.

WOMEN WHO SHOULD CONSIDER HAVING THIS TEST DONE:
Women over age 35.
Women who have previously given birth to a baby with a genetic defect.
Women who have a genetic disease or have a history in their family of genetic diseases.
Women carrying the baby of a man who has a genetic disease or whose family has a history of genetic disease.

DISEASES WHICH CAN BE DETECTED BY THIS TEST:
Erythroblastosis fetalis—Blood incompatibility between mother and fetus (p. 46).
Down's syndrome.
Sickle cell anemia (p. 82).
Hemophilia.
Tay-Sachs disease (p. 60).
Spina bifida.

COST: approximately $600, including analysis of the cells.

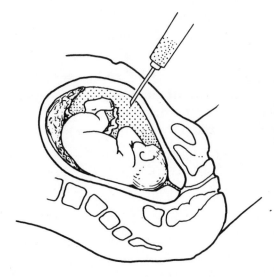

Position of the needle and fetus during amniocentesis. The site at which the needle is placed will be determined by an ultrasound examination (p. 151) that is done during the amniocentesis. This will allow the physician to keep the needle as far away as possible from the fetus and placenta.

ARTERIAL BLOOD GASES

OTHER NAMES: ABGs, arterial blood gas analysis, blood gases.

PURPOSE OF THE TEST: To measure the level of oxygen, carbon dioxide, and acid in the blood.

BACKGROUND: As your heart pumps blood through your lungs, carbon dioxide that has accumulated in the body is expelled and exchanged for fresh oxygen from the air. Any change in the efficiency of the heart or lungs will result in an abnormal level of one or both of these gases in the blood as well as a change in the acid content.

HOW THE TEST IS DONE: The test for arterial blood gases is different from other blood tests in that the blood specimen is obtained from an artery and not a vein. The one most commonly used is the radial artery found in the wrist. Occasionally, if this artery cannot be used, the blood will be taken from the brachial artery (inside surface of the elbow) or the femoral artery (groin area). The person drawing the blood (usually a physician, but sometimes a nurse, respiratory therapist, or blood gas technician) will feel the area with the hand and locate the pulse. This indicates the exact location of the artery. The skin over the artery is cleaned with an antiseptic and a needle is inserted. A small amount of blood (usually ¼ ounce) is collected in a syringe and sent to the laboratory, where it is analyzed on a blood gas machine. This equipment is highly automated and the results can be obtained within 15 minutes.

HOW THE RESULTS ARE GIVEN: The blood gas analysis consists of three measurements: the amount of carbon dioxide in the blood, the amount of oxygen in the blood, and the amount of acid in the blood. This last measurement is called the pH of the blood.

NORMAL RANGE: oxygen level—80–100mm Hg.
              carbon dioxide level—35–45mm Hg.
              pH—7.35–7.45.

PATIENT PREPARATION: None.

RISKS AND DISCOMFORTS: Arteries are located more deeply beneath the skin surface than veins and consequently are not seen as easily. Therefore, drawing blood from an artery is more difficult and distinctly more painful than obtaining blood from a vein because the needle must be placed more deeply into the tissues than it is into a vein. Often, it is difficult to determine the exact location of the artery and the patient must be pricked with the needle several times before blood is successfully drawn. The amount of blood taken is small and its loss is of no danger to the patient. There is a risk of continued bleeding from the site where the blood is obtained, but this is minimized when the person drawing the blood applies pressure to the area for five minutes.

SYMPTOMS FOR WHICH THIS TEST IS COMMONLY OBTAINED:
These symptoms can all be accompanied by abnormalities in lung function. The arterial blood gas analysis will be useful in determining both the specific diagnosis and the severity of the problem:
Shortness of breath (p. 290).
Chest pain (p. 291).
Rapid or abnormal breathing (p. 290).
Cyanosis (bluish discoloration of the skin caused by low levels of oxygen in the blood).

DISEASES FOR WHICH THIS TEST IS COMMONLY OBTAINED:
Lung disease of all kinds—The arterial blood gases will help determine the severity of the lung disease:
Bronchitis (p. 315).
Emphysema (p. 315).
Asthma (p. 312).

Pneumonia (p. 321).

Pulmonary embolus.

Diabetes (p. 318)—The blood of patients with severe diabetes is often more acidic than normal. This test will reveal if that complication is present.

Congestive heart failure (fluid in the lungs)—If the heart does not pump the blood adequately, fluid will accumulate in the lungs. As a consequence, the lungs will not be able to exchange oxygen and carbon dioxide as well as they should, and, in addition, the blood may become more acidic.

SPECIAL SITUATIONS IN WHICH THIS TEST IS COMMONLY OBTAINED: In addition to testing patients with the symptoms and diseases described above, arterial blood gas analysis is sometimes done in four special circumstances:

Before surgery—By measuring the function of the lungs before surgery, this test will help determine which anesthesia to use and how risky the anesthesia will be for the patient.

After surgery—to evaluate how the patient handled the anesthesia. This blood gas analysis will be studied in comparison to the presurgery test to see if the surgery or anesthesia produced any decrease in lung function.

Industrial exposure—Workers in industries in which a dust or fume hazard exists (i.e., miners, asbestos workers, powder manufacturers) will be tested to determine if these exposures have decreased the lung function.

Smoke inhalation—After a person has suffered smoke inhalation, this test will determine the severity of any lung damage. Such people will usually have a carboxyhemoglobin measurement (p. 49) done as well.

COST: approximately $80.

AUDIOGRAM

OTHER NAMES:: audiometry, hearing test.

PURPOSE OF THE TEST: to test the patient's hearing.

BACKGROUND: Hearing is a complex function that involves the brain as well as the ear. Abnormalities anywhere along the hearing pathway can produce a hearing loss. Most hearing loss affects one ear more than the other and is a greater problem with some tones (high or low frequency) than with others. For instance, it is not uncommon for a patient to complain that he cannot hear the doorbell but can hear normal speech without difficulty. When he complains of a hearing problem, an audiogram is performed to identify the exact nature of the problem: (1) which ear, (2) which type of sound, and (3) the severity of the hearing loss. This will allow the doctor to diagnose the specific problem as well as determine later on if the problem is worsening so that appropriate therapy can be planned.

HOW THE TEST IS DONE: The patient sits at a desk in a soundproof room and puts on a pair of headphones. A series of tones is then played—varying in loudness and pitch—for either one or both ears. The patient is asked to state if a sound was heard and, if so, in which ear. In the second half of the test, the patient listens to a series of spoken words that vary in loudness and is asked to identify the word as well as the ear in which it was heard. The test takes about 30 minutes to complete.

HOW THE RESULTS ARE GIVEN: The audiologist—a trained professional who has generally received an M.A. degree in the field and conducts the study—prepares a graph showing the results from each ear, giving the lowest volume that could be heard at each pitch. This information is available immediately after the test, and at that time the audiologist or physician will usually discuss the results with the patient. A copy of these results is kept in the patient's medical chart for comparison with future audiograms.

RISKS AND DISCOMFORTS: For most patients there are no risks or discomforts to this test. But for others, listening to certain frequencies may be slightly painful because of their hearing problem.

PATIENT PREPARATION: None.

SYMPTOMS FOR WHICH THIS TEST IS COMMONLY OBTAINED:
Hearing loss—to identify the extent and nature of the problem.
Ringing in the ears (tinnitus).
Dizziness (p. 293)—to see if an ear or brain abnormality is causing the problem.

DISEASES FOR WHICH THIS TEST IS COMMONLY OBTAINED:
Brain tumor.

Otitis media (ear infection)—to determine whether hearing loss has resulted from the infection.

COST: approximately $50.

BIOPSY

PURPOSE OF THE TEST: To study tissues in the body under a microscope for the presence of cancer, inflammation, or other abnormality.

BACKGROUND: Sometimes, no matter how many other tests are performed, the doctor needs to see the actual tissue that is abnormal. This is frequently true with liver and kidney disease as well as any lumps or tumors in the body. Biopsies, which are taken of these suspicious tissues and then studied under the microscope, give the doctor a much greater understanding about the actual disease that is occurring.

HOW THE TEST IS DONE: Biopsies can be taken from almost any site in the body: breast, lung, liver, kidney, lymph node, intestines, cervix, and skin are but a few. The actual procedure varies. Biopsies can be performed as separate medical procedures or during the course of surgery, but in this part we will discuss biopsies that are done as separate tests. Those done during surgery are processed in a similar fashion.

There are generally two approaches. The first type of biopsy is usually performed in conjunction with endoscopy (p. 153) for the stomach, small intestine, colon, cervix, and lung. The second biopsy procedure is done when endoscopy is not easily applicable; for example, when the liver, kidney, or breast needs to be biopsied. In those situations the general approach to performing the biopsy is the same. The skin over the biopsy site is cleaned thoroughly with antiseptic and a local anesthetic given with a small needle. The doctor performing the biopsy—often a surgeon, but other specialists as well—then removes the biopsy tissue. If he's removing the tissue from the kidney or liver, he inserts a special needle through the skin and into those organs. For cutting breast tissue he may actually use a scalpel. A dressing is applied and the specimen is sent to the laboratory for analysis.

HOW THE RESULTS ARE GIVEN: A final biopsy report takes at least one day, and often two to three, for the pathologist to prepare. If necessary, when biopsies are performed during surgery, an immediate report is given. This latter report, called a frozen section, can occasionally prove to be wrong upon further study and should be done only when absolutely necessary. The report usually will be sent to the referring physician, who will discuss the results with his patient. Those results will indicate, as best as can be determined by the microscopic examination, what the tissue looks like and whether it is malignant or abnormal in any other way.

PATIENT PREPARATION: Usually none, depending upon the type of biopsy to be done. A sedative or general anesthetic may be given to the patient.

RISKS AND DISCOMFORTS: All biopsies will involve some discomfort from the local anesthetic and the biopsy technique. In addition, some biopsies have certain specific risks associated with them. Both kidney and liver biopsies can cause internal hemorrhage and infection; skin biopsies will leave a small scar; lung biopsies can sometimes cause a punctured or collapsed lung.

SYMPTOMS FOR WHICH THIS TEST IS COMMONLY OBTAINED:
Kidney biopsy—blood, cells, or protein in the urine.
Liver biopsy—jaundice (p. 300), abdominal pain (p. 285).
Breast—breast mass or lump (p. 302), nipple discharge.
Intestine—blood in stool (p. 289), weight loss (p. 306), change in bowel habits.
Lungs—shortness of breath (p. 290), cough (p. 292), bloody sputum.
Skin—unusual rash.

DISEASES FOR WHICH THIS TEST IS COMMONLY OBTAINED:
Pneumonia (p. 321).
Colitis.
Hepatitis.
Kidney failure.
Cancer (p. 313).

COST: approximately $50–200.

BONE MARROW ASPIRATE AND BIOPSY

PURPOSE OF THE TEST: to obtain bone marrow for examination under a microscope.

BACKGROUND: The bone marrow is the site of production for the different kinds of blood cells: red, white, and platelets. If these cells are abnormal in number (either too many or too few) or in appearance, the problem may be due to a disease in the bone marrow. Based on the patient's history, physical examination, and other laboratory tests—especially a complete blood count (CBC, p. 51)—the doctor may decide that a bone marrow aspirate and biopsy are indicated.

HOW THE TEST IS DONE: Not all bones contain bone marrow. The usual site for the bone marrow test is the back side of the pelvic bone above the buttocks. Other sites that can be used if necessary are the front side of the pelvic bone and the breastbone. The skin over the bone is cleaned thoroughly with an antiseptic, and sterile clothes are placed around the site to be biopsied so that only a small area of skin is visible. A local anesthetic is given in the skin with a small needle, and with a longer needle, a small amount of anesthetic is applied to the actual bone as well. The anesthetic needle is removed and the bone marrow needle is passed through the skin and down to the surface of the bone. Sometimes, a tiny incision, about 1/16th of an inch in length, is made in the surface of the skin to ease the entry of the needle. Using pressure, the bone marrow needle is forced through the bone surface and into the bone marrow. A syringe is attached to the needle and a small specimen of bone marrow is sucked up. The bone marrow needle is removed and a tight bandage placed over the site to stop bleeding. The bone marrow sample is sent to the lab for processing and examination.

HOW THE RESULTS ARE GIVEN: The bone marrow specimen is sent to the laboratory for examination. The doctor—usually a hematologist (blood specialist) or oncologist (cancer specialist)—will determine if the various blood cells are being made in sufficient numbers, and if they are normal in appearance. In addition, the bone marrow will be examined for the presence of any cells or bacteria that should not normally be there.

PATIENT PREPARATION: None is required. If the patient is very apprehensive, a sedative and analgesic can be given before the procedure.

RISKS AND DISCOMFORTS: The injection of the local anesthetic can cause some slight pain and burning, but if it has been properly administered, the incision in the skin and the initial entry of the bone marrow needle should cause no pain. The pressure of the needle as it enters the bone will be felt, however. When the bone marrow is sucked into the syringe, there will be moderate pain that will last for only a moment. This is due to the bone marrow specimen breaking off from the bone. Some patients will describe this sensation as feeling that the bone cracked. Bleeding or infection at the site of the bone marrow test may result but is a rare complication.

SYMPTOMS FOR WHICH THIS TEST IS COMMONLY OBTAINED:
Recurrent bruising or bleeding (p. 288)—might be due to insufficient numbers of platelets.
Fatigue (p. 295)—may be due to anemia (insufficient numbers of red blood cells).
Fever (p. 296)—may be due to insufficient numbers of white blood cells to fight off infection.

DISEASES FOR WHICH THIS TEST IS COMMONLY OBTAINED:
Anemia (p. 309)—to see if the red cells are being made and, if not, what is the reason; also, to examine the size and shape of the various red cells in the bone marrow.
Thrombocytopenia (too few platelets)—to see if the platelets are being made and, if not, the reason why.
Leukemia—to diagnose leukemia, which is cancer of the blood cells that grow in the bone marrow. The test will also be done frequently in a patient with leukemia to determine if the treatment is successful and to monitor for return of the disease.
Cancer (p. 313)—to see if the tumor has spread to the bone marrow.

COST: approximately $100.

CELLOPHANE TAPE TEST

OTHER NAMES: pinworm test, Scotch tape test.

PURPOSE OF THE TEST: to detect pinworm infection.

BACKGROUND: Pinworm is one of the most common parasitic infections of the intestine. It almost always occurs in children and is usually transmitted through dirt or contaminated clothing. Unlike most parasites, it is more common in areas of temperate climate.

Pinworm infection is characterized by intense anal itching, especially at night, which may be of sufficient intensity to wake the child repeatedly, leading to loss of sleep, restlessness, and irritability. Most other parasites are detected by examination of the stool for parasites and their eggs (ova, p. 96). Pinworm, however, is not diagnosed in this manner, as the worms and eggs are not found in the stool. Instead, the worms crawl out from the anus and deposit the eggs outside on the skin surrounding the anus, then crawl back inside. The best way to detect these worms and eggs is with the cellophane tape test.

HOW THE TEST IS DONE: Because the eggs are deposited at night, the test is best done in the early morning before the child bathes and dresses. A piece of standard cellophane tape, ½ inch wide and 3 inches long, is folded over a tongue depressor, the wooden stick used by the doctor when he examines a patient's throat. The tape is placed with the sticky side facing out, away from the wood. The stick is pressed down between the buttock crease, as far as possible, until the anus is reached. After the tape and stick are removed, they are brought to the doctor, who will then examine the tape under a microscope to see if any worms or eggs were "caught" on its sticky surface. Usually, the test is repeated on three consecutive mornings. Some doctors will recommend using one of the commercially available kits for this test (although the "homemade" materials work just as well).

HOW THE RESULTS ARE GIVEN: Each time a tape is obtained, the doctor or laboratory technician will examine it under a microscope to see if any worms or eggs are present. If they are, the diagnosis of pinworm is made and the patient will be treated. If none of the three tape tests reveals any worms or eggs, it is assumed that the parasites are not present.

PATIENT PREPARATION: The test is best performed while the child is still in bed, before he bathes and dresses.

RISKS AND DISCOMFORTS: None.

SYMPTOMS FOR WHICH THIS TEST IS COMMONLY OBTAINED:
These symptoms can be caused by pinworm infection, and the tape test is done to see if the parasite is present:
Anal or rectal itching.
Vaginal itching.

DISEASES FOR WHICH THIS TEST IS COMMONLY OBTAINED:
Pinworm—Once treatment has been given, the test is usually repeated to be sure that the parasite has not returned.

COST: approximately $15.

CYTOLOGY

PURPOSE OF THE TEST: to examine various cells found in the body for cancer or inflammation.

BACKGROUND: The examination of cells in the body can give the doctor a great deal of information. Cells can be found in many collections of body fluid that are normally present (cerebrospinal fluid) as well as some that are present only during illness (fluid around the lungs). These cells can reflect the presence of infection, malignancy, or inflammation. Examination and study of these cells can be useful in the diagnosis of these conditions.

HOW THE TEST IS DONE: The cells to be studied are collected in a variety of ways. Sometimes the tissue is scraped (Pap smear (p. 212), or buccal smear), other times it is collected from fluid (thoracentesis, arthrocentesis, or paracentesis, p. 222), and still other times the cells are collected from sputum. See the separate listings under these tests for a discussion of how the actual procedure is done. Once the cells are sent to the laboratory, they are studied under a microscope and the size, shape, and nature of the cells are determined.

HOW THE RESULTS ARE GIVEN: The pathologist studies the cells and writes the report. He will say if the cells are related to an infection, inflammation, or malignancy. If malignancy is present, he will often diagnose the specific kind of cancer that is found.

PATIENT PREPARATION: None, except for the actual procedure in which the cells are collected.

RISKS AND DISCOMFORTS: The actual cytological study is done in the laboratory and is without risk to the patient. The collection of cells, on the other hand, can involve a procedure, such as thoracentesis, that is slightly painful or risky.

SYMPTOMS FOR WHICH THIS TEST IS COMMONLY OBTAINED:
Shortness of breath (p. 290).
Abdominal pain (p. 285).

Cough (p. 292).
Fever (p. 296).
Weight loss (p. 306).
Breast mass (p. 302).

DISEASES FOR WHICH THIS TEST IS COMMONLY OBTAINED:
Pneumonia (p. 321).
Cancer (p. 313).
Liver disease.
Ascites (fluid in the abdomen).
Pleural effusion (fluid around the lungs).

COST: approximately $20–100, depending upon which cells are being examined.

ELECTROCARDIOGRAM

OTHER NAMES: EKG, ECG, cardiogram, electrocardiograph, heart tracing.

PURPOSE OF THE TEST: to evaluate heart function and diagnose heart disease.

BACKGROUND: The heart has four chambers: right atrium, left atrium, right ventricle, and left ventricle (as can be seen in the illustration). Each normal heartbeat originates with an electrical impulse from a specialized part of the right atrium called the sinoatrial (S-A) node. The S-A node functions as a battery for the heart, discharging approximately one to two times a second; therefore, it is called the pacemaker. The electrical impulse leaves the S-A node and travels in an orderly fashion throughout the heart, causing the heart muscle to contract and pump the blood throughout the body. The right and left atriums contract first, followed by the ventricles.

This electrical activity taking place throughout the heart is transmitted outward and can be detected on the skin surface. The EKG measures these electrical impulses, picking up first the discharge in the S-A node and the contraction of the atriums, followed by the contraction of the ventricles. Lastly, the EKG demonstrates the electrical activity that occurs as the heart is at rest and filling for the next contraction. Most heart disease, including heart attacks, heart enlargement, abnormal heart rhythms, heart inflammation, and abnormalities in the minerals that control the heart's electrical activity (potassium, calcium, magnesium) will cause abnormalities on the EKG. It is important to remember that it is still possible to have serious heart disease that will go undetected by the EKG unless it affects the electrical impulses traveling throughout the heart.

The heart has four chambers: right atrium (RA), right ventricle (RV), left atrium (LA), and left ventricle (LV). The sinoatrial (s-A) node, located in the right atrium, is the heart's natural battery. From it will come the electrical current necessary to trigger the contraction of the heart chambers and the resultant pumping of the blood through the aorta (Ao).

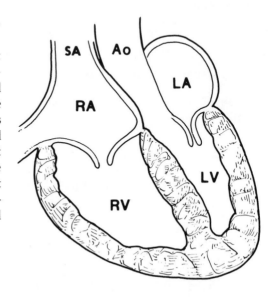

HOW THE TEST IS DONE: The test can be done in the hospital or in the physician's office. The patient lies on a table and electrodes are attached to each limb at the wrists and ankles. These are small pieces of metal, 1 by 1½ inches, that are held to the skin with rubber strips. A paste that conducts electricity is applied between the electrode and the skin to help in picking up the heart's electrical activity. In addition, a fifth electrode—called the chest electrode—is applied sequentially to various locations on the chest. This electrode consists of a small metal cup that is held to the skin by suction, again with electrically conducting paste placed between it and the skin. The electrodes are connected by wires to the EKG machine, which records the impulses detected by the leads on a moving piece of graph paper. The four limb electrodes plus the chest electrode, placed in various positions, look at the heart from 12 different directions (called leads) from which the heart can be evaluated. A routine EKG will collect information from all 12 leads and takes about 15 minutes.

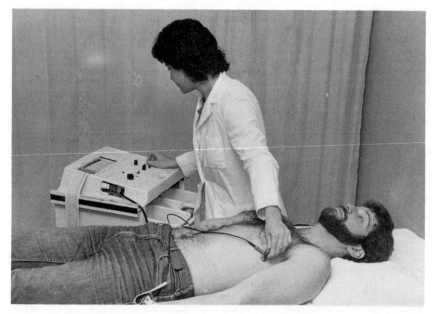

Patient having an electrocardiogram (EKG). Wires are attached to each limb, and a fifth wire is attached to a suction cup that is placed on the chest.

HOW THE RESULTS ARE GIVEN: The physician looks at the electrical patterns from the 12 leads and interprets the EKG. Generally, the patient will be told that either the EKG is normal or that certain abnormalities were seen. These abnormalities correlate with various kinds of heart disease.

PATIENT PREPARATION: None is required. Occasionally, if a male patient's chest is very hairy, a small area must be shaved to enable the chest electrode to stick properly.

RISKS AND DISCOMFORTS: The test causes no pain, but the patient does have to lie still for the duration of the EKG. The machines are safe so there is no risk of electric shock to the patient. Following the EKG the conduction paste must be washed off.

SYMPTOMS FOR WHICH THIS TEST IS COMMONLY OBTAINED:
All of these symptoms can be due to various forms of heart disease. When these symptoms are present, the EKG is obtained to detect if the heart is abnormal:
Chest pain (p. 291).

Shortness of breath or trouble breathing (p. 290).

Palpitations, pounding heart beat, or tachycardia (fast heart beat).

Fainting spells—to see if the heart beat is irregular or stopping periodically, causing the patient to pass out.

DISEASES FOR WHICH THIS TEST IS COMMONLY OBTAINED:

Each of these diseases produces a specific abnormality on the EKG that will aid in the diagnosis or monitoring of that particular illness:

Arrhythmias (abnormal cardiac rhythms).

Myocardial infarction (heart attack) (p. 319).

Hypertrophy (cardiac enlargement).

Rheumatic fever.

Pulmonary embolus.

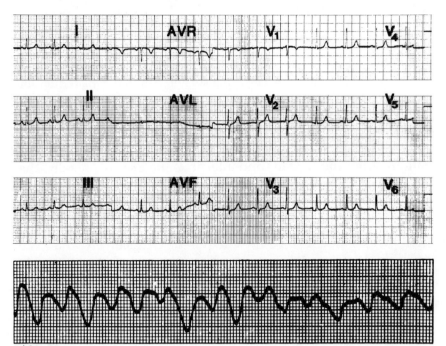

LEAD II

Electrocardiogram (EKG) tracings from a normal patient and one who has a cardiac arrhythmia, or abnormal heart rate. The normal EKG consists of 12 leads, each identified by a Roman numeral or letters. The abnormal EKG is of lead II in a patient with ventricular fibrillation, a severe disorder of heart rhythm that prevents the heart from pumping blood normally and will be fatal if not corrected.

Congestive heart failure.

Inflammation of the heart (endocarditis, myocarditis, and pericarditis).

Angina pectoris and cardiac ischemia—decreased oxygen supply to the heart muscle.

Drug overdose—If two common heart drugs, digitalis and quinidine are taken in excess, they can produce EKG changes.

Blood mineral abnormalities—abnormal levels of potassium, calcium, and magnesium.

COST: approximately $40.

ELECTROENCEPHALOGRAPHY

OTHER NAMES: EEG, brain wave test.

PURPOSE OF THE TEST: To measure the electrical impulses produced by the brain waves in order to diagnose illnesses and abnormalities of the brain.

BACKGROUND: In many ways your brain operates like a complex and sophisticated computer. In fact, the cells of your brain communicate with each other by electrical impulses. This electrical activity is very slight, much less than the electrical impulses that occur in the heart. Many abnormalities or illnesses within the brain, including epilepsy, tumors, blood clots, stroke, and infections, will alter this pattern of electrical impulses. An EEG is a test that measures the electrical activity of the brain and records it on paper for analysis and diagnosis. The EEG does not measure intelligence, nor can it "read the mind" of the patient. It is not at all related to electrical shock therapy; in an EEG electrical activity flows only from the patient to the machine, not the other way.

Another purpose of the EEG—one that has become important only in the last few years—is to diagnose brain death. The definition of death is complicated and controversial when a patient is being kept alive by a respirator and other sophisticated equipment. In many states there are laws that define death as brain death, meaning that even though the patient has a heart beat, he is pronounced dead if all the electrical activity in the brain has ceased. This is critical in obtaining organs for donation from such patients. Brain death will occur hours (sometimes days) before the heart stops beating. It is during this time, when the blood flow to the organ to be donated is maintained, even though the patient is dead, that it is best to remove organs for transplantation.

HOW THE TEST IS DONE: The patient lies on a table or sits in a reclining chair. The EEG technician applies from 16 to 30 electrodes to the scalp. These are small pads, ½ inch in diameter, and are attached to the scalp with either adhesive that conducts electrical impulses or small needles. The hair does not have to be trimmed or cut. The patient lies still while the brain wave tracing is made. He will not feel anything when the machine is switched on and the waves are actually being recorded. Sometimes, it is important for the doctor to have a tracing when the patient is asleep (the patient will be given a sedative), being stimulated by bright lights (flashing lights similar to a rapid series of flashes from a photograph camera), or breathing quickly (the patient will be instructed to do so). Altogether, the tracing is made for 30 to 60 minutes.

HOW THE RESULTS ARE GIVEN: An EEG is interpreted by a neurologist, and the results will be discussed with the patient. Although it is rarely necessary, an immediate reading can be obtained. If the EEG was being done to determine if brain death had occurred,

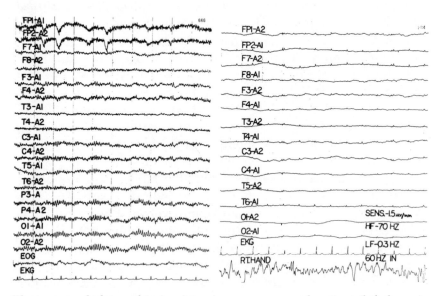

Electroencephalographic (EEG) tracings on a normal patient (left figure), and one (right figure) who has been declared "brain dead" because of the flat line tracing. (Courtesy of Beaver Spooner, R.EEGT.)

the reading would simply state that brain waves are present or absent. If they are absent (sometimes referred to as a "flat line" or "straight line" pattern), the diagnosis of brain death will be confirmed.

PATIENT PREPARATION: Food should be eaten before the test so that the patient is not hypoglycemic (low in blood sugar), a condition that might influence the test result. There is one exception to this: foods containing caffeine (coffee, chocolate, tea) should be avoided. The hair should be shampooed the night before the test so that the electrodes will stick better. If the EEG is to include a portion with the subject asleep, he should get only four to five hours of sleep the night before by postponing the usual bedtime and awakening early. Many patients who will have an EEG are already taking medication for a neurological problem and should discuss this with the doctor at least a week before the test so the drug can be discontinued if necessary. Following the procedure, the patient can resume normal activity (unless a sedative was given that must wear off) and can shampoo to remove any electrode adhesive paste.

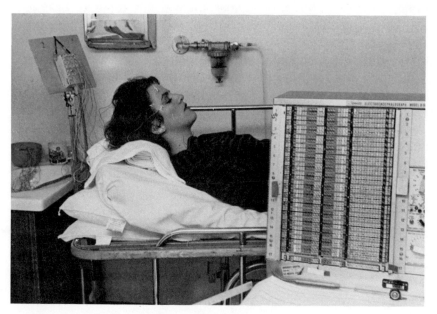

A patient having an electroencephalogram (EEG) done. The wire leads are attached to her scalp with adhesive paste and are connected to the EEG machine. (Courtesy of Beaver Spooner, R.EEGT.)

RISKS AND DISCOMFORTS: If the electrodes are connected with adhesive, they are not painful at all. If small needles are used, they will cause a pinprick sensation as they are being placed. The flashing bright lights are momentarily annoying.

SYMPTOMS FOR WHICH THIS TEST IS COMMONLY OBTAINED:
An EEG will frequently be obtained if any of these symptoms is present to determine if a brain tumor, stroke, blood clot, infection, or epilepsy is the cause. The EEG will also help to pinpoint the location of the abnormality within the brain.
Headache (p. 297).
Convulsions (epileptic fits, seizures).
Paralysis.
Recurrent vomiting (p. 303).
Abnormal or strange behavior.
Unconsciousness.

DISEASES FOR WHICH THIS TEST IS COMMONLY OBTAINED:
Cancer (p. 313) or brain tumor—to detect if it has spread to the brain and, if so, to what locations in the brain.
Stroke (p. 324)—to locate the parts of the brain that are involved.
Epilepsy—used both to diagnose the various types of epilepsy and, once treatment has been started, to see if the drugs are controlling it.
Meningitis—to determine if the meningitis is causing any abnormalities in the brain wave conduction, especially if the patient had a seizure as a result of the meningitis.
Head injury—to evaluate the location and extent of the injury.
Coma—to see if electrical waves are still present, or if brain death has occurred.
Dementia (p. 316)

COST: approximately $165.

ELECTROMYOGRAPHY

OTHER NAMES: EMG, electromyogram, nerve conduction tests.

PURPOSE OF THE TEST: to test the function of the muscles and nerves.

BACKGROUND: Nerve cells in your body communicate with one another by electrical impulses. Your muscles, which are controlled by nerves, are activated by these electrical impulses as well.

In many diseases the conduction of these electrical impulses along the nerve and to the muscle is abnormal. This test measures these electrical waves and is useful in diagnosing the specific diseases that can cause muscle weakness, paralysis, or abnormal nerve sensations (tingling or pain).

HOW THE TEST IS DONE: The test is done in a special room that screens out any extraneous electrical activity that could interfere with the result. The patient lies on his back on a table, and electrodes are taped on the area to be tested. These are small white pads (approximately ½ inch in diameter) connected with wires to the recording machine. In the first half of the procedure electrical conduction in the nerves is tested. The technician will ask the patient to contract or relax certain muscles. In addition, a small current of electricity is passed between two of the electrodes. The second half of the test measures electrical conduction by the muscles. Small needle electrodes are placed through the skin and into the muscles to be tested. The patient is asked to contract and relax certain muscles, and again a small electrical current is passed through the electrodes. The entire EMG takes about one hour.

HOW THE RESULTS ARE GIVEN: The test records the electrical waves from the nerves and muscles in three ways: on moving paper (as in an EKG), on a television screen, and over a loudspeaker. The activity over the loudspeaker will be heard by the patient and sound like machine-gun fire (rapid popping noises). The doctor—usually a neurologist—interprets these three collections of information. This usually takes a few days, although an immediate reading can be made if it is important to do so.

PATIENT PREPARATION: Sometimes, if the patient is very apprehensive or worried, a mild sedative or analgesic will be administered prior to the test.

RISKS AND DISCOMFORTS: The test can cause short periods of burning pain when the electrical currents are passed. In addition, there can be slight discomfort when the needle electrodes are inserted. The patient should tell the technician if muscle pain is experienced so that the test can be momentarily stopped and the electrodes replaced or reimplanted.

SYMPTOMS FOR WHICH THIS TEST IS COMMONLY OBTAINED:
The EMG will determine if these symptoms are caused by nerve or muscle disease:

Muscle weakness.
Muscle pain.
Abnormal sensations (tingling, numbness, or pain).

DISEASES FOR WHICH THIS TEST IS COMMONLY OBTAINED:
Myopathy—these diseases (muscular dystrophy is an example)
cause muscle weakness. The EMG is used to see if the muscles
alone are affected, or if the problem involves the nerves as well.
Diabetes (p. 318)—Since many patients with severe diabetes develop neuropathy or nerve disease, this test is used to distinguish
the different kinds of nerve illness that can be present and determine which nerves are involved.
Polio—This test can help make this diagnosis since the disease
causes a specific abnormal pattern in the EMG test.
Amyotrophic lateral sclerosis (Lou Gehrig's disease)—The EMG
helps make this diagnosis because a uniquely abnormal pattern is
seen.
Neuropathy (nerve illness)—This test can detect abnormal nerve
function and pinpoint which nerves are affected and which specific nerve disease is present.
Alcoholism—Severe alcoholism can cause nerve disease that will
be diagnosed by this test.
Myasthenia gravis—This disease causes muscle weakness that will
be detected by the EMG.
Multiple sclerosis—Although the results of the EMG in this disease
are usually normal, this test helps in making the diagnosis of multiple sclerosis because it rules out the possibility of other diseases
with similar symptoms that give positive electromyographic findings.

COST: approximately $200.

EXERCISE TOLERANCE TEST

OTHER NAMES: cardiac stress test, stress test, exercise test.

PURPOSE OF THE TEST: to test heart function and efficiency during
periods of increased stress on the heart.

BACKGROUND: The demands placed on the heart when a person is
exercising are far greater than when he is resting. The standard
EKG is done with the patient at rest; thus, it may not detect abnormalities that are apparent only when the body is exercising or

stressed. The cardiac stress test is intended to study the heart when the patient is exercising. It is very useful in evaluating a patient who has suffered a heart attack in the past, and it determines how much exercise he can tolerate. Also, the test determines if heart disease is present in a patient who has symptoms that are suggestive of heart disease when he exercises. But this test is probably not necessary for a person who has no symptoms and has never had heart disease unless he is over 40 years of age, has been physically inactive previously, and is about to embark on a strenuous program of exercise and physical activity (running, swimming, jogging). The use of the exercise stress test for the screening of healthy people is controversial and is discussed on page 243.

HOW THE TEST IS DONE: Stress tests are conducted under the direct supervision of a physician. The patient is attached to an EKG machine using chest electrodes only. A resting (base line) blood pressure, heart rate, and EKG are obtained. The patient then begins to exercise. Most medical centers have the patient walk on a treadmill, although a few centers will do a stress test having the patient pedal a bicycle. The patient walks on the treadmill and the EKG, heart rate, and blood pressure are monitored constantly. The treadmill is adjusted to move faster and at an angle, so that the patient must walk and then jog and run increasingly faster. He will periodically be asked to rest, to determine how quickly the heart rate and blood pressure return to base line levels. The entire test takes about 30 minutes to perform. Frequently, immediately after the patient stops the exercise test, a thallium scan (p. 138) is performed to determine if any part of the heart is getting insufficient oxygen.

HOW THE RESULTS ARE GIVEN: The test is often done in a cardiologist's office but may be done in the outpatient clinic of a hospital. The doctor conducting the test will determine if any abnormalities in the EKG pattern, blood pressure, or heart rate occurred while the patient was exercising. These results are available after the test but are usually given to the patient later, after the doctor has had sufficient time to analyze all the information collected during the test.

PATIENT PREPARATION: Only a light breakfast should be eaten the morning of the test. The hair on a male patient's chest may have to be shaved slightly to allow for good attachment of the elec-

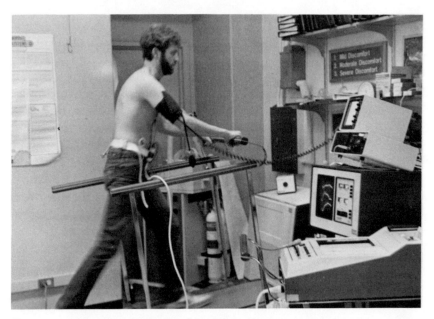

Patient undergoing exercise tolerance testing.

trodes. The patient should come to the examining room dressed comfortably, wearing sneakers and shorts or slacks.

RISKS AND DISCOMFORTS: The test can be risky for a person with a recent heart attack and should be postponed in that case. Anyone with symptoms of heart disease undergoing a stress test should alert the examining doctor immediately if chest pain, shortness of breath, or other similar symptoms develop during the test. Similarly, the examining doctor will terminate the test if the patient develops an abnormal heart rhythm, EKG changes, or abnormal increases in blood pressure. Equipment is always nearby so that if a patient develops complications during a stress test, the proper medical care can be given.

SYMPTOMS FOR WHICH THIS TEST IS COMMONLY OBTAINED:
The test is used to determine if the following symptoms are related to heart abnormalities brought on by exercise:
Chest pain (p. 291).
Heart palpitations.
Dizziness or fatigue during exercise.

DISEASES FOR WHICH THIS TEST IS COMMONLY OBTAINED:
Myocardial infarction (heart attack) (p. 319)—Although this test is not performed for several weeks after an actual heart attack, it is

a good indicator of how much exercise can be tolerated by the recovered patient.

Angina pectoris—This disease, characterized by periodic chest pain due to insufficient oxygen supply to the heart muscle, can be diagnosed by changes in the EKG that will occur with exercise.

COST: approximately $140.

GASTRIC ANALYSIS

PURPOSE OF THE TEST: to measure the amount and composition of the digestive juices made by the stomach.

BACKGROUND: When the stomach is stimulated by the presence of food, it will secrete digestive juices, the major component of which is hydrochloric acid. There are conditions in which too much acid is made (ulcers) as well as other diseases in which too little acid is made (stomach cancer, pernicious anemia). If any of these illnesses are suspected, the patient may have a gastric analysis performed to measure how much acid is produced. Since different foods stimulate varying amounts of acid, the stomach is stimulated chemically so that a standardized amount of acid can be expected.

HOW THE TEST IS DONE: The patient fasts for eight hours before the test. A narrow plastic tube, ¼ inch in diameter, is placed into the patient's nose and down the esophagus into the stomach. Sometimes, an x-ray will be taken to be sure that the tip of the tube is in the stomach. Otherwise, if digestive juices are found, it is assumed that the tube is in the proper location and an x-ray is not done. When the tube is in place, the physician or nurse conducting the test uses a syringe to draw out the stomach juices every 15 minutes; these are then stored in separate tubes. After four such measurements (one hour after the start of the test), the patient receives an intramuscular injection of Histalog, a chemical that will cause the stomach to make acid. Four more samples are collected, 15 minutes apart. At the conclusion of that time the nasogastric tube is removed, and the tubes with digestive juices are sent to the laboratory for analysis.

HOW THE RESULTS ARE GIVEN: The tubes containing the digestive juices are assayed in the laboratory for the acid content. The physician will receive a report describing the acid production in both the resting (before Histalog injection) and stimulated (after Histalog injection) phases of the test. The physician—usually a gastroenterologist—will discuss these results with the patient.

PATIENT PREPARATION: Eating, drinking, and smoking are prohibited for at least 8 and preferably 12 hours before the test.

RISKS AND DISCOMFORTS: The placing of the nasogastric tube can be slightly painful and is uncomfortable, causing most patients to experience a gagging or choking sensation. This uncomfortable feeling will lessen once the tube is in place. The intramuscular injection of Histalog is also slightly painful.

SYMPTOMS FOR WHICH THIS TEST IS COMMONLY OBTAINED:
Bleeding in the gastrointestinal tract or blood in the stool (p. 289)—the amount of acid produced will help distinguish between ulcers (excessive acid production) and gastric cancer (decreased acid production).
Abdominal pain (p. 285)—can be caused by ulcers or stomach cancer. The amount of acid produced will help determine if either is the cause.

DISEASES FOR WHICH THIS TEST IS COMMONLY OBTAINED:
Recurrent ulcers (p. 325)—can often be caused by excessive acid production; the patient diagnosed as having duodenal ulcers and being treated with medications such as cimetidine or antacids may have this test done to see if the acid production has decreased.
Pernicious anemia—can be accompanied by the absence of gastric acid production.
Vitamin deficiency (lack of vitamin B12)—associated with decreased acid production.
Anemia—can be due to pernicious anemia, bleeding from ulcers, or gastric cancer. The amount of acid produced will help in determining the specific cause of the anemia.

COST: approximately $100.

HOLTER MONITOR

OTHER NAMES: 24-hour EKG.

PURPOSE OF THE TEST: to evaluate the functioning of the heart over a 24-hour period.

BACKGROUND: Certain heart disease only shows itself intermittently. A routine EKG, which traces the heart for several minutes, may not pick up abnormalities in heart rhythm that come only once or twice in a day. A Holter monitor (named after the company that manufactures the device) is intended to screen the heart for an entire day, so that any abnormality in heart rhythm that is occurring periodically will be likely to be found.

HOW THE TEST IS DONE: Chest leads are attached to the patient and connected to a small machine (Holter monitor) that the patient carries with him for the next 24 hours. The monitor—which resembles a small radio or tape recorder—weighs only a couple of pounds and is worn around the waist. The patient is encouraged to follow his usual schedule and pattern of activity and, as best as possible, forget that he is wearing the monitor. At the end of the measuring day, the monitor is returned to the doctor and the 24 hours of electrocardiogram analyzed by a computer. The patient records any symptoms and the time they occurred so they can be correlated with the EKG tracing on the machine.

HOW THE RESULTS ARE GIVEN: The results of a Holter monitoring are not available for a few days after the test is completed for the computer must first analyze the cardiogram. The result will be either normal (no abnormalities seen during the entire 24-hour monitoring period), or abnormal. The doctor will discuss with the patient the specific abnormality and its implications to his health.

PATIENT PREPARATION: Sometimes the hair on the chest must be shaved so the electrodes will stick well.

RISKS AND DISCOMFORTS: The patient must wear the monitor all day. Although not heavy, it can be a nuisance. There are no risks to this test.

SYMPTOMS FOR WHICH THIS TEST IS COMMONLY OBTAINED:
With all these symptoms, the purpose of the test is to detect any changes in heart rhythm that did not show up on the routine EKG but are apparent when monitored over a 24-hour period.
Dizziness (p. 293).
Fainting (p. 294).
Sudden fatigue
Heart or chest palpitations
Chest pain (p. 291).

DISEASES FOR WHICH THIS TEST IS COMMONLY OBTAINED:
Heart arrhythmia—to detect if irregular heart beats are present, to determine which part of the heart they came from, and to check

if treatment is effective in preventing them from recurring.
Mitral valve prolapse—to determine if this abnormality in one of
the heart valves is causing any problems in heart rate or rhythm.

COST: approximately $240.

KARYOTYPING AND CHROMOSOME STUDIES

OTHER NAMES: gene studies.

PURPOSE OF THE TEST: To study the number and appearance of a
patient's chromosomes.

BACKGROUND: Genes—the part of the cell composed of deoxyribonucleic acid (DNA), the chemical in the body that carries hered-
itary information—are arranged in structures within the cell called
chromosomes. Abnormalities in the number or structure of the
chromosomes can result in genetic or inherited diseases, including Down's syndrome (mongolism), abnormal genitalia, and certain kinds of leukemia. When patients have symptoms suggestive
of a genetic disease, the doctor will often order a chromosomal
analysis (karyotyping) to see if the chromosomes are normal. The
other common reason to do chromosomal analysis is for pregnant
women who are over 35. In these women there is a significant
increase in the chance of having a baby with Down's syndrome.
In this situation, the woman undergoes an amniocentesis (discussed in greater detail on p. 180), and the actual karyotyping is
done on the baby's cells.

HOW THE TEST IS DONE: Almost every cell in the body can be used
for chromosomal analysis, but the easiest to obtain are white blood
cells. The doctor will draw a small amount of blood (less than 1
ounce) from the vein in the routine manner (p. 43) and send the
blood to the lab. Other cells that are occasionally studied are bone
marrow cells, skin cells, or cells scraped from the inside of the
mouth. In addition, as mentioned above, amniocentesis is performed to obtain fetal cells for analysis.

HOW THE RESULTS ARE GIVEN: A normal human cell has 23 pairs of
chromosomes—46 in all. The pairs are identified by number, 1
through 22. The 23rd and last pair are the chromosomes that
determine sex and are identified by the letters: X and Y. A person
with two X chromosomes is female; a person with 1 X and 1 Y is

male. A chromosomal analysis will count the chromosomes, study their structure, and determine the makeup of the sex chromosomes. Abnormal results include having 3 instead of 2 chromosomes in a "pair"—as is the case with Down's syndrome, which has 3 chromosomes in the 21st pair (hence its other name: trisomy 21). Abnormalities in the sex chromosomes can also be identified. Klinefelter's syndrome, for instance, leads to infertility and small genitalia in otherwise healthy males. This disease is characterized by the presence of 3 sex chromosomes: XXY. This test is used by genetic counselors to help them advise patients and families about family planning and the risk of certain genetic diseases.

PATIENT PREPARATION: None.

RISKS AND DISCOMFORTS: The only risk with this test comes from the collection of the cells, as the entire test itself is done in the

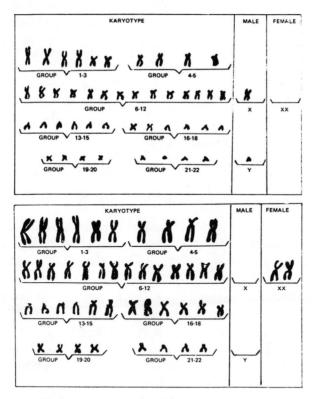

Normal karyotypes showing the 23 pairs of chromosomes. The upper one has an X and Y chromosome and is from a male. The bottom one, which has two X chromosomes, is from a female.

laboratory. If the cells are collected from the blood, the only discomfort is the slight pain of venipuncture. The risk from amniocentesis is discussed separately (p. 180).

SYMPTOMS FOR WHICH THIS TEST IS COMMONLY OBTAINED:
All these symptoms suggest a possible chromosomal (genetic) disease. The test is done to detect such a problem.
Mental retardation.
Abnormal or small genitalia.
Infertility.
Birth defects.

DISEASES FOR WHICH THIS TEST IS COMMONLY OBTAINED:
All these diseases are associated with chromosomal abnormalities. Any patient thought to have one of these diseases will have this test done to detect the presence of these abnormalities.
Turner syndrome—This is a disease in which the patient has only one X chromosome. These women have female genitalia but are sterile.
Klinefelter's syndrome—In this disease males have XXY chromosomes.

COST: approximately $250.

LUMBAR PUNCTURE

OTHER NAMES: spinal tap, LP.

PURPOSE OF THE TEST: to examine the spinal fluid.

BACKGROUND: Spinal fluid (also called cerebrospinal fluid or CSF) bathes the brain and spinal cord. In an adult there is almost a cup of spinal fluid (6 ounces), of which more than half is made daily. The most important purpose of the CSF is to act as a "water" cushion for the brain and spinal cord. Normally, the CSF contains no cells, only some sugar and protein. In various diseases, injuries, or other abnormal conditions, the spinal fluid may contain white or red blood cells, increased amounts of protein, and elevated or lowered levels of sugar. In addition, many diseases will cause the pressure of the CSF to be higher than usual. When any abnormality of the brain or spinal cord is suspected, a lumbar puncture almost always is performed because examination of the CSF often provides valuable information about possible problems.

HOW THE TEST IS DONE: The spinal fluid is sampled from the lower back, where there is the least danger of injury to the spinal cord or brain. The patient either sits on a table with his head down on his knees, or he lies on a table with his knees and head tucked together (the fetal position)—both positions forcing open the spaces between the spinal vertebrae so the needle can be inserted into the spinal fluid. The site to be used is selected and the overlying skin cleaned with soap and an antiseptic. Sterile drapes are placed so that only the puncture site is exposed. A local anesthetic is injected into the skin and the hollow spinal tap needle then inserted through the skin and into the spinal fluid. When spinal fluid begins to flow through the needle, the doctor measures the CSF pressure and then collects some of the fluid for analysis in the laboratory. Some of the fluid is sent for spinal fluid culture (p. 171) as well. When enough fluid has been collected, usually a teaspoonful, the spinal needle is withdrawn and the patient allowed to relax. The patient is generally told to lie flat in bed without a pillow for a few hours.

HOW THE RESULTS ARE GIVEN: Numerous measurements are made on the CSF:

Pressure—Elevated pressure can be a sign of brain tumor, meningitis, or cancer that has spread to the brain.

Color—CSF is normally clear. The following colors are abnormal: (1) red CSF is usually due to the presence of blood and is a sign of a hemorrhage in the brain, (2) yellow CSF is usually due to the presence of bilirubin (p. 45) and can be related to previous bleeding that occurred in the brain, (3) white CSF can be due to infection.

Clarity—Normal CSF is clear. Cloudy fluid is due to the presence of white blood cells or bacteria—both worrisome signs of serious infection in the brain (meningitis or a brain abscess).

Cells—Normal CSF has no cells. Red blood cells are a sign of hemorrhage in the brain or spinal cord. White blood cells are a sign of infection (meningitis, encephalitis, abscess) or inflammation (from tumors, lupus erythematosus, or multiple sclerosis).

Protein—Elevated levels of protein in the CSF are usually due to infection (meningitis) or inflammation (from cancer or brain tumor).

Glucose—Decreased levels of glucose in the CSF are usually due to infection (meningitis). Increased glucose levels can be found in a diabetic or in a person who has suffered brain injury.

PATIENT PREPARATION: None.

RISKS AND DISCOMFORTS: A spinal tap is moderately painful, and the local anesthetic can itself cause slight burning when it is given. The placing of the spinal needle can hurt as well. Frequently, the doctor does not successfully get spinal fluid the first time and the needle must be replaced until he does. This can be painful, especially if the vertebrae (bones in the back) become irritated from the needle. Following the tap, many patients develop "spinal headaches," which are thought to be related to slight leakage of CSF from the puncture site. Lying flat will decrease this leakage and diminish the headache.

SYMPTOMS FOR WHICH THIS TEST IS COMMONLY OBTAINED:
All of these symptoms are suggestive of diseases within the brain or spinal cord. The lumbar puncture will provide information helpful in determining the exact problem.
Fever (p. 296).
Headache (p. 297).
Vomiting (p. 303).
Seizures (convulsions, epilepsy).
Dizziness (p. 293).
Unconsciousness or coma.

DISEASES FOR WHICH THIS TEST IS COMMONLY OBTAINED:
This test is helpful in the diagnosis as well as monitoring of these various diseases:
Cancer (leukemia and brain tumor) (p. 313).
Multiple sclerosis.
Stroke (p 324).
Bleeding or hemorrhage into the brain.
Brain infection (meningitis, encephalitis, or abscess).
Dementia (p. 316).

COST: approximately $100.

PAP SMEAR

OTHER NAMES: cervical cytology, Papanicolaou smear.

PURPOSE OF THE TEST: to detect cervical cancer, especially early cancer and precancerous lesions.

BACKGROUND: One of the basic tenets of cancer medicine is that early detection substantially increases the patient's chances to be cured of the disease. This has proven to be the case in cervical cancer. At one time cancer of the cervix was almost always fatal. Diagnosis was made only when a woman began complaining of abnormal vaginal bleeding or other symptoms that did not occur until the tumor was far advanced. At that point there was little that could be done. The Pap smear has changed all that. Now, when cervical cancer is suspected on the Pap smear, further testing will be done to confirm the diagnosis. If cancer is present, the patient will be treated accordingly. Pap smear allows for detection of cancer of the cervix many years before other symptoms appear, and it is this difference that has greatly reduced the death rate from the disease.

The Pap smear was first described in 1928 by Dr. George Papanicolaou, after whom the procedure is named. It was only in the 1950s, however, that the test began to be used routinely. Pap smears are most frequently performed on healthy women who have no symptoms suggestive of cervical cancer. How often the Pap smear should be done is discussed on page 244. In addition, medical research has shown that women with genital herpes infection may have a higher incidence of cervical cancer than the rest of the population. Pap smears may be done more frequently for these women since they appear to be at higher risk of developing this malignancy.

HOW THE TEST IS DONE: The woman to be examined prepares in the same way as for a routine pelvic examination; in fact, the Pap smear is most often done as part of a patient's gynecologic examination. The woman lies on the table with legs in stirrups and a speculum is inserted into the vagina to allow the doctor to see the cervix. Using a small wooden spatula, he gently scrapes the cervix as well as any abnormal areas that are evident and immediately smears the scraping on a glass microscope slide that is sprayed with a fixative to preserve the cells. The entire test takes 10 minutes.

HOW THE RESULTS ARE GIVEN: Pap smears are examined to see if any abnormal or malignant cells are pesent. The smear is scored from I through V as below:

I—Normal smear with no atypical cells evident.

II—Few atypical cells present but not suggestive of malignancy.

III—Many atypical cells present, suggesting the presence of malignancy.

IV—Strong evidence of malignancy.

V—Malignancy definitely present.

Most patients are not told the number of the interpretation but are simply informed that the test was normal or abnormal. Patients with a truly abnormal result (Classes III, IV, and V) will be asked to return immediately to their gynecologist for further evaluation, frequently beginning with colposcopy (p. 159). Patients with Grade II will be asked to have another Pap smear done in a few weeks time. The results from a Pap smear are not available for at least 48 and usually 72 hours after the specimen is obtained.

PATIENT PREPARATION: Optimally, this test should be done approximately five days after the end of the last menstrual cycle. Douching, suppositories, and sexual intercourse should be avoided for 24 hours before the test.

RISKS AND DISCOMFORTS: The scraping of the cervix is not painful, but slight bleeding may occur. The only discomfort associated with this test is that which accompanies a standard gynecologic examination.

SYMPTOMS FOR WHICH THIS TEST IS COMMONLY OBTAINED:
Abnormal vaginal bleeding.
Pain in vaginal area or lower abdomen.

DISEASES FOR WHICH THIS TEST IS COMMONLY OBTAINED:
Cervical cancer—After treatment for the cancer, the patient will have frequent Pap smears to be sure that the tumor has not recurred.

COST: approximately $20.

PREGNANCY TESTS

PURPOSE OF THE TEST: to determine if a woman is pregnant.

BACKGROUND: Within days of becoming pregnant, a woman will have elevated levels in her blood and urine of human chorionic gonadotropin (HCG), a hormone associated with the growth of the placenta and fetus. All pregnancy tests measure, by one means or another, the presence of this hormone. In years past, from the 1930s to the 50s, pregnancy testing was a cumbersome procedure that involved injection of urine into an animal—usually a rabbit.

The animal was subsequently killed and its tissues examined for the changes induced by the presence of HCG. In the 1960s the rabbit population of this country could breathe a sigh of relief with the development of immunological methods to test for HCG that use an antibody directed against the hormone. This has become even more simplified, so that today pregnancy tests have been developed for home use (p. 343) as well.

HOW THE TEST IS DONE: The test can be done on either blood or urine. The choice between the urine and blood test is a classic trade-off between quality and cost. The blood test—also known as a beta-1 subunit test—is more accurate and will be positive earlier in pregnancy than the urine test. It is also more expensive, however, and requires the patient to go to the laboratory for the blood to be drawn. If the blood is to be examined, a small specimen is obtained from the vein by the routine manner (p. 43). If a urine test is performed, a specimen is collected: the first specimen of the day is optimal because the concentration of HCG will be highest. The urine or blood specimen is brought to the doctor's office or laboratory. Occasionally, the urine test will be negative early in the pregnancy even though the woman is pregnant. Home pregnancy tests are discussed on p. 343.

HOW THE RESULTS ARE GIVEN: Both the blood and urine tests give a simple answer—either pregnancy is detected or it is not. It is important to remember, however, that a negative result may be due to testing too early. Therefore, if the woman continues to be suspicious that she is pregnant, the test should be repeated in two-weeks time.

RISKS AND DISCOMFORTS: None.

PATIENT PREPARATION: None

SYMPTOMS FOR WHICH THIS TEST IS COMMONLY OBTAINED:
All these symptoms are suggestive of pregnancy and, if present—especially in combination—a woman should have a pregnancy test done.
Missed menstrual period.
Breast swelling and tenderness.
Frequent urination.
Vomiting (p. 303).

COST: urine—approximately $10.
     blood—approximately—$50.

Pulmonary Function Tests

OTHER NAMES: PFTS, lung tests, spirometry, breathing tests.

PURPOSE OF THE TEST: to test the function of the lungs.

BACKGROUND: The lungs are constantly inflating (when we inhale) or deflating (when we exhale). The various diseases that affect the lungs, including bronchitis, asthma, emphysema, and cancer, change this pattern of breathing. In some of these diseases a patient will not be able to inhale as much as usual; in other cases, the expiration of air is obstructed and delayed. The pulmonary function tests are a series of measurements based on the patient's breathing abilities that will be useful in diagnosing and monitoring various lung diseases.

HOW THE TEST IS DONE: The patient sits or stands in the testing room, and a mouthpiece is placed between his lips. He closes his nose either with noseclips or with his fingers. The patient then breathes when instructed to do so by the technician. At times he will be asked to inhale or exhale as deeply and as quickly as possible; at other times, to breathe normally. The entire test takes from 15 to 30 minutes. Sometimes, the test is conducted while the patient is breathing 100% pure oxygen. Occasionally, the test will be repeated a few minutes after medicine is sprayed or inhaled into the lungs to see if this treatment improves the lung function. Often, arterial blood gases (p. 183) are performed during or immediately after pulmonary function tests are conducted.

HOW THE RESULTS ARE GIVEN: The volume of air that is exhaled is measured by a machine connected to the mouthpiece. In addition, this volume is recorded on a moving piece of paper resulting in a "picture" of lung function called a spirogram. Numerous measurements are made from this spirogram. Some of the more important ones are: the total capacity of the lung, the quantity of air that can be exhaled within one second, the quickest rate of exhaling air, and the size of the usual breath. All of these, plus other lung function measurements, will be used by the doctor to interpret the overall function of the lungs.

RISKS AND DISCOMFORTS: This test causes little or no discomfort. For some patients with lung diseases, it might be difficult to inhale and exhale deeply.

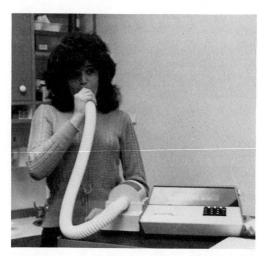

A patient having pulmonary function testing (PFTS) performed. The patient breathes into the machine, which automatically records a variety of measurements concerning the lungs.

PATIENT PREPARATION: If necessary, the patient should urinate or defecate before the test so the breathing can be done as deeply as possible. For the same reason the test should not be conducted immediately after the patient eats a large meal.

SYMPTOMS FOR WHICH THIS TEST IS COMMONLY OBTAINED:
For all of these symptoms, the purpose of the pulmonary function tests is to determine the nature and severity of the lung problem and diagnose the specific illness.
Shortness of breath (p. 290).
Breathing difficulty (p. 290).
Wheezing.
Coughing (p. 292).

DISEASES FOR WHICH THIS TEST IS COMMONLY OBTAINED:
For all of these diseases, pulmonary function tests will be abnormal. But the patterns of abnormality will be different, so that the test is used both to diagnose these diseases and to judge their severity as well as to monitor them once the diagnosis has been made and treatment started.
Pneumonia (p. 321)—to determine the extent to which the lung infection has altered the patient's ability to breathe normally.
Asthma (p. 312)—to see the extent and severity of the illness and test whether various medications are useful in opening up the lungs.
Bronchitis and emphysema (p. 315)—to detect the extent and severity

of the illness and to test the usefulness of certain medications in improving the lung's function.

Cancer (p. 313)—If the cancer originated in the lung or spread there from another organ, this test will be used to determine how much the cancer has impaired normal breathing.

Smoking—to see if lung damage has resulted from heavy smoking.

COST: approximately $40–200.

SEMEN ANALYSIS

OTHER NAMES: semen examination, sperm analysis, sperm count.

PURPOSE OF THE TEST: to help determine the cause of infertility or the effectiveness of a vasectomy.

BACKGROUND: Infertility is thought to affect approximately 10% of all couples. At one time it was assumed that all infertility was due to a problem with the woman. In fact, we now recognize that nearly half of all infertility results from problems with the male, the most common being insufficient numbers of healthy sperm in the semen. When this abnormality is supected, a semen analysis is ordered to test the semen carefully for the number and function of healthy sperm. In addition, in males who have had a vasectomy, it is important to document that sperm are not present before relying upon the vasectomy for safe birth control.

HOW THE TEST IS DONE: Semen is collected by one of three methods: masturbation, coitus interruptus, or intercourse with a condom (the inside of which has been washed). With the first two methods, the specimen should be collected in a clean, dry container. If a condom is used, it also should be placed in a clean, dry container. The specimen should be refrigerated as quickly as possible and brought to the laboratory within two hours.

HOW THE RESULTS ARE GIVEN: In the laboratory, four essential measurements are made on the semen: volume of semen, number of sperm, percentage of mature healthy sperm, and percentage of sperm that move properly and are able to "swim" up the vagina, uterus, and fallopian tube to fertilize the egg. This last measurement is called the motility. The doctor informs the patient of any abnormal values. When the semen analysis is being done to test the efficiency of a vasectomy, the doctor will tell the patient if the sperm count is now low enough so that no other form of birth control is necessary.

Normal range for a semen analysis:

Semen volume—2.0–5.0 ml.

sperm number—80–150 million/ml.

% of healthy sperm—greater than 75%.

% motility—75–100% motile.

PATIENT PREPARATION: Frequent ejaculations as well as significant alcohol intake can cause a decrease in the sperm count. Therefore, for three days prior to semen collection and analysis, the patient should abstain from sexual intercourse and alcoholic beverages.

RISKS AND DISCOMFORTS: It has been our experience that semen collection sometimes will raise religious or ethical issues with certain patients, especially with regard to masturbation or coitus interruptus. In such situations we make sure that the patient has the opportunity to discuss the method of collection with a clergyman.

DISEASES FOR WHICH THIS TEST IS COMMONLY OBTAINED:

Infertility (p. 299).

After vasectomy—to see if the sperm count is low enough so that no other birth control is necessary.

After cancer chemotherapy or radiation therapy—to see if the treatment left the patient sterile.

COST: approximately $35.

SWEAT TEST

PURPOSE OF THE TEST: To test the level of minerals in the sweat. Elevated levels are almost always due to cystic fibrosis.

BACKGROUND: The most common inherited disease in Caucasians is cystic fibrosis, with approximately 1 in 20 people carrying the gene for this disease. In contrast, only 1 in 15,000 nonwhites carry the gene. A person who carries the gene for cystic fibrosis has no symptoms or evidence of the disease; if both parents have the gene, however, their children will have a 25% chance of inheriting the actual disease. Children with cystic fibrosis do not digest or absorb food properly and, consequently, are small and malnourished in appearance. Also, they make abnormally high amounts of secretions in their lungs and are thus susceptible to colds and pneumonia. In addition, the sweat of children with cystic fibrosis contains excessive amounts of minerals (chloride, sodium, and potassium).

Infants and children with symptoms suggestive of cystic fibrosis, such as being small for their age and undernourished as well as suffering from frequent colds, pneumonia, coughing, and wheezing, will often have a sweat test to see if the disease is, in fact, present. The test can only detect those who actually have the disease—a person who only carries the gene for the disease will have a normal sweat test. Very recently, some new tests have been reported that claim to have the ability to detect the gene for cystic fibrosis in healthy carriers. It is too early to know if these tests will turn out to be accurate and sensitive enough to be useful. If they do prove to be reliable tests, they will enable physicians to identify situations in which both parents carry the gene, and if children are planned, appropriate genetic counseling can be given.

HOW THE TEST IS DONE: The usual site for the collection of sweat is the inner surface of the lower arm, although in very small infants the thigh may be used. The area to be used is washed and dried thoroughly with distilled water (water without any mineral content). A few drops of a drug that induces sweat—pilocarpine—is applied to a 1-inch square area of skin and covered with a small piece of copper (electrode). Another electrode is attached elsewhere on the limb and a small electrical current—a few volts at very low amperage—is passed between the electrodes. This will cause the drug to enter the skin and induce sweating. After a few minutes the electrodes are removed, and the skin where the drug was placed is again washed with distilled water and dried. A piece of absorbent paper is placed over the area and taped in place, and the sweat being produced is collected for 30 to 45 minutes. The paper is sent to the laboratory for analysis. Sweating will continue for a couple of hours at the test site.

HOW THE RESULTS ARE GIVEN: The mineral content of the sweat is measured in the laboratory. The only disease that causes an elevation in the mineral content is cystic fibrosis. The test does not detect carriers of the gene for cystic fibrosis but only patients who actually have the disease. If the test is positive (high mineral content), the diagnosis of cystic fibrosis is confirmed. If the result is negative (normal mineral content) but the patient has symptoms strongly suggestive of the disease, the physician will often repeat the test.

PATIENT PREPARATION: None.

RISKS AND DISCOMFORTS: The passing of the electrical current is slightly uncomfortable. In addition, the infant or child must be kept quiet and still for the duration of the test.

SYMPTOMS FOR WHICH THIS TEST IS COMMONLY OBTAINED:
All of these symptoms, especially when occurring together, suggest cystic fibrosis. The test is used to diagnose the presence or absence of that disease.
Poor weight gain in an infant.
Frequent colds.
Recurrent pneumonia.
Recurrent coughing or wheezing.

COST: approximately $10.

THERMOGRAPHY

PURPOSE OF THE TEST: to detect breast cancer.

BACKGROUND: Malignant tumors generally have increased blood flowing through them and, consequently, give off more heat than does normal tissue. Thermography measures the temperature of the skin on the surface of the breast and is used to detect "hot spots" of increased temperature suggestive of an underlying malignant tumor.

HOW THE TEST IS DONE: The woman undresses to the waist and puts on a hospital gown that opens in the front. While sitting still, a camera that detects infrared radiation (temperature) takes a series of "pictures" of each breast—usually three on each side.

HOW THE RESULTS ARE GIVEN: The pictures are developed immediately and interpreted by a radiologist or gynecologist, who sends a report to the woman's doctor. The report will state if any "hot spots" were seen and, if so, give their size and location. The test provides less accurate information than does mammography but it is risk-free. Since the results are sometimes ambiguous, this test must always be interpreted in light of the breast examination.

PATIENT PREPARATION: None.

RISKS AND DISCOMFORTS: None.

SYMPTOMS FOR WHICH THIS TEST IS COMMONLY OBTAINED:
Breast mass or lump (p. 302).
Nipple discharge.

COST: approximately $100.

THORACENTESIS, PARACENTESIS, ARTHROCENTESIS

PURPOSE OF THE TEST: to withdraw fluid for analysis from various sites in the body as well as to collect any cells that are present for cytology (p. 192).

BACKGROUND: The abdomen, chest, and joints will sometimes collect fluid in response to a variety of conditions, including infection, inflammation, or malignancy. When these fluid collections are present (called effusions in the chest and joint, ascites in the abdomen) the doctor will often order some of the fluid to be withdrawn and analyzed. In addition, cytology will be performed on any cells that are present.

HOW THE TEST IS DONE: In all three tests—thoracentesis (chest), paracentesis (abdomen), and arthrocentesis (joint)—the skin is cleaned thoroughly with an antiseptic and sterile cloths placed so that only a small area of skin is exposed. A local anesthetic is injected with a small needle into the skin, then a bigger needle is inserted through the skin and some of the fluid is withdrawn. This collection needle is removed and a dressing is applied over the site.

HOW THE RESULTS ARE GIVEN: The fluid and cells are analyzed in the laboratory. The report that comes back to the doctor, usually after one day, will give the protein and glucose content of the fluid as well as the type and number of any cells that were present, including cancer cells. In addition, the fluid is usually sent for culture (p. 167) to see if any bacteria are present.

PATIENT PREPARATION: A sedative may sometimes be given before the procedure if the patient is very nervous.

RISKS AND DISCOMFORTS: The injection of a local anesthetic can be slightly painful. Thoracentesis can occasionally result in a punctured lung, and x-rays will often be taken after the procedure to check for this possibility as well as to see how much fluid was removed. Paracentesis can occasionally cause perforation of an abdominal organ. All of these procedures can lead to infection, but this is exceedingly rare.

SYMPTOMS FOR WHICH THIS TEST IS COMMONLY OBTAINED:
Breathing difficulty (p. 290).
Joint pain or swelling.
Coughing (p. 292).
Abdominal pain (p. 285).
Abdominal swelling.

DISEASES FOR WHICH THIS TEST IS COMMONLY OBTAINED:
Ascites (collection of fluid in the abdomen).
Pneumonia (p. 321).
Cancer (p. 313).
Pleural effusion (collection of fluid around the lungs).
Arthritis (p. 310).

COST: approximately $30–100.

TONOMETRY

PURPOSE OF THE TEST: to measure the pressure within the eye and screen for glaucoma.

BACKGROUND: Glaucoma is one of the leading causes of blindness. The patient with glaucoma develops increasing pressure within the eye, which eventually causes damage to the optic nerve that connects the eye to the brain and conducts vision. The end result is blurriness, loss of vision, and eventual blindness. Fortunately, most patients with glaucoma can be treated if the problem is identified early enough. Tonometry measures the pressure within the eye (intraocular pressure) and, therefore, can detect the presence of glaucoma. Tonometry is performed on patients suspected of having glaucoma and on healthy adults as a screening test (p. 246).

HOW THE TEST IS DONE: Tonometry is usually performed by an opthalmologist or optometrist. There are three methods that are used:

1. A drop of local anesthetic is placed in both eyes, and after a few minutes the tonometer, a small, delicate instrument that detects

pressure, is applied against the surface of the eye and the pressure reading is made.

2. A small machine blows a puff of air against the surface of the eye to measure the pressure.

3. The tonometry is done as part of the total ophthalmologic exam. A piece of equipment called a slit lamp is used. The patient places his or her head on a chinrest, and the doctor looks into the eye through a special lens while he records the pressure.

With any of the three methods, the entire procedure takes 10 minutes.

HOW THE RESULTS ARE GIVEN: The opthalmologist or optometrist doing the test will have the results immediately and will discuss them with the patient at that time.

PATIENT PREPARATION: None. But if a patient drinks large quantities of water or any liquid immediately prior to the test, the pressure value may be falsely elevated.

RISKS AND DISCOMFORTS: Putting drops into the eye is mildly uncomfortable; once they are there, however, the eye is anesthetized and the actual tonometry is not felt by the patient.

SYMPTOMS WHEN THIS TEST IS COMMONLY OBTAINED:
All of these symptoms could be signs of glaucoma. The test is done to detect the presence of this disease.
Blurriness.
Loss of vision.
Eye pain.
Red eyes.

COST: approximately $30.

TUBERCULOSIS SKIN TEST

OTHER NAMES: PPD, tine test, TB test.

PURPOSE OF THE TEST: to determine if a patient has been exposed to tuberculosis.

BACKGROUND: When a person has an infection with tuberculosis bacteria, the immune system is stimulated to respond. Subsequently, when a small amount of tuberculosis bacteria is injected into the skin, an immunological reaction occurs over the next 48 to 72 hours, characterized by swelling and redness. This skin test for tuberculosis does not distinguish between a patient who has an active tuberculosis infection and one who has a dormant one. Nevertheless, the test remains the most important screening test available to identify people with tuberculosis.

HOW THE TEST IS DONE: There are two ways for the test to be done. In both a small amount of tuberculosis bacteria is injected into the top layer of skin and reexamined at 48 hours to see if the swelling or redness has occurred.

1. The tine test is a small white button with four sharp tines (little needles) protruding from its base, each coated with tuberculosis extract. The button is pushed down on the skin of the forearm, leaving behind a pattern of four small holes.

2. The PPD test injects with a single needle a small quantity of the tuberculosis extract under the skin, raising a small blister. The tine test is quicker and preferred when a large number of patients are screened (for example, in a school). The PPD is done when a more accurate test is desired.

HOW THE RESULTS ARE GIVEN: The doctor or nurse examines the injection site 48 hours later and measures the diameter of the red swelling, if any. The interpretation is as follows:

If the diameter is:

Less than ¼ inch (5 mm)—negative reaction; patient does not and never has had tuberculosis infection.

Greater than ¼ inch but less than ⅜ inch (between 5 and 10 mm)—questionable response and should be repeated.

Greater than ⅜ inch (10mm)—positive result; patient definitely has tuberculosis, but it is impossible to distinguish between an active infection and one that is dormant.

Many physicians, including ourselves, will ask patients to examine the tine or PPD site in 48 hours and let us know if there is any swelling present. If there is, we will ask them to come to the office so we can see the test ourselves since the actual interpretation of tuberculosis skin tests is complex and should never be done by the patient alone.

PATIENT PREPARATION: None. If the patient has had immunization with BCG (cow tuberculosis vaccine—commonly used in much of the world except the United States and Canada), it will give a positive reaction that is not due to TB. Therefore, the doctor should be told if the patient has had this immunization in the past.

RISKS AND DISCOMFORTS: Both the tine and PPD cause slight pain when the implantation into the skin is made. In a few patients with active tuberculosis, the reaction to the skin test is so severe that a small permanent scar may remain. However, this is uncommon.

SYMPTOMS FOR WHICH THIS TEST IS COMMONLY OBTAINED:
For all of these symptoms, the purpose of the test is to determine if tuberculosis infection is the cause:
Cough (p. 292).
Fever (p. 296).
Weight loss (p. 306).
Anemia (p. 309).
Fatigue (p. 295).

DISEASES FOR WHICH THIS TEST IS COMMONLY OBTAINED:
Tuberculosis.

COST: approximately $5.

PART III

The Use of Medical Tests on Healthy Patients

12

Medical Tests for Healthy People

WHY DO MEDICAL TESTS ON HEALTHY PEOPLE?

Americans have become obsessed with health maintenance. We fill the jogging paths in an effort to get into shape. We read the packages of food that we buy for the content of fiber (hopefully high), cholesterol, and salt (hopefully low). A glance at the best-seller list illustrates the popularity of books on nutrition and exercise. It seems that finally we have taken to heart the adage: "an ounce of prevention is worth a pound of cure."

This revolution in the way we think about health has changed the way we use our doctors as well. More people than ever before visit their doctor for a regular checkup while they are healthy, rather than wait until they have a medical problem. During that checkup, the doctor—who might be a family practitioner, general practitioner, internist, gynecologist, or, in the case of children, a pediatrician—should talk to you about your medical history and perform a physical examination. Even if the exam is entirely normal, the visit is worthwhile. A relationship will develop that will make it easier for the doctor to care for you if you become sick at some time in the future. The information the doctor obtains will be helpful in the evaluation of symptoms and diseases that may develop later. So we can all agree that visiting a doctor is important even when you are well.

Nevertheless, there is considerable disagreement as to the appropriate frequency of such visits. Doctors are questioning whether an exam should be performed annually or whether on people without any symptoms longer intervals are sufficient. When an unexpected abnormality is found in someone who is feeling well, it is very easy to justify the value of that visit to the doctor.

When the exam is normal—and on young people without any symptoms it usually will be—it is more difficult to measure the benefits. The peace of mind that the patient obtains when the exam and test results are normal is important, but a person can also develop a false sense of security and may choose to ignore symptoms that develop later and assume that all is well. Although much controversy exists in medical literature as to the appropriate frequency of regular exams on healthy individuals, fewer and fewer doctors and patients believe that yearly exams are necessary for good medical care.

Not only is the frequency of visits to your doctor in question, but what should take place during that visit is controversial as well. When a healthy individual visits the doctor, the major goal is health maintenance, including exploration with the patient of any internal or external stress or concerns that might affect their physical health. In addition, the visit should have as a goal the early detection of potentially dangerous disease. What is the role of medical tests in this process? Which tests should be performed and how often? Many doctors automatically include a number of medical tests as part of the regular checkup in order to detect a previous unrecognized disease. It is important to remember, however, that medical tests, if performed indiscriminately, can sometimes create more problems than they solve. Twenty tests are not necessarily an improvement over two tests.

This point can best be illustrated by the example of John R., a healthy 42-year-old man. As part of this patient's annual checkup, his doctor obtained a series of 20 blood tests. One of these tests came back with an abnormal result. Only after an extensive battery of costly and risky additional tests was John's doctor able to conclude that the original abnormal result was a "false-positive." This term is used to describe an abnormal test result that occurs even though the patient is truly healthy. The more tests that are done, the higher the chance of one test giving a false-positive result. This is not a rare occurrence. In fact, studies have shown that if you perform screening tests in healthy people without medical complaints, false-positive results are actually very common.

Knowing about this possibility, what should the doctor do about an abnormal test result in a healthy patient? Perhaps the abnormal test is not a false-positive, and a potentially serious disease is present and could be treated early. Should the doctor therefore order additional tests looking for this "hidden" disease? This approach could be costly and potentially dangerous. Perhaps, then, the doctor should tell the patient but do nothing more about it. This would create needless worry and concern in the patient. So should the doctor do nothing at all and not even tell the patient? This goes against the belief of most doctors that patients have the right to know everything about their medical condition. The bottom line is that there is no good course of action for the doctor to follow when test results are abnormal if those tests were ordered indiscriminately.

The answer, then, is to be very selective and discreet in the use of medical tests on healthy patients. How does a doctor decide which tests should be used to screen people for potential disease when they are presently healthy?

There are four factors the doctor takes into account in deciding which tests are appropriate to order:

1. *The diseases for which the patient is tested should be likely to occur in his particular age group.* It makes little sense to test a healthy 20-year-old man for colon cancer, since that disease generally does not occur in healthy men of this young age group. Besides, such screening tests would be considerably expensive and uncomfortable for the patients. In addition, false-positive results might occur, which would require additional and potentially dangerous tests to confirm or deny the initial findings.

2. *The screening test should be inexpensive and easy to perform with little discomfort and risk to the patient.* Even though 60-year-old men should be screened for colon cancer, it would not be practical for this screening to be conducted by a colonoscopy (p. 158) and barium enema (p. 109) since these tests are expensive, uncomfortable, and potentially dangerous. Most important, the hemoccult test for blood in the stool (p. 246) can provide almost the same information, is easy to perform, and is relatively inexpensive with low risk to the patient. Given these factors, it makes sense to include this test for blood in the stool as a screening test at the regular checkup of men in this age group. It is important to remember that we are talking now about healthy people without symptoms. In people with black stools (a sign of bleeding in the intestines) or abdominal pain, more complicated tests, such as sigmoidoscopy or x-ray studies, may be appropriate.

3. *The treatment for the disease implicated by an abnormal test result must be available and necessary.* Clearly, if someone is found to have blood in his or her stool on a screening test and is diagnosed as having an early curable cancer, an operation will be performed to treat the problem. This screening test was appropriate because an effective treatment plan is available for that disease. On the other hand, to do an antinuclear antibody (ANA, p. 45) on healthy people and screen for systemic lupus erythematosus would be of little value. Even if the test were positive, in the absence of symptoms, no treatment would be required. In fact, there would be no value to this healthy patient in knowing that the test is abnormal.

4. *There should not be an excessive number of false-negative results (normal tests in people who have the disease) and a manageable number of false-positive results.*

Based on these four concerns, the following pages contain a listing for healthy patients of various ages of what we believe to be the appropriate frequency of visits to the doctor as well as a reasonable group of tests that should be performed at this checkup. These recommendations are only for healthy patients who do not have symptoms or medical complaints. A patient with specific symptoms or a medical and family history suggestive of a particular disease will probably require additional tests.

The Complete Physical

If the purpose of all medical tests is to gather information about your health, then the most important medical test that you will ever have done is the complete physical. This consists of the doctor taking your medical history as well as doing a physical examination.

The information gained from this complete physical will aid your doctor in deciding what other tests are necessary to evaluate your health fully. Although the emphasis that he will place on the different parts of this process will vary, depending upon the purpose of your visit with him, the essential sequence will remain the same. Since the complete physical is a part of every visit with your doctor, we will discuss this in detail first, before giving our recommendations for the other tests that should be conducted at that time.

Preparation should start a few days before visiting the doctor.

It is natural for patients to feel nervous when they are having their complete physical. As a result, it is not uncommon that they will forget to tell their doctor important facts or neglect to ask the questions that are on their mind. The solution to this problem is to write down questions and facts so you will have them on hand when you go to the doctor's office. This will be appreciated by your doctor as well, so that he knows you are asking him about all your concerns. In addition to keeping this list of questions and facts, be sure you bring to the visit a copy of your Medical Test Diary (p. 361). Finally, if this is the first time you are seeing this particular doctor, be sure to gather all available medical records from your previous physician.

Once you are at your doctor's office, he will start your visit with taking a medical history. If you have gone to this doctor before, he will merely review your medical history from the time he last met with you. If it is a first visit, he will begin this process by giving you a history form to complete. Although not commonly done, what we find most effective is to mail this form to our patients a few days before their first appointment. In this way they can spend time filling out these questions accurately and not feel rushed or pressured.

Once we actually meet with our patient, we begin by asking if there is anything in particular that prompted this appointment with us. Do not be afraid or embarrassed about telling your doctor the specific reason. Perhaps this story will illustrate the point. A few weeks ago we saw in our office Mary F., a 27-year-old secretary. When asked the question, "What can we do for you today?" she replied, "Nothing special, I'm here for a routine checkup." As she was walking out the door at the conclusion of her visit, she turned, lifted up her hand and asked us what we thought of this mole on her wrist. It turns out that this was the actual reason why she had scheduled an appointment with the office, but she had been nervous about mentioning it before. So, again—when your doctor asks what brought you to the office that day, be sure to tell the reason, no matter how inconseqential or unimportant it may seem. Sometimes, there will not actually be a specific reason, and the purpose of the visit is a routine checkup.

If our patient has told us about a particular problem or reason for coming to see us, the next group of questions that we will ask will focus on that specific concern. If, on the other hand, our patient has told us that this visit is only routine, we will go on to the next part of the medical history—reviewing the various parts of the body and asking if there have been any problems or symptoms associated with them. For example, when it comes to the lungs, we will ask our patients the following list of questions:

Have you ever had pneumonia, tuberculosis, or other lung infections in the past?

Do you currently have a cough, shortness of breath, wheezing, sputum, or phlegm?

Do you smoke now, or did you smoke in the past? If so, how much?

Here is a good time to make the point that you must be wholly honest with your doctor. Many patients are embarrassed by a history of smoking and will not tell the doctor they smoke, or, if they do, they may not be truthful about the amount. Providing the doctor with misleading information can only be harmful in the end. We hope you will establish from the very beginning a relationship with your doctor in which you will find it comfortable to reveal the most intimate details of your life with complete honesty.

Similar questions will be asked about all the organs and parts of your body including the head, eyes, ears, nose, throat, mouth, neck, lungs, heart, breasts, abdomen and gastrointestinal tract, urinary tract, genitalia and sexual organs, nervous system, skin, lymph nodes, blood, bones and joints, endocrine glands and hormones, and allergies. If the answers to any of these questions are suspicious or suggestive of a problem, we will ask more comprehensive questions about that particular organ.

At the end of the history we will ask a series of questions about the patient's previous health, including any infectious illnesses he or she may have had and previous hospitalizations and surgery. We will also inquire about the health of close relatives including parents, grandparents, siblings, and children. Finally, we will ask a series of questions about the patient's life in general—occupation, residence, any habits (smoking, drinking), hobbies, travel history, and perception of the major stresses in his life. Some of these questions may not seem relevant to the acute problem but, in fact, they all are. For example, if the patient had recently been to Mexico and was now suffering from diarrhea, we would consider a completely different list of possible diagnoses than if that person had never left the country. If you are not certain why your doctor is asking a particular question, be sure to ask him the reason. He is not prying but is simply trying to understand, as best he can, who you are as a person and what are the possible medical problems that should concern him.

Once the history is completed, we will give the patient a gown to put on. When he or she is ready, we will perform the physical examination. In the next few pages we are going to describe a typical physical examination that we would perform on an adult patient who has come for a routine physical.

The first, and one of the most important parts of the physical, is our observation of the patient as we take the history and perform the physical. There is much information that we gain simply by carefully watching the patient. During this time we are evaluating the patient's mood and general condition. In addition, we will be looking at the patient's ability to speak, listen, walk, move, stand, and sit. A hallmark of a good physician is that he must first and foremost be an excellent observer. When we teach medical students how to do a physical examination, we always make the point that they must constantly look at the patient to detect subtle abnormalities. No matter what else they are doing—taking a history, talking to the patient as they enter and leave the room—there is valuable information to be learned by careful study of the patient. Interestingly, this skill, once learned, is sometimes difficult to "turn off." We have both had the experience of observing someone on the street or in the elevator and remarking to each other about some subtle physical abnormality that he has, such as an unusual gait or a swollen joint in the hand.

Once we start the actual physical, the first thing we do is "take the vital signs"; sometimes, our nurse will perform the task before we come back into the examination room. In addition, the patient will be weighed and the height obtained.

The vital signs consist of four measurements:

1. Blood pressure—When we take the blood pressure, we have the patient sit comfortably on the examining table. The blood pressure consists of two numbers: the higher, called the systolic pressure, is a measurement of the pressure generated by the heart when it contracts; the lower, called the diastolic pressure, is a measurement of the pressure in the arteries when the heart is at rest. Often, especially if the blood pressure is elevated, we will take it again at some later point in the examination.

2. Heart rate—The pulse is usually taken at the wrist. In addition to measuring the pulse rate, we pay careful attention to whether the pulse has a regular rhythm.

3. Respiratory rate—We measure the respiratory rate by watching the patient's breathing and, at the same time, we evaluate whether the patient has any difficulty in breathing.

4. Temperature—The temperature is taken orally and the value recorded.

Once the weight and height as well as the vital signs are measured, we perform the rest of the physical examination, moving from head to toe.

We begin by examining the patient's head, studying it for any abnormalities in its size or shape. We will then feel it all over, paying attention to any tender spots or lumps.

Next we study the eyes, first testing whether the patient can move his eyes in all directions and then checking the vision. We observe the color of the white of the eye and test to be sure that the pupils get smaller when we shine a light on them. Finally, we will use the ophthalmoscope to look into the eye, enabling us to see the retina at the rear of the eye and to look for any abnormalities in it as well as in the delicate blood vessels that run within it. Abnormalities of these blood vessels, if present, will be a sign of diabetes or hypertension. In addition, with the ophthalmoscope we will be able to see the optic nerve—which connects the eye to the brain—and check it for any problems.

Next we examine the ears using the otoscope. With this instrument we can see the ear drum (tympanic membrane) and observe if there is an infection in the ear or collection of fluid or wax in the ear canal.

When we examine the nose, we pay special attention to the patient's ability to breathe easily through both nostrils, and we look inside the nose for any obstruction or inflammation that may be present, such as that cause by an allergic condition.

With a light and tongue depressor we study the mouth and throat, looking at the condition of the teeth, gums, tonsils (if present), and the throat itself.

We next feel the neck, paying careful attention to the presence of any enlarged lymph nodes or an enlarged thyroid gland. Sometimes, when we are concerned about the thyroid gland, we may ask the patient to swallow repeatedly by sipping a glass of water, for this makes it easier for us to feel the thyroid gland.

Next we examine the chest and lungs, looking again at the patient's breathing pattern and the ease with which he inhales and exhales. We will sometimes tap on the back of the chest with our finger to hear the resonance from the lung. Finally, with our stethoscope we will listen to the patient breathe, checking for the possible presence of any wheezing (a sign of asthma) or crackling noises called rales, suggestive of pneumonia or fluid buildup in the lungs.

The examination of the heart is best done with the patient lying down on the examining table. First, we carefully observe the movement of the heart that can be seen on the left side of the chest and then feel the heart beat by placing our hand over it. With our stethoscope we will listen to the sounds the heart valves make as the organ beats. Normally, there are two such sounds with each beat, called S1 and S2. We listen for other sounds besides these two and for a heart murmur, suggestive of heart disease.

With the patient still lying down we examine the abdomen. Again, we first observe, looking for any unusual movement in the abdomen as well as its overall shape. With the stethoscope we listen for the noises that the bowel makes as it moves food along. With our hands we will now carefully examine the abdomen, feeling for the liver in its right upper portion and the spleen in its left upper portion. Normally, neither of these organs can be felt unless they are enlarged. In addition, we will feel throughout the abdomen for any unusual masses or tumors and note if the patient has any tenderness there during the examination.

Next, we examine the nervous system. This consists of testing muscle strength, the ability of the patient to perceive touch and pain and perform a series of tasks such as walking in a straight line. Finally, a reflex hammer is used to tap various tendons. When tendons are tapped in this manner, a reflex is elicited if the nerves to and from the spinal cord are normal, and the muscle contracts causing a jerking motion. Reflexes can be abnormal if they are either too slow or too strong in their muscle contraction.

The skin is examined at this point. We will judge its color, looking for jaundice (yellow) or cyanosis (dusky blue) as well as any rashes, infections, or other abnormalities. In addition, we will judge its texture for unusual dryness or moisture.

Next, we will feel for any enlarged lymph nodes that may be

present. In addition to those in the neck, we will carefully examine the armpit and groin region, two common sites of enlarged nodes.

Finally, if required, a rectal or pelvic exam will be done to conclude the examination.

RECOMMENDED TESTS FOR ADULTS

Recommended Tests for Females between Ages 18–40
A visit to your doctor should be made every three years. This is more frequent than for men of the same age group because of the need for Pap smears. In addition to a history and physical examination, the following tests should be performed:
1. Hematocrit.
2. Urinalysis.
3. Pap smear.
4. Blood glucose—once during these years.
5. Mammography—once only between ages 35 and 40.

Recommended Tests for Females between Ages 41–50
A visit to your doctor should be made every year. This is more frequent than for men of the same age group because of the need for yearly breast exams. In addition to a history and physical examination, the following tests should be performed:
1. Mammography—every one or two years.
2. Complete blood count—every three years.
3. Pap smear—every three years.
4. Blood glucose—every three years.
5. Urinalysis—every three years.
6. Test for blood in stool.
7. Tonometry—every three years.

Recommended Tests for Females between Ages 51–60
A visit to your doctor should be made every year. This is more frequent than for men of the same age group because of the need for annual mammography. In addition to a history and physical examination, the following tests should be performed:
1. CBC.
2. Urinalysis.
3. Blood glucose—once every three years.

4. Pap smear—every three years.
5. Mammography.
6. Sigmoidoscopy—every five years.
7. Cholesterol—once during the decade.
8. Triglycerides—once during the decade.
9. EKG—once during the decade.
10. Test for blood in stool.
11. Tonometry—every two years.

Recommended Tests for Females between Ages 61–70

A visit to your doctor should be made every year. In addition to a history and physical examination, the following tests should be performed:

1. CBC.
2. Urinalysis.
3. Blood glucose—every two years.
4. Pap smear—every three years.
5. Mammography.
6. Sigmoidoscopy—every five years.
7. EKG—twice during the decade.
8. Chest x-ray—once during the decade.
9. Test for blood in stool.
10. BUN—once during the decade.
11. Tonometry—every two years.

Recommended Tests for Females from Ages 71 and Over

A visit to your doctor should be made every year. In addition to a history and physical examination, the following tests should be performed:

1. CBC.
2. Urinalysis.
3. Blood glucose—every two years.
4. BUN—every three years.
5. Pap smear—once during each decade.
6. Mammography.
7. Sigmoidoscopy—every five years.
8. EKG—every three years.
9. Test for blood in stool.
10. Chest x-ray—once a decade.
11. Tonometry—every two years.

Recommended Tests for Males between Ages 18–40

A visit to your doctor should be made every five years. In addition to a history and physical examination, the following tests should be performed:

1. Hematocrit.
2. Urinalysis.
3. Blood glucose—once during these years.

Recommended Tests for Males between Ages 41–50

A visit to your doctor should be made every three years. In addition to a history and physical examination, the following tests should be performed:

1. Complete blood count.
2. Urinalysis.
3. Blood glucose.
4. Test for blood in stool.
5. Cholesterol—once during the decade.
6. Triglycerides—once during the decade.
7. Tonometry.
8. EKG—once during the decade.

Recommended Tests for Males between Ages 51–60

A visit to your doctor should be made every three years. In addition to a history and physical examination, the following tests should be performed:

1. CBC.
2. Urinalysis.
3. Blood glucose.
4. Test for blood in stool.
5. Sigmoidoscopy—every five years.
6. Cholesterol—once during the decade.
7. Triglycerides—once during the decade.
8. EKG—twice during the decade.
9. Tonometry.

Recommended Tests for Males between Ages 61–70

A visit to your doctor should be made every year. In addition to a history and physical examination, the following tests should be performed:

1. CBC.
2. Urinalysis.

3. Blood glucose.
4. Test for blood in stool.
5. Sigmoidoscopy—every five years.
6. EKG—twice during the decade.
7. BUN—once during the decade.
8. Chest x-ray—once during the decade.
9. Tonometry—every two years.

Recommended Tests for Males from Ages 71 and Over

A visit to your doctor should be made every year. In addition to a history and physical examination, the following tests should be performed:

1. CBC.
2. Urinalysis.
3. Blood glucose.
4. Test for blood in stool.
5. Sigmoidoscopy—every five years.
6. BUN—once during the decade.
7. Chest x-ray—once during the decade.
8. EKG—every five years.
9. Tonometry—every two years.

EXPLANATION OF TESTS PERFORMED ON HEALTHY PEOPLE

Blood Glucose (p. 61)

Diabetes can harm the body in many ways. It can cause blindness, heart disease, kidney disease, intestinal disease, and nervous system problems. Early detection of diabetes is essential so that effective treatment can be started and these complications avoided. Unfortunately, in the early stage of diabetes a person can feel perfectly healthy. Although a urinalysis can screen for diabetes, it is easier for a doctor to detect this common disease— even in the absence of symptoms—if a blood glucose is obtained. An elevated level will alert the doctor to the possibility that the patient has diabetes.

Blood Urea Nitrogen (BUN, p. 74)

This test will measure in an imprecise fashion how well the kidney is functioning. Although the urinalysis also suggests if kidney disease is present, frequently the BUN will be abnormal even though the urinalysis is normal. It is necessary to know renal function in older people since kidney failure can develop in the absence of any symptoms. Early detection of renal failure may prevent the need for dialysis.

Chest X-Ray (p. 113)

Until recently, a yearly chest x-ray was a routine part of the complete physical, even if the patient was in good health and without symptoms. Now doctors believe that this practice is in error. The radiation risks from chest x-rays are thought to be greater than previously recognized. Also, the major disease that this test used to diagnose—tuberculosis—is much less common than before, and can be detected as readily with safe skin tests (p. 224). Finally, doctors now realize that lung cancer, the other disease that this test was used for, is rarely detected at an early stage with a chest x-ray. The result of all this new information is that the policy on chest x-rays as a screening test has been substantially revised. Currently, we recommend chest x-rays only once per decade for a healthy patient over the age of 60. Prior to that age, the risks simply outweigh any benefit that may result.

Cholesterol and Triglycerides (p. 76)

These tests help to indicate whether your blood vessels are at risk for becoming clogged with fat deposits (arteriosclerosis). Many doctors feel that these tests are a good indicator of whether someone will develop heart disease. What is uncertain, however, is the proper treatment for patients with an elevated cholesterol and triglyceride level. Although treatment with drugs can lower cholesterol and triglycerides, it has risks. The best treatment for those with high cholesterol is a diet low in cholesterol and high in polyunsaturated fats.

Since this diet should be recommended to everyone regardless of the blood cholesterol and triglyceride levels, measurement of these values will not change therapy in the healthy patient. In addition, yearly cholesterol and trigylceride measurements are of little value to healthy people, since these values do not change frequently. Measuring these levels intermittently will, however, help patients know how well they have been regulating their diet and emphasize to them and their doctor the continued need for eating a diet low in harmful fats.

Complete Blood Count, Hematocrit (p. 51)

Checking the hematocrit is a simple test that screens for many different diseases in a healthy person. Iron-deficiency anemia is a very common problem in women because of blood loss from their menstrual cycles. This test will identify people who might be anemic even though they do not have any symptoms. In healthy older men and women, a low hematocrit will suggest occult bleeding from the intestines and raise the possibility of cancer. An abnormally low hematocrit will also indicate poor nutritional status, while a high hematocrit might be a sign that the patient's lungs have been damaged from too much smoking.

Electrocardiogram (EKG, p. 193)

Although the EKG provides a lot of information about the size of the heart and whether any damage has occurred, it does not tell whether a heart attack is likely to occur in someone who has no symptoms. We have all heard the story about the 50-year-old executive who, after being told his routine EKG was normal, suffered a massive heart attack two days later. Because it does not screen for potential heart attacks, yearly EKGS are not necessary in an otherwise healthy person. EKGS performed occasionally in a healthy person will provide base-line information that may be helpful to compare with an EKG obtained later if the person develops heart symptoms. For this reason an EKG performed periodically is appropriate for people who are at increased risk for heart disease because of their age. Those with high blood pressure or symptoms related to heart disease will, on the other hand, benefit from more frequent use of this test because it will detect heart damage that has occurred from these problems.

Exercise Tolerance Test (ETT, p. 202)

The use of the exercise tolerance test has received wide publicity in recent years in the news media. What role does it have as part of a routine checkup for someone who has never had symptoms of heart disease? When a typical person with no symptoms of heart disease goes to the doctor for a checkup, an exercise tolerance test serves little value. More often than not, an abnormal test is not due to the presence of heart disease but is rather falsely-positive. Unfortunately, once the doctor is faced with this abnormal result, he can not simply ignore it but must do other tests—

some of which can be dangerous—to prove conclusively that the patient's heart is healthy. This will create unnecessary worry and anxiety for both patient and his doctor. Besides, even if heart disease is documented, in the absence of symptoms, no change in treatment would be necessary.

For these reasons we do not routinely recommend the exercise tolerance test as a screening test for heart disease as part of a routine checkup. The use of the exercise tolerance test in a healthy sedentary person who is about to begin a strenuous exercise program is controversial. Ordinarily, men and women under 40 do not benefit from this test even in this situation. On the other hand, for people who have symptoms of heart disease or have already had a heart attack, the exercise tolerance test can provide useful information.

Mammography (p. 124)

Breast cancer is by far the most feared disease a woman can have. When not detected early by screening, it is often not curable by the time it is discovered. There is increasing evidence that breast exams by the doctor during every office visit as well as monthly breast self-exams (p. 345) by the woman help to discover breast cancer earlier and enable better treatment and cure of the cancer. Even with frequent examinations, however, some early breast cancers are missed. Mammography will detect many of these. For a woman without breast problems or family history of the disease, one mammogram should be obtained between ages 35 and 40, then every one or two years in her 40s, and annually after age 50. Mammograms expose a woman to radiation, and frequent exams at a young age are unwarranted because the risks of mammography outweigh the benefits. This is not true, however, for women with a history of breast lumps, even if benign; they should have earlier and more frequent mammograms since in these cases the benefits of detecting a problem early outweigh the risks of the mammogram. After age 40, however, when the risk of cancer is high, the benefits of screening far outweigh the risk of radiation.

Pap Smear (p. 212)

Before the use of the Pap smear, cervical cancer was one of the common causes of death in women. By the time this cancer was detected, it would often be too late for the disease to be cured. Screening for cervical cancer with a Pap smear enables the disease to be diagnosed very early in its course so that a complete cure can be obtained. Until very recently, doctors recommended a yearly Pap smear in all women. We now know that it is not necessary to perform a Pap smear that frequently. Cervical cancer takes many years to develop and if your pap smear is now normal, it would take several years for cancerous changes to occur. Yearly Pap smears do not add significantly more information than Pap smears obtained every three years.

Sigmoidoscopy (p. 165)

Some colon cancers bleed intermittently and occult blood will not always be present in the stool, even though a cancer is present. In addition, many colon polyps, although initially benign, can become malignant over a period of years. Because many colon cancers occur in the part of the intestines that can be seen by sigmoidoscopy, additional cancers and polyps might be detected by this test and removed. The sigmoidoscopy does not need to be performed as often as the test for stool blood, however. This is because benign polyps, which may become malignant, take more than 10 years to undergo this change to cancer. This provides plenty of time for sigmoidoscopy—if done every five years—to detect and remove them.

Multiple Blood Chemistry Testing

In this chapter we have listed tests that should be performed because of their value in screening for potential disease. Medical laboratories often perform automated multiple chemistry tests on a tube of blood. One such machine is called a Sequential Multiple Analyzer (SMA-12). Even if the doctor wants only one test, the laboratory will do 12 or more because it costs the same to do 12 tests as it does to do one. This creates a problem for the doctor and the patient. What do you do with the information that you did not ask for? Superficially, it would seem to be a bargain: the more tests that are done for the same price, the better it is. As we have discussed earlier, however, the tests that you did not want in the first place may be falsely positive and additional blood tests may have to be performed to evaluate the results. These additional tests are expensive and may expose the patient to further risks.

In fact, if 12 tests are performed on a healthy person, the risk of a false-positive test may be as high as 40%. Therefore, we discourage use of these multiple blood chemistry testing machines and recommend that each blood test be ordered individually as needed. We realize, however, that this is not always possible because some medical laboratories automatically provide a whole series of test results on one blood sample, even though the doctor requested only a single test. In addition, some laboratories charge less for a set of 12 tests than they do for only a few of them to further encourage getting the battery of tests.

Test for Blood in Stool (p. 96)

Colon cancer is the second most common malignancy in the United States. If detected early, the cancer can be completely removed and the person will have an excellent chance of being cured. If, however, the cancer is detected only after abdominal pain or obvious rectal bleeding is noticed, the chance of a complete cure is much lower. Frequently, people with early colon cancer will have "occult" blood in their stool. Although the stool looks normal, evidence of small amounts of blood will be detected when it is tested with chemicals. Therefore, the stool of men and women at risk for colon cancer is tested frequently for the presence of occult blood. This test is simple to perform, causes little discomfort to the patient, and should be done yearly in all people over 40. During years when a complete physical is not being performed, the test for blood in stool can be done at home (p. 340).

Tonometry (p. 223)

Glaucoma is a condition in the eye caused by increased eye pressure, which if left untreated will cause blindness. Tonometry measurements detect people who have elevated eye pressures and are at risk for developing glaucoma. Treatment can then be started that will prevent blindness. It is therefore important that frequent measurements be made in people who are over 40 since this is the age group most susceptible to glaucoma. Sometimes, your regular doctor will be able to perform tonometry, but, if he does not, this can be performed by an optometrist or opthalmologist. In addition, local health groups often offer free screening tests for glaucoma.

Urinalysis (p. 87)

The urinalysis is an inexpensive test that provides the doctor with a lot of useful information. The urine examination will screen for the presence of glucose (diabetes); protein and kidney cells (kidney disease); white cells, red cells, and bacteria (urinary tract infection); bilirubin and urobilinogen (liver disease); and urine pH (acidity). If one of these tests is abnormal, additional tests would then be obtained.

Recommended Tests for Newborns, Infants, and Children

We said earlier that visiting a doctor, when you are healthy, has two main goals: health maintenance and early detection of potentially serious disease. Infants and children are in a continual state of growth and development. For them, the most important part of visiting a doctor when healthy is for the physician to be sure that this growth and development is proceeding normally: physically, psychologically, intellectually, and emotionally. With only very few exceptions, however, there are no laboratory tests available for the detection of abnormal growth and development. Therefore, a critical part of a healthy infant's or child's visit to the doctor is the medical history and physical examination. The following pages discuss the complete physical that should be done during your child's visit to the doctor and tests that should be done at that time. In addition, we have included the immunizations that should be given at each pediatric visit as well.

The Complete Physical

Earlier in this chapter we detailed the medical history and physical examination that are done during an adult patient's visit to his or her physician. There are certain differences between that procedure and the complete physical that will be done when the patient is a child. These differences are described below:

1. The doctor organizes the physical examination of an adult from head to toe; for a child the examination is organized from what the child finds least bothersome to most bothersome. In an adult patient the physician will examine the head first and look in the eyes, ears, and throat. In a child, doing any of those manipulations, as well as using the stethoscope and reflex hammer, can frequently lead to crying, thereby ending a useful examination. For this reason we will first do those parts of the exam that the child will find least annoying. We start with detailed and careful observation. It has been our experience that the most valuable

part of the physical examination is simply observing the child before we actually touch him or her. This will give us much information concerning the child's development and health: speech patterns, level of physical activity, emotional behavior, degree of illness (if present), and intellectual skills. Next, we will do those parts of the exam that require touching the child—for example, feeling the abdomen. Finally, we will finish the physical examination by using any instruments that are necessary.

2. The physician will devote considerable effort to decreasing the child's stress during the exam. Although adults can feel stress when they visit a doctor and undergo a physical examination, a child's stress can lead to poor cooperation and crying, causing an inaccurate physical. There are a number of ways in which we can decrease the child's stress—many of which require the parent's cooperation in order to be successful.

First, and perhaps easiest, is to be sure that the child is in as secure an environment as possible. Usually, a baby will be examined while sitting on the parent's lap, not on an examining table. Even for an older, bigger child, the parent should remain in the room and close to the patient. The parent should reassure the child frequently that he or she will not be left alone. Many times it is useful for the parent to actually touch the child. For example, when the doctor looks in the child's ears, he will often have the parent hold the baby while he pushes the head against the parent's shoulder to keep it still.

Second, a basic rule of good pediatric care is "no surprises." Children do not like the feeling of suddenness and surprise that can sometimes accompany a physical examination. Even a young child will benefit by having the parent discuss with him or her the upcoming visit to the doctor's office a few days before it actually occurs. The parent should explain to the child what the doctor is going to do ("look in your ears, ask you to open your mouth . . .") and even mention those parts of the visit that may be uncomfortable or painful ("You probably will receive an immunization this visit. This will hurt . . ."). As part of the principle of "no surprises," it is important to stress that it never helps to lie to a child. We always find it ironic when parents tell children not to worry because the injection or blood test that they are going to have "doesn't hurt." The parent well knows that the procedure will cause the child pain. And once children realize the physician or parent has lied, they will become angry and not cooperate further. Instead of telling a child that the immunization will not hurt, it is more productive to explain why it is being done and why it is necessary.

3. The parent and physician must work together to restore to the child as much control over the situation as possible. Numerous studies have shown that what bothers and frightens children most about going to the physician or hospital is the loss of control that they experience. Children are told what to do, have painful or uncomfortable procedures done with little choice, and, overall, have an overwhelming sense that they have lost control of their world. The parent and doctor can help the child to a significant degree by restoring as much control as possible to the child.

For example, if a child needs a blood test, there is no sense in lying to six-year-old Billy and saying that it will not hurt. Similarly, it will be counter-productive to spring the test suddenly upon him. What is much more effective at decreasing his stress and increasing cooperation is to give him as much choice (control) as possible with the "painful" situation. Let him choose the arm from which the blood will be taken ("Billy, you have to have this injection now. Which arm would you prefer—right or left?"). If possible, let him decide the order of tests ("Billy, the doctor has to do a blood test and give you an immunization. Which do you want first—the blood test or the shot?"). Let the child make decisions as much as possible. While insignificant to our perspective, it helps restore the child's sense of controlling his world.

4. In the physical examination of an adult patient, the doctor is concerned mainly with finding abnormalities; in a child's physical, he must focus as well on the patient's growth and development. For example, when a child's height and weight is measured, it is not sufficient—as it might be in an adult—to determine only if the patient is overweight or underweight. The child's physician must also be concerned with the growth pattern: is the child gaining height and weight at the correct pace, or is the process occurring too rapidly or too slowly? The child, at almost all ages, is undergoing change at a tremendous rate. The doctor must determine if this is happening appropriately or abnormally. It should be made clear that the doctor or nurse–practitioner cannot make a thorough assessment of the child, especially regarding the emotional, psychological, and social development in a 15- or 20-min-

ute visit every few months. Parents must bring to the attention of the medical team any abnormalities that they believe the child has.

In addition to a thorough medical history and physical examination, we recommend the following medical tests as well.

RECOMMENDED TESTS

Newborn Infant

These are the tests that are done in a standard hospital nursery before the infant is discharged. Even if the birth took place at home or a birthing center, many of these tests will still be required.

Hematocrit (p. 51): A variety of diseases that occur in the uterus or immediately after birth can cause anemia to be present at this time. It is important to detect it now and treat it so that the newborn has an ample amount of red blood cells for proper growth to occur.

Blood test for phenylketonuria (PKU, p. 60): This disease, if untreated, can cause severe mental retardation. In many states this test is mandated by law. Because it is possible for a baby to have a normal blood test for PKU at birth yet still have the disease, it is recommended that the urine be tested as well on the first visit to the doctor.

Blood test for galactosemia: This test can detect galactosemia, a disease caused by the lack of the enzyme necessary to digest certain carbohydrates in the body. Untreated, it can cause retardation, liver disease, and blindness.

Blood test for hypothyroidism (p. 69): Although few infants have hypothyroidism, those that do, if untreated, will suffer severe abnormalities in their mental and physical growth and development.

Blood test for sickle cell anemia (black children only): Although there is no treatment for sickle cell anemia, early detection of the disease can allow for optimal family counseling and preparation for raising a child with this chronic and sometimes serious illness.

Blood test for G6PD deficiency (black and Oriental children only): Red blood cells deficient in this enzyme can be destroyed if the patient takes certain medications, including aspirin. Detection of the disease in the nursery will prevent, as much as possible, the use of these medications during the infants' first few years of life.

Two Months Old

A *complete physical* (physical examination and medical history) should be performed. In addition:

Immunization: diphtheria, pertussis (whooping cough), and tetanus (DPT) injection; oral polio (OPV).

Four Months Old

Besides a *complete physical:*

Immunization: diptheria, pertussis, tetanus (DPT) injection; oral polio (OPV).

Six Months Old

Besides a *complete physical:*

Immunization: diptheria, pertussis, tetanus (DPT) injection; oral polio (OPV).

Nine Months Old

Besides a *complete physical:*

Complete blood count (CBC, p. 51): Most anemia that develops in children (e.g., iron deficiency, sickle cell anemia, thalassemia,) will be evident by this age. Studies have shown that yearly testing for anemia does not improve health care; screening at this age, however, does detect almost all children who will develop anemia during childhood. The red blood cell indices (p. 52) will indicate if the red blood cells are smaller than normal. If they are, and anemia is present, the most likely cause is iron deficiency.

Blood test for lead (p. 75) (only in those children exposed to lead-based paints): Children at this age might be eating lead paint, which, if undetected, can cause lead poisoning, a serious medical problem that can be corrected by early detection and prompt medical treatment.

One Year Old

Besides a *complete physical:*

Tuberculosis test (p. 224): The frequency of tuberculosis testing in the pediatric age group is controversial. Everyone should be screened at ages one and five. Those children living in an area where tuberculosis infection is common should have annual screening throughout their childhood and adolescence. In areas where tuberculosis is virtually unknown, additional screening beyond those two times may be unnecessary.

Fifteen Months Old
   Besides a *complete physical:*
   Immunization with measles, mumps, rubella (German measles) injection (MMR).

Eighteen Months Old
   Besides a *complete physical:*
   Blood test for lead (p. 224) (only in those children exposed to lead-based paints).
   Immunization: diptheria, pertussis, tetanus (DPT) injection; oral polio (OPV).

Two to Four Years Old
   Yearly visits consisting of *complete physical* only; no further tests are required except for a blood test for lead every six months in those children exposed to lead-based paints

Five Years Old (or Before Entry to School)
   Complete physical, with special emphasis on:
   Hearing test (p. 185): The best test for hearing is audiometry. Some doctors will rely instead on a good history and some simple office tests (e.g., a child's ability to hear a whisper or a ticking watch) to screen for hearing problems. The health department of many municipalities runs hearing clinics that provide audiometry testing to the preschool child.
   Vision test: Most doctors will perform an eye chart exam in their own office; others will recommend a visit to an opthalomogist or optometrist at ages 4 to 5 to detect any vision problem before the start of school. Either screening is acceptable.
   Blood pressure: It is rare for a child to have hypertension. On the other hand, some children do have blood pressure readings that are higher than normal. These children should be monitored throughout life for the development later of true hypertension. (Some pediatricians will start blood pressure monitoring when the child is three years of age.)
   Routine urinalysis (p. 87): The dipstick detection of glucose or protein is a good screen to pick up diabetes or kidney disease in this age group.
   Urine culture (p. 175) (girls only): Approximately 5% of girls will have bacteria growing in the urine although they will not have symptoms. It is controversial if this bacteriuria without symptoms

(asymptomatic bacteriuria) can lead to serious kidney disease in later life; nevertheless, its detection and treatment at this pre-school age will avoid any question later on. Therefore, we recommend that this test be done. Some physicians screen for this problem by using a special dipstick that detects high levels of nitrites in the urine, a chemical that is only there if certain bacteria are present.

Tuberculosis test (p. 224)

Immunization: diphtheria, pertussis, tetanus (DPT) injection; oral polio (OPV).

Six to Eighteen Years Old (through High School)

Yearly visits consisting of a *complete physical* (physical examination and medical history) and the following additional medical tests:

Urinalysis (p. 87): At ages 10 and 15 to detect glucose (diabetes)

RECOMMENDED SCHEDULE FOR IMMUNIZATIONS

Age	Vaccine
Two months	Diphtheria, pertussis, tetanus (DPT). Oral polio (OPV).
Four months	DPT. OPV.
Six months	DPT. (OPV optional for those areas where there is a higher-than-usual incidence of polio; at this time, this would be limited to the southwestern portions of the United States.)
Fifteen months	Measles, mumps, rubella (MMR).
Eighteen months	DPT. OPV.
Five years (preschool)	DPT. OPV.
Fourteen to sixteen years and every ten years for lifetime	Tetanus, diphtheria (Td) injection.

or protein (kidney disease); in addition, dipstick test for nitrites to detect urinary tract infection is useful for girls.

Complete blood count (CBC, (p. 51) (for girls, only after onset of menstruation): Every other year the hematocrit should be performed to detect iron-deficiency anemia in this group, a common problem due to the combination of menstrual blood loss and poor adolescent nutrition. The hematocrit will determine if anemia is present, and the red blood cell indices will determine if the red cells are small, a sign of iron-deficiency anemia.

Vision test: Age 12; most children who develop nearsightedness (myopia) do so at around this age. Screening by eye chart at this time will detect those children in need of glasses.

Immunizations: tetanus, diphtheria (Td) injection at age 15.

PART IV

The Use of Medical Tests in Special Situations

13

Tests during Pregnancy

THE results of medical tests for pregnant women require special interpretation because the body of a pregnant woman undergoes tremendous changes in response to the growing fetus within her. By the time the baby is due, the mother's heart must supply nearly twice the blood flow that it did before pregnancy in order to deliver blood to the placenta and baby as well as to herself. Her kidneys must filter far more waste materials than before. The weight of the uterus—which gains 20 pounds or more in many women—places enormous strain on the back as well as the adjacent nerves and blood vessels. The purpose of the complete physical and other medical tests that will be conducted when the woman visits her doctor or other health care provider (nurse-midwife) is to monitor her health during these months. But that is not all. For in addition to caring for the expectant mother, the medical team must begin to care for a new patient—the fetus. Thus, the purpose of medical tests during pregnancy are multifold: to monitor the health of the mother, to monitor the health of the fetus, and to ensure that the fetus is developing properly. In fact, the entire process of caring for a pregnant woman and the fetus has become a medical "mini-specialty" called perinatal medicine or perinatology.

There are many acceptable alternative styles of prenatal care and birth of the baby. Regardless of where this care is obtained, and whether the mother gives birth in a hospital, a birthing center, or even at home, certain medical tests must be done during pregnancy and at the time of delivery in order to safeguard the health of both mother and child.

When discussing the nature and frequency of medical tests during pregnancy, it is important to recognize that there are two different kinds of pregnancy:

1. Uncomplicated pregnancy in which both mother and fetus should have no problems during the nine months.

2. Pregnancy in which there is a higher risk that complications may develop. These may involve the mother only and not affect the health of the fetus; or the fetus itself may not be normal because of a congenital or genetic defect. Women whose prognosis falls into this high-risk group will need to have additional medical tests performed.

There are many different criteria we use to place a woman in the high-risk pregnancy group. If one or more of the following are present, then we consider the pregnancy to be high risk, and in addition to the medical tests described on the next few pages, you should read the pages at the end of the chapter for the special testing that this group will require.

Age: Women who are under 16 or over 35.

Height and weight: (at the time the pregnancy starts): Women who are very underweight or overweight for their height.

Previous problem with pregnancy: Cesarean section in the past; difficult forceps delivery; previous pregnancy that ended in premature birth; previous pregnancy with prolonged labor; difficulty conceiving in the past; previous history of one or more spontaneous abortions, miscarriages, or stillborn births; previous pregnancy complicated by uterine bleeding at any time.

Previous birth of an infant with cerebral palsy, mental retardation, or birth defect.

Previous medical history in the mother of serious illness, such as high blood pressure, heart disease, thyroid disease, diabetes, drug use or addiction, and alcoholism.

Unusual pregnancy: It is very important to stress that frequently women whom we expect to have an uncomplicated pregnancy will develop problems or symptoms at some later point and are then placed in the high-risk group. Examples of this are: women who develop diabetes or hypertension during pregnancy (even though it was not there at the start), who show unusual weight gain (too rapid, too slow, or sudden fluctuations), who do not deliver by two weeks after their due date, or who experience any uterine or vaginal bleeding. If any of these develop, additional medical tests will be required, which are described at the end of this chapter.

A pregnant woman can develop diseases unrelated to pregnancy, such as pneumonia or asthma, or an injury. Medical tests

HIGH-RISK PREGNANCIES

I. *Mother has a medical history of:*
Heart disease.
High blood pressure.
Diabetes.
Anemia.
Cancer.
Thyroid condition.
Autoimmune disease (rheumatoid arthritis, systemic lupus erythe-
matosus).
Drug abuse or alcoholism.

II. *Mother is:*
Over 35 years of age.
Under 16 years of age.
Very overweight or underweight for height.

III. *Mother has previous obstetrical history notable for:*
Cesarean section.
Difficult forceps delivery.
Miscarriage.
Spontaneous abortion.
Stillborn.
Premature live birth.
Prolonged labor.
Uterine bleeding during pregnancy.
Multiple births.
Difficulty in conceiving.

IV. *This current pregnancy is unusual because of:*
High blood pressure in the mother.
Multiple fetuses are present.
Uterine bleeding.
Viral infection during the pregnancy.
Abnormal fetal heart rate.
Unusual weight gain.
Diabetes.

are often done in these women—not because of the pregnancy—
but to evaluate the nonobstetrical problem. The use of x-rays in
pregnant women is highly discouraged because radiation can cause
damage to the developing fetus. Consequently, x-rays should be
used with great caution and only in those situations where the
benefit of the x-ray to the mother clearly outweighs the risk to
herself or the fetus. Pregnant women should bear in mind that

our recommendation for x-rays made elsewhere in this book is intended for those women who are not pregnant and may not apply to the expectant mother.

MEDICAL TESTS FOR ALL PREGNANCIES

Pre-pregnancy Visit to the Obstetrician
The first visit to the obstetrician or nurse-midwife should not be made after the woman is pregnant but at the time she decides to become pregnant. This first visit will allow the obstetrician to evaluate her and determine the likely course of her pregnancy. Possible problems that might arise can be discussed, and the physician can ascertain if any special treatment or counseling is required. This pre-pregnancy visit should include:

Complete physical (physical examination and medical history): In addition to a thorough medical history—including that of any diseases or genetic problems that run in either the mother's or father's family—the physical examination will place special emphasis on:
Anatomy of the birth canal.
Blood pressure.
Weight.
Possible presence of any sexually transmitted diseases.

Complete blood count (CBC, p. 51): If anemia is present, the doctor will try to determine its specific cause. If iron deficiency is the problem, he will try to correct it before the woman becomes pregnant since it is very difficult to do so once pregnancy has occurred.

Rubella titer (p. 262): Infection during the first trimester with rubella (German measles) can result in catastrophic birth defects, including blindness, deafness, and physical deformity. If the woman has antibodies against the rubella virus, she will be protected against developing the infection. If she does not have antibody titers, her obstetrician will recommend that she become immunized with the rubella vaccine before attempting pregnancy.

Genetic screening: If the family history reveals the presence of any genetic-associated diseases, appropriate screening might be performed. Even without a family history, this should include testing for sickle cell anemia in blacks, (p. 263), Tay-Sachs disease in Jews, (p. 263), and thalassemia in people of Mediterranean descent, (p. 264).

X-rays: All x-rays, even dental films, are dangerous during pregnancy. The doctor will keep in mind that if any x-rays are likely to be indicated within the next few months, they should be ordered at this time, before pregnancy has occurred.

First Visit

Many medical tests should be performed during a woman's first visit to the obstetrician or nurse-midwife. The time for a patient's first visit will vary, depending upon when she finds out she is pregnant. This first visit should be made as soon as she has a positive pregnancy test (p. 214). Some of these tests may have been done at the time the woman had a pre-pregnancy visit to her obstetrician. If not, they should be done now.

Complete physical: In addition to a thorough medical history, the physical examination will place special emphasis on:

Anatomy of the birth canal—The birth canal—the passage from the uterus through the vagina to the outside—of some women will be too small to allow for a usual vaginal birth and will require that a Cesarean section be performed. Recognizing this problem now will allow the obstetrician and patient to plan for this procedure.

Blood pressure—Hypertension can exist prior to pregnancy or result as a complication of pregnancy. In either case it can lead to problems for the mother and fetus and should be diagnosed and treated early on.

The mother's weight.

The presence in the mother of any sexually transmitted disease, including gonorrhea, syphilis, and herpes.

Complete blood count (CBC, p. 51): This test will check on the hematocrit level. Anemia, especially iron-deficiency anemia, is common during pregnancy. The earlier it is detected, the quicker treatment can be initiated.

Blood glucose (p. 61): Diabetes can be present before pregnancy, or it can develop in some mothers during pregnancy. In either case it is one of the most important causes of maternal and fetal complications. The best screening test for pregnant women is a two-hour postprandial blood glucose. This means that a routine blood glucose is done approximately two hours after the woman eats a meal. If diabetes is present, the glucose level will be much higher (greater than 120 mg / dl), while in a nondiabetic, the glucose will have returned to normal levels (less than 100 mg / dl). Patients with a high blood glucose level should have the test repeated in the morning after fasting or have a glucose tolerance test (p. 61) done as well.

Syphilis tests (p. 83): Syphilis can cause serious birth defects. Recognition of infection early in pregnancy can allow for successful treatment and prevention of complications.

Routine urinalysis (p. 87): This test will include testing for sugar, protein, white cells, and bacteria in the urine. Sugar in the urine might be an indication of diabetes. If present, the woman should have a fasting blood sugar (p. 61) and glucose tolerance test (p. 61) done. Protein in the urine is an early sign of hypertension or kidney disease, which complicates pregnancy. Bacteria and white cells in the urine—indicating most probably a urinary tract infection—are a frequent complication of pregnancy that needs treatment.

Urine culture (p. 175): If the urinalysis is abnormal, this will be done as a further test to detect the presence of bacteria in the urine.

Gonorrhea cultures (p. 172): A cervical culture will be sent to the lab if the doctor suspects the presence of gonorrhea so that the disease can be treated immediately and lessen any risk of infection to the fetus.

Rubella antibody titer (p. 72): Infection with rubella (German measles) during pregnancy, especially in the first trimester, can cause catastrophic birth defects. If the woman has rubella antibody present in sufficient amounts, it means that she is immune to the disease and exposure to an active case will not be dangerous. If, on the other hand, the rubella antibody titer test is negative, she is not protected against the disease. Exposure to rubella will require her to receive gamma globulin in an attempt to prevent the disease. If she actually develops the infection, she should discuss the consequences with her obstetrician. Once she has been exposed to the disease, rubella antibody titers rarely change during a woman's lifetime. If this test has been performed in the past, it need not be repeated. Many pediatricians are now doing this test on young adolescents so that if the rubella titer is low they can be reimmunized with rubella vaccine. The pediatrician may be one person to check with to see if the test was ever done before.

Blood typing (p. 46) and Coombs' test (p. 55): The patient should have her blood typed with regard to ABO and Rh blood groups. The Coombs' test will screen her blood for the presence of antibodies directed against blood cells that could cross through the placenta and cause problems for the fetus. Women who are Rh negative will possibly require additional tests.

Pap smear: In addition to checking for cervical cancer, this test can also reveal the presence of an active genital herpes infection. This disease can cause serious problems—even death—to the newborn baby if the mother has a vaginal delivery when the herpes is in an active phase. This risk is so great that if the mother has active genital herpes, she should have a Cesarean section performed.

Genetic screening: The tests described above should be done on every pregnant woman. In addition, there are three tests that are available to screen women of particular ethnic backgrounds for particular genes that, if present in both her and the baby's father, place the fetus at risk of being born with certain serious diseases. It is important to remember that women who only carry the gene for the disease are themselves not affected and lead a fully normal life. It is only if both parents have the gene that the baby is at risk. Consequently, if the mother tests positive for the gene, the father should also be tested.

Screening for genetic diseases remains highly controversial and involves many moral, ethical, and religious issues beyond the scope of this book. Nevertheless, we think it is important to mention these tests, as many pregnant women will want to have them done.

A woman's genes never change during her lifetime. If these tests have been done in the past, the results will not change and the test need not be repeated. Of course, if the woman carries another baby fathered by a different man, the tests might have to be repeated, depending upon that man's genetic background and family history.

If a pregnant woman decides to have these screening tests done and both she and the baby's father carry a gene that transmits a disease or condition, the results should be discussed with the doctor and a genetics counselor.

Sickle cell test (p. 82): Sickle cell anemia is a serious disease that can cause severe anemia and other related complications. Many black women have this test done because approximately 10% of American blacks carry this gene.

Tay-Sachs test (p. 60): This disease is caused by a deficiency of an enzyme necessary to the nervous system. Lack of the enzyme causes the buildup in the nervous tissue of toxic materials that will eventually be fatal. The gene is carried by approximately 5% of Jews of Ashkenazi (Eastern Europe) background.

Thalassemia test: This disease is a genetic inability to make hemoglobin, the protein within red blood cells that carries oxygen. Thalassemia can range from a minor problem to a serious and even fatal disease. The gene is most common in people of Mediterranean descent (Greeks, Italians, Portuguese, Spanish, Sephardic Jews, Arabs) as well as Orientals, especially Chinese. Approximately 10 to 25% of these people might carry the gene for thalassemia.

Remainder of Pregnancy

Visits to the medical team should be made at the following frequency:

Fourth to sixth month (12 to 26 weeks): once a month.

Seventh and eighth month (27 to 35 weeks): every two weeks.

Ninth month (36 to 40 weeks): weekly.

Visits to the obstetrician or nurse-midwife for a woman with an uncomplicated pregnancy will generally involve the same tests done each time.

Complete physical: In addition to a medical history, the physical examination will emphasize the following:

Blood pressure—Hypertension can develop at any time during pregnancy and must be recognized as early as possible.

Weight—There are many different opinions as to what is the optimal amount of weight to be gained during pregnancy. Some doctors believe that a woman should gain as much weight as she wishes and in this way the baby will be well nourished. Other doctors believe in a strict policy of weight gain, recommending that their patients gain a certain amount—usually 15 to 20 pounds—and no more. We take the middle ground and recommend that a woman be allowed to gain a reasonable amount of weight, perhaps 20 to 30 pounds. Regardless of whose opinion is followed, it is important to document the patient's weight so that changes—up or down—can be recognized.

Fundus examination—The woman's abdomen should be examined and the location of the top of the uterus (fundus) determined. Uterine growth that is too rapid or too slow may indicate abnormal fetal development and must be investigated further.

Fetal heart rate—The rate will be taken to determine if it is normal, about 120 to 150 beats per minute. If more than one heart is heard, it implies a multiple birth (such as twins or triplets).

Hematocrit (p. 51): Many women become anemic during pregnancy. The hematocrit will detect this problem so that appropriate treatment can be initiated. The blood for this test might be obtained by fingerstick or venipuncture. Even if not done at every visit, this test should be performed at the start of the fourth, seventh, and ninth months of pregnancy.

Routine urinalysis (p. 87): Many pregnant women will have small amounts of sugar or protein in their urine. Persistent and significant amounts of sugar may suggest diabetes, while protein in the urine may be an early sign of hypertension or kidney disease.

In addition to those tests done at every visit, the following tests are likely to be done during the ninth month:

Vaginal-cervical culture (p. 167): Infection with a bacteria called Group B strep (a "cousin" of the bacteria that cause strep throat) can cause pneumonia, meningitis, and even death in the newborn. During delivery it is transmitted from the mother to the baby. If the culture reveals the presence of the bacteria in the mother, she should receive treatment with penicillin or other antibiotics. In addition, the physician will culture for gonorrhea at this time if he suspects that the mother may be infected.

Pap smear (p. 212): If the first Pap smear during pregnancy revealed the presence of a genital herpes infection, or if the physician thinks that the woman has herpes, a Pap smear will now be done to determine if the infection is in an active stage. If it is, plans must be made for a Cesarean section.

Delivery

Labor and birth are a very complex process during which a series of physiological changes are accomplished by the mother and baby. In addition to a *complete physical* (physical examination and medical history) when a woman enters the hospital for the delivery, various medical tests will frequently be done at the time of delivery to monitor this important moment. Women who choose to give birth in a birthing center or at home will probably not have all of these tests performed. A good compromise between the cold and sterile environment of a conventional hospital birth and the warm, yet potentially unsafe home birth is a hospital that has established birthing rooms within its own walls. In these settings women may give birth in an environment that is comfortable and warm, with other family members or friends present, yet they will still have immediate access to the facilities of a major medical center if an emergency suddenly develops. The issue in evaluating an alternative birth location is not the tests that can or cannot be performed; it is the availability of emergency care should problems arise.

The following three tests are done routinely on any pregnant woman who is admitted to the hospital:

Complete blood count (p. 51).

Urinalysis (p. 87).

Blood typing (p.46).

In addition, these tests may also be done:

Fetal monitoring: There are many different ways to monitor the fetus, but the usual fetal monitoring during delivery involves the simultaneous measurement of the baby's heart rate together with the frequency and intensity of maternal uterine contractions. There are two ways in which this can be done. The usual monitoring device will consist of a large (2-inch-wide) rubber strap placed around the mother's abdomen, attached to a Doppler ultrasound (p. 149), which detects the fetal heart rate. The strap itself detects the frequency and relative intensity of maternal contractions. Recently, more sophisticated monitoring has become available using probes that are inserted through the cervix. One probe attaches to the baby's scalp and records the fetal heart rate; the other lies within the uterus and is a sensitive monitor for the pressure of the uterine contractions.

In either system the actual measurements are recorded on a slowly moving piece of graph paper (similar to an EKG). The fetal heart rate may slow down during maternal contractions; if, however, the fetal heart rate is too late in returning to normal after a contraction, or if it is abnormally slow between contractions, it may be a sign of fetal distress and require a Cesarean section or forceps to deliver the baby more quickly.

The use of fetal monitoring is controversial. Some obstetricians think that almost every woman should be monitored in order to detect fetal distress. Other doctors, as well as many nurse-midwives, think that in an uncomplicated routine pregnancy the problems associated with fetal monitoring outweigh any possible benefits that might result. There are two major problems. First, fetal monitoring is uncomfortable for the woman. She must lie flat on her back and not walk around during labor. Second, and perhaps most important, the use of fetal monitoring has been shown to be associated with an increased number of Cesarean sections. One such study estimated that in the United States indiscriminate use of fetal monitoring resulted in 100,000 extra Cesarean sections being performed. Were all of these operations necessary? No one can be certain, but it is likely that many were not medically essential but were done only because the obstetrician interpreted the fetal monitoring result to be suggestive of fetal distress.

We recommend a middle approach. Uncomplicated, routine pregnancy should not be monitored at all, or there should be only a short period (about 10 minutes) of monitoring with the external strap device to be sure that everything is proceeding normally. However, women with increased risk during pregnancy (see the Table on p. 259) as well as women having an unusual labor should be monitored throughout labor. Unusual labor includes prolonged labor, premature rupture of membranes (breaking the bag of water), use of Pitocin (a synthetic hormone that stimulates the uterus) to augment or initiate good uterine contractions, and use of certain kinds of anesthetics and analgesics during labor (e.g., epidural block). If monitoring is being done by the obstetrician as a routine procedure and abnormal labor is not suspected, then the easy-to-use external strap monitoring is sufficient. If, on the other hand, the labor is truly unusual, or the obstetrician has reason to believe that the baby is truly distressed, the accurate, but riskier internal monitoring should be performed. If the obstetrician recommends a Cesarean section on the basis of the fetal monitoring, the woman in labor should find out exactly what the monitoring showed that prompted his decision.

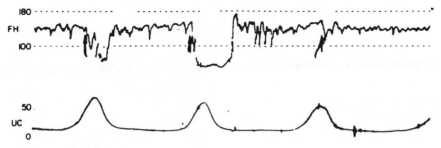

Tracing obtained during external fetal monitoring. The top line (FH) demonstrates the *Fetal Heart* rate, while the bottom line (UC) shows *Uterine* Contractions.

Cervical measurement: During labor, in preparation for the passage of the baby through the birth canal, the cervix thins (effaces) as well as opens (dilates). Frequent cervical measurements are made by the health care team during labor to ensure that this process is occurring, as the baby cannot be delivered until it has occurred. Effacement will be measured in percentage—100% effacement means the cervix is fully thinned out. Dilation is measured from 0 to 10 centimeters in diameter.

MEDICAL TESTS FOR HIGH-RISK PREGNANCIES

Women with high-risk pregnancies (see the table at the beginning of this chapter) will visit their obstetrician more frequently than a woman with an uncomplicated pregnancy. In addition, further tests might be done to monitor the health of the woman as well as that of the fetus. Many of these tests are not unique to pregnancy but are identical (with the exception of x-rays, see p. 90) to those obtained in women with comparable health problems who are not pregnant. Five tests, however, are unique to pregnancy, and many women with a high-risk pregnancy will have these tests done.

Nonstress testing: This test, which has nothing to do with stress testing for the heart, is used by obstetricians as a screening test to evaluate the function of the placenta and the overall status of the pregnancy in any woman who is suspected of having an obstetrical problem. The woman lies on her back in the doctor's office and has the external fetal monitoring equipment described earlier (p. 266) placed on her. In this instance, however, the strap around her abdomen is not meant to detect uterine contractions (there should not be any) but fetal movement. When the baby moves or "kicks," the abdomen moves and the strap records that movement. The Doppler ultrasound (p. 149), a part of the monitor equipment, records the baby's heart rate. The test is usually conducted for 20 minutes. The interpretation of the nonstress test is based on the relationship between the fetal heart rate and fetal movement. A normal nonstress test will show fetal movement occurring two or more times during the 20-minute test period. Moreover, during these periods of fetal activity, the heart rate must increase. Even if fetal movement occurs, if the heart rate stays the same or decreases during that activity, it is a worrisome sign.

Like all of us, the fetus sometimes sleeps. If it is not showing any movements during this nonstress test, the doctor may try to arouse him by gently poking at the mother's abdomen or by making loud noises, which are transmitted within the uterus and will awaken the fetus.

Oxytocin stress test (OTC): Another test that may be done late in pregnancy, if the doctor is worried about the status of the fetus and placenta, is the oxytocin stress test. Like the nonstress test, this one has a fetal monitor that evalutes the mother. In this test, however, a small amount of the hormone oxytocin is given to the mother (usually intravenously), and the monitor will record the uterine contractions that result. As with external fetal monitoring at the time of delivery, the number and intensity of uterine contractions and their relationship to the baby's heart rate will be used to evaluate the health of the pregnancy.

Estriol: This hormone is secreted by the placenta and passed into the urine of a pregnant woman, where it can be measured (p. 92), usually as a 24-hour collection. The estriol level will slowly increase throughout pregnancy. If the placenta is not functioning properly, as can happen in pregnant women over 35 or those with diabetes, hypertension, or other problems, the obstetrician will do frequent urine estriol measurements. As long as the concentration of the hormone is appropriate for that stage of pregnancy, the placenta is functioning properly and the baby is probably fine. If the level of estriol drops, however, the placenta is no longer working well, and the baby is probably at serious risk. Labor might have to be induced or a Cesarean section performed. This test may also be done in a woman who has not delivered by her due date. As long as the estriol remains elevated, the pregnancy is probably normal and the baby is fine. If, however, the estriol drops, it is time for the baby to emerge and labor will be induced. From 32 to 40 weeks of gestation, the normal 24-hour urine value is 10–40 mg / 24 hours.

Obstetrical ultrasound (p. 151): This is a very useful test and reveals tremendous information about the fetus (its size, shape, and presence of any birth defects). It is a good indicator of fetal age and maturity and is often used to determine more accurately the expected due date of the baby. In any pregnancy with an increased risk for whatever cause, ultrasound will be done as a screen to be sure that the baby is developing normally and growing at the right pace and that the placenta is functioning normally. It can also be used to diagnose the presence of multiple fetuses, suspected by the size of the woman or by the sound of more than one fetal heart beat. In addition, ultrasound is often done early in pregnancy when there is some question if the fetus is viable at all.

When a woman has a positive pregnancy test, but the obstetrician has reason to doubt that the pregnancy is progressing normally, ultrasound may be done in an effort to see: if the baby is present and normal; or, if the woman has an ectopic pregnancy (in which the fetus starts to grow in the fallopian tube and not in the uterus) or molar pregnancy (in which there is no fetus at all, but growth in the uterine wall of abnormal tissue), conditions that can mimic real pregnancy. Some obstetricians recommend ultrasound as a screening test for every pregnant woman. Although at this time it does not appear that there are risks to ultrasound, intensive research is currently underway to judge the long-term effects on the fetus. Until such research is concluded, we do not recommend ultrasound for pregnant women as a routine screening procedure.

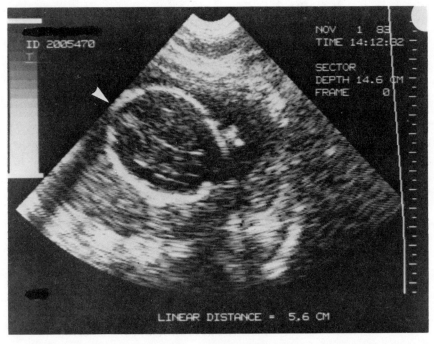

Normal obstetrical ultrasound of a woman in the twenty-third week of pregnancy. The arrow points to the fetal head.

Amniocentesis (p. 180): This medical test provides important information about the possible presence of birth defects or other complications during pregnancy. Amniocentesis is recommended for pregnant women who are: over age 35; have previously had a baby with a serious birth defect; have a family history of genetic disease; or a positive screening test for various genetic diseases or birth defects. If a woman is suspected of having a specific genetic disease (e.g., a positive test for Tay-Sachs or sickle cell), amniocentesis should probably be performed to screen for the presence of those genes in the fetus. The procedure may also be done late in pregnancy when the obstetrician is considering inducing early labor or doing a Cesarean section and when a woman has diabetes or hypertension. One of the tests that can be measured by amniocentesis is the L / S ratio, a measurement of two chemicals in the amniotic fluid—lecithin and sphingomyelin. This measurement can be used to judge the maturity of the fetal lungs, the organ of greatest concern when premature birth is possible.

It should be made clear that amniocentesis is not a benign procedure. Approximately one in two hundred women undergoing the test will have a miscarriage as a result. Other complications, including bleeding by the fetus, placenta, or mother, are possible as well. The decision to have amniocentesis should not be taken lightly but should be discussed seriously between the woman and her physician. Amniocentesis should be performed only when the information gained will alter the woman's medical care. For example, a woman who does not believe in abortion should not have an amniocentesis done to screen for trisomy 21 (Down's syndrome) since finding the presence of that problem in the fetus will not alter her decision.

14

The Use of Medical Tests on Hospitalized Patients

MANY people complain that when they were in the hospital, they were bombarded with tests. It seemed as if every other minute someone was drawing blood (". . . and so many tubes"), taking the temperature (". . . just when I fell asleep"), sending them down for an x-ray ("Didn't I just have this x-ray taken yesterday?"), or performing some other test. When a patient is admitted to the hospital, which medical tests should be done? How can a patient tell if those blood tests are needed every morning? Why are so many more tests done in the hospital? To answer these questions, let's look at a few examples of people admitted to the hospital.

When a patient goes to the emergency room of a hospital and is acutely ill, it will almost always be necessary to do some medical tests at that time. For example, if a 50-year-old male patient of ours comes to the hospital by ambulance because he has had crushing chest pain for two hours, we will immediately order an electrocardiogram (EKG, p. 193) to determine if a heart attack is occurring. If, following the EKG, we suspect the diagnosis of a heart attack, additional tests will be necessary: heart enzymes (p. 63) and a chest x-ray (p. 113). While in the cardiac care unit during the next few days, the patient will have frequent EKGS and blood tests done to determine the extent of the heart damage. So the first group of tests that a patient has in the emergency room of the hospital will always be related to the specific problem he had when he was admitted.

In addition, however, it is usual in almost all hospitals for certain standard tests to be performed regardless of the patient's particular diagnosis. These tests are useful to the medical staff as base-line information that will be helpful in evaluating any changes that may occur to the patient during the course of the hospitalization. This list of tests ordered on every patient admitted to the hospital has been undergoing critical analysis in the last few years and has appropriately gotten smaller. Here are the tests that we recommend for every adult patient admitted to the hospital:

Complete blood count (CBC, p. 51).

Urinalysis (p. 87).

Electrolytes (p. 58).

Electrocardiogram (for patients over the age of 35).

In addition, once the patient is actually in the regular hospital room, the nurses will periodically perform four tests: respiratory rate, temperature, blood pressure, and pulse. These four—which are sometimes grouped together and called vital signs—are monitored often, sometimes every four hours, or even more frequently if a problem is suspected to make sure the patient has not developed a fever, infection, or other medical problem while in the hospital.

It is also worthwhile to mention two tests that we do not recommend, although they were once done routinely for all admitted patients and are still common practice in some hospitals. The first of these is a chest x-ray, which used to be required of every person admitted to a hospital. This practice developed when tuberculosis was common and hospitals wanted to be sure that newly admitted patients were not contagious with that disease. Studies have now proven that chest x-rays obtained on patients without symptoms of heart or lung disease have such a low yield that they are a waste of time and money and not worth the risk of radiation exposure. Who should get a chest x-ray when admitted to the hospital? Only the patient who has a disease that affects the heart or lungs or has symptoms suggestive of such a problem. Even for these patients, however, if an x-ray has been obtained within the past six months or so, it may not be necessary to repeat it.

Here's an example: Last winter Mary W., a 72-year-old patient of ours, came to us complaining of fever and coughing. When we examined her, we thought she had pneumonia. We sent her to a radiologist's office and a chest x-ray revealed the presence of the disease. We decided to admit her to the hospital and sent her to the admitting office. The intern on the floor, seeing the diagnosis of pneumonia, ordered a chest x-ray, not realizing that Mary just had one done in the last few hours. It is the responsibility of every patient to know when his last chest x-ray (or any medical test for that matter) was performed so that unnecessary tests can be avoided during the hospital stay. Keeping an accurate Medical Test Diary (p. 361) will help in this regard.

The other test that we no longer order routinely for our hospitalized patients is a prothrombin time (PT or protime, p. 80). This test was once used to screen patients who may develop bleeding problems during their hospitalization. Again, this is no longer done, since several studies have shown that the protime provides no additional information as long as the patient's history and physical examination do not suggest that a bleeding problem is likely.

In addition to the patients described above who were admitted to the hospital for an acute medical problem, further medical tests may be ordered routinely for patients admitted to the hospital for elective surgery. In that situation, in addition to our list above (CBC, urinalysis, electrolytes and EKG), the surgeon will order blood typing (p. 46) so that if a transfusion is necessary as a result of the surgery the blood bank will already have the patient's blood type identified. Patients who are undergoing general anesthesia will be evaluated by the anesthesiologist prior to the surgery. If he has any question about the status of the lungs or the patient's ability to tolerate the anesthesia, pulmonary function tests (p. 216) and arterial blood gases (p. 183) may be obtained as well. After surgery vital signs will be obtained frequently as will complete blood counts and electrolytes to be sure that no postsurgical complications— infection, bleeding, kidney problems—have developed. Electrolytes are especially important when the patient is not eating or drinking and will be receiving all of his fluid and nourishment intravenously.

Are medical tests performed more frequently in a teaching hospital where residents, interns, and medical students are being trained? Many patients assume that in such a hospital they will have more tests done simply to satisfy the educational needs of teaching the young students and doctors. In fact, this is probably true to a limited degree. Students, interns, residents, and occasionally even senior staff physicians do order more tests than are sometimes necessary. It is one of the trade-offs that a patient must make when admitted to a teaching hospital. Medical care in such a center is probably the best that can be obtained, but, in return, patients may have to "suffer" from being examined a few more times by a student or intern or from having an extra tube of blood drawn.

Nevertheless, whether in a university medical center, teaching hospital, or small community hospital, we believe that patients have certain rights concerning the use of tests during their hospital stay:

1. *You have the right to know why tests are being done.* As we have stressed throughout this book, ask your physician if you have any questions about why certain tests are being done. If an appropriate explanation is not provided, then you can legitimately raise the issue of whether the test should be done at all.

2. *You have the right not to be disturbed for tests, unless there is a legitimate reason.* Many patients complain that they are continually being disturbed in the hospital—awakened for blood tests in the morning, sent to x-ray during lunch, and so on—and they don't understand why. Unless there is good reason, such disturbances are inappropriate. Often, however, there is good reason, and patients aren't aware of it. For example, in almost all hospitals blood tests are drawn first thing in the morning. This has two consequences. First, many patients are awakened in order for their blood to be drawn; and second, even if they have awakened early by themselves, they are not allowed to have breakfast until the blood is taken.

But there is good reason for both of these practices. Blood is drawn first thing in the morning so that the laboratory can have results back early enough for the patient's doctor to act on them: changing therapy if necessary, altering medication orders, or arranging for additional tests. Also, almost without exception, blood tests are more accurate if the patient has not eaten breakfast but has been fasting since the previous night. So for these two reasons, blood is best drawn early, even if patients must be awakened or kept from their breakfast.

Other tests that appear to be disturbing are often appropriate. If a patient is in the hospital with a serious infection, the nurse will probably be ordered to take his temperature every few hours, even throughout the night. That will mean, of course, that the patient will be disturbed from his sleep. Is it necessary? Yes, if the doctor is concerned enough about the infection to have the patient in the hospital in the first place. To be honest, however, there are many instances when disturbing the patient for a test is unjustified and avoidable.

Take x-rays for example. When the doctor sends a request for an x-ray down to the radiology department, he is not given any choice about the timing of that test. In most hospitals the radiology department is so busy that patients must be scheduled throughout the day, even during meal times. When the department is ready for a patient, it will call the floor and tell the nurses to send him down. If a test is being done at a time when it is disturbing to you (during meals, visiting hours, your nap), you have the right to find out from the nursing staff if it must be done right at that moment or if it can be postponed until a more convenient time.

3. *You have the right not to have unnecessary tests performed.* Again, frequently during a hospital stay some unnecessary tests will be performed. How does a patient know if a certain test is necessary? A good rule of thumb to follow is this: If the test has been ordered routinely—for example, a complete blood count every morning or an electrocardiogram every day—there is a chance that the test is unnecessary, and those are the tests that you should question.

15

Medical Tests, Athletes, and Physical Fitness

OUR country is in the midst of a physical fitness boom never experienced before. The signs are everywhere: early morning finds the streets dotted with joggers and runners of all ages and both sexes; stores devoted solely to selling equipment, books, and clothing for the physical-fitness-minded consumer are in numerous shopping malls; health and exercise clubs are mushrooming in every city and most suburbs; and bookstores are filled with books and magazines devoted to exercise and physical fitness.

This revolution in our approach to physical fitness has had an impact on the field of medical testing as well. The body of a person involved in a rigorous physical fitness program, including that of aerobically conditioned athletes—cyclists, swimmers, runners—undergoes significant changes in its physiological function. While most everyone is aware that the heart of a well-conditioned athlete is stronger, there are many additional changes in other parts of the body as well, including hormones, blood counts, kidney function, and temperature. Consequently, athletes and people who exercise vigorously will give different results to a variety of medical tests compared to nonathletes.

We believe it is important for an athlete or well-conditioned person to be aware of the changes that are present in his or her body so that if medical testing is done, they can work with the doctor to evaluate the results accurately. In fact, although sports medicine is becoming a medical specialty in its own right, most physicians in practice—unless they have a number of physically active patients—are unaware of the numerous changes that exercise can cause in medical test results. This chapter will review some of the more important of these. Remember that not every person who exercises will show all of these alterations. They are highly variable; some people who do even minimal exercise on a regular basis will display significant changes in their medical test results, while world-class athletes show little difference. The important thing is to share your exercise history with your physician and be aware of the changes that physical conditioning can induce, so if medical tests are done, the interpretation will be accurate and appropriate.

Pulse (p. 332)

One of the earliest and most consistent changes induced in the body by regular aerobic exercise is improvement in the function of the heart. The heart muscle enlarges and pumps more efficiently. The amount of blood pumped with each beat—called the stroke volume—increases, and, consequently, the heart does not have to beat quite so often. The resting pulse of most people with a regular exercise program is 40 to 60, 15 to 20 beats per minute less than average. During exercise the heart rate of athletes will still rise to the level of 150 to 180, but at rest the heart is able to accomplish what it needs to at a slower rate.

Blood Pressure (p. 330)

Another consequence of the effect of exercise on the heart is lowering of blood pressure. This, too, is highly variable, but on the average regular exercising can cause a decrease of 20 points in both the systolic and diastolic measurements.

Electrocardiogram (ekg, p. 193)

The enlarged heart of a well-conditioned athlete will give a different electrocardiographic tracing than that of the average person. There are many changes that can occur on the ekg, most related to the heart being larger than normal and beating at a slower rate. Since some of the changes can mimic the patterns seen in a person suffering a heart attack, it is important for the doctor to know if the person having an ekg is an athlete.

Chest X-Ray (p. 113)

In addition to causing changes on the EKG, the enlarged heart will show up on a chest x-ray. The radiologist—unless alerted to the situation—will be unable to distinguish easily the enlarged heart of a person who exercises regularly from that of a person who has heart disease or other illness.

Temperature (p. 335)

The energy needed during intense exercise generates tremendous amounts of heat within the body, heat that must be disposed of. The temperature regulatory system of an athlete or person who exercises regularly is different from that of the nonathlete. One difference is that the athlete can exercise with less chance of suffering heat stroke or heat exhaustion than other people. Nevertheless, it is not uncommon for someone who exercises strenuously or runs long distances to have a temperature of 103° immediately afterwards.

Anemia (p. 309)

One additional effect of the enlarged heart and the requirement for good temperature control is that the physically fit patient has within his or her blood more of the fluid component (plasma) and less of the cells (red blood cells or erythrocytes). Consequently, some of these people will have a hematocrit or red blood cell count that is slightly less than average. This lower hematocrit in the athlete is appropriate and is not a sign of anemia, nor does it require any treatment.

Proteinuria and Hematuria (p. 87)

Following exercise, the urine will often contain protein as well as red blood cells. These are not dangerous but reflect, instead, changes in the kidney associated with physical activity. In addition to actual red blood cells, the urine of someone who has just exercised may contain hemoglobin (a chemical found in red blood cells) or myoglobin (a related chemical found within muscle). The presence of both of these will lead to a urine dipstick analysis that is positive for blood—when, in fact, it is these proteins and not actual blood that is present. One word of caution is necessary here. Although red blood cells or hemoglobin found after exercise in small, microscopic amounts is almost always benign, the presence of bright red blood in the urine, especially after a sport with physical contact (e.g., football or soccer), should always alert the patient and physician to the possibility that a more serious injury to the kidney has occurred.

LIVER FUNCTION TESTS (P. 77) AND HEART ENZYMES (P. 63)

Muscles and red blood cells contain a variety of enzymes. One of these, lactic dehydrogenase (LDH) is also found within cells of the liver and heart; another enzyme, serum glutamic-oxaloacetic transaminase (SGOT), is found within liver cells only; a third, creatine phosphokinase (CPK), is found in both muscles and the heart. Following exercise, the level of any or all of these enzymes may be elevated in the blood because of the stress placed on the muscles and red blood cells during intense physical activity. Unfortunately, elevations in these enzymes are also signs of hepatitis or heart attack. It is important for the active person who has these tests done to alert the physician of his exercise program so that an erroneous diagnosis of hepatitis or heart attack is not made.

SERUM LIPIDS (P. 76)

One of the serum lipids, high-density lipoproteins (HDL), is thought to be protective against the development of atherosclerosis (hardening of the arteries). The level of HDL is elevated in a conditioned patient, probably further evidence of the benefits of exercise.

ELECTROLYTES (P. 58)

People who exercise regularly will often have decreased potassium levels (hypokalemia). This will sometimes require them to take potassium supplements, especially when they sweat profusely, since sweat contains large amounts of potassium.

As you can see, the athlete or person with a rigorous and regular exercise program could walk into a physician's office and be wrongly diagnosed for any number of diseases because of the unusual results from several medical tests. Basing his information on an inaccurate assessment of these test results, the physician may want to initiate treatment or order additional tests—some dangerous and costly. The patient, however, must alert his physician to these changes that may occur in an athlete or well-conditioned person so that medical tests can be interpreted wisely and correctly.

PART V

The Use of Medical Tests in Illness

16

The Use of Medical Tests for Twenty-One Common Symptoms

ABDOMINAL PAIN

BACKGROUND: For many reasons, determining the cause of abdominal pain is among the most difficult tasks we face in medicine. Abdominal pain can begin suddenly and require immediate surgery or develop slowly over many months. The causes of abdominal pain include problems that are serious (colon cancer, appendicitis, ulcer, and hepatitis) or trivial (overeating and excessive gas). Complicating matters further is the fact that the abdomen contains many organs that are not readily accessible to examination, such as the liver, intestines, pancreas, stomach, kidneys, and gallbladder. When we are faced with a patient complaining of abdominal pain, our thinking is directed towards answering three questions: (1) Which of the many organs in the abdomen is causing the pain? (2) What is the specific nature of the problem with that organ? (3) Is surgery required? Clues can be obtained from the history and physical exam, but frequently medical tests are still necessary to determine the specific diagnosis.

TESTS COMMONLY OBTAINED FOR A PATIENT WITH ABDOMINAL PAIN

Complete blood count (CBC, p. 51): An elevated white blood cell count will frequently accompany hepatitis, pancreatitis, appendicitis, diverticulitis, cholecystitis (inflamed gallbladder) or other diseases caused by the inflammation or infection of abdominal organs. This test, however, is not specific for any one of these diseases. In addition, a low hematocrit (p. 52) will suggest bleeding from a site within the abdomen, including ulcers, tumors, and diverticula.

Abdominal x-ray (KUB, p. 105): If there is obstruction of the intestines, the x-ray will show that this normally air-filled organ has become distended and filled with fluid. In addition, gallstones and kidney stones are occasionally visible.

Urinalysis (p. 87): Red blood cells in the urine may indicate a kidney stone; white blood cells may indicate a urinary tract infection.

Amylase (p. 44): Although it is not always the case, an elevation in the level of amylase is most often due to pancreatitis.

Liver function tests (p. 77): Abnormalities in this series of tests will accompany diseases of the liver and gallbladder.

Upper GI series (p. 128): This test can reveal the presence of an ulcer or cancer (in the stomach or intestines), either of which can cause abdominal pain.

Barium enema (p. 109): This test can indicate the presence of cancer, polyps, and diverticulitis in the colon and rectum.

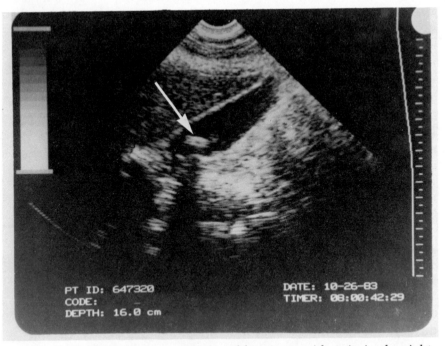

Abdominal ultrasound in a 54-year-old woman with pain in the right upper side of her abdomen. The arrow points to a stone in her gallbladder.

OTHER TESTS:
Test for blood in stool (p. 96).
Gastroscopy (p. 162).
Sigmoidoscopy (p. 165).
Colonoscopy (p. 158).
Liver-spleen scan (p. 141).
Abdominal ultrasound (p. 147).
Abdominal CT scan (p. 115).
Electrolytes (p. 58).

BACKACHE

BACKGROUND: If an engineer were given the task of redesigning the human body, one part that definitely would be altered is the back. It is better suited for an animal walking on four limbs than a human standing upright on only two legs. The spine is made up of a long column of bones along the back called vertebrae as well as cushions between the vertebrae (discs). These are needed to support man while he is standing. In addition, the vertebral column encloses and protects the spinal cord and nerves that emanate from it. Not surprisingly, because of the stress placed on these structures, almost everyone at some time in his life will experience back pain. Most often, this pain is due to strained muscles and ligaments of the lower back and will subside without medical treatment. Other causes of pain are more serious and include vertebral disc herniation (protrusion of the disc between two vertebrae), osteomyelitis (infection of the vertebrae), fractures of the vertebrae, and tumors. Most episodes of back pain can be diagnosed from the patient's medical history and physical exam and do not require medical tests. If tests are ordered, the patient should be sure to find out from the physician why he thinks this particular case of back pain is more than the usual muscle spasm or ligament pull in the lower back.

TESTS COMMONLY OBTAINED FOR A PATIENT WITH A BACKACHE
X-rays (p. 98): X-rays of the lower back (lumbosacral area) visualize the vertebrae in that portion of the spine. Unfortunately, protrusion of a disc or strain of muscles and ligaments cannot be seen by these x-rays.
Bone scan (p. 133): This test can corroborate abnormalities seen on lumbosacral x-rays. In addition, a bone scan can clearly show small areas of infection and cancer before they appear on x-rays.

Myelogram (p. 126): This test is useful to define better the anatomic relationship between the vertebral column and the spinal cord running within it. Therefore, it is often done for patients with persistent back pain when surgery is being considered.

OTHER TESTS:
Electromyography (p. 200).
HLA B27 (p. 66).
Erythrocyte sedimentation rate (p. 58).
CT scan (p. 115).

BLEEDING AND BRUISING

BACKGROUND: Clotting of your blood when you are cut or injured is achieved through a complex series of reactions by various proteins in the blood called clotting factors as well as by the help of platelets, a type of blood cell. If the levels of the clotting factors or platelets in the blood are low, then the blood will not clot as it should and excessive bleeding or bruising will result. A deficiency of clotting factors can be congenital (hemophilia) or accompany other diseases such as liver failure and malnutrition. In addition, certain drugs, such as Coumadin, are specifically used to lower the amount of clotting factors in the blood, and bleeding can result from taking too much of these medications. Platelet deficiencies can occur following a viral infection (idiopathic thrombocytopenic purpura) or as a result of various serious diseases in the bone marrow (leukemia, aplastic anemia), the site where platelets are produced.

TESTS COMMONLY OBTAINED FOR A PATIENT WITH BLEEDING AND
BRUISING
Prothrombin time (PT, p. 80) and partial thromboplastin time (PTT, p. 80):
These two tests measure whether the various clotting factors are present in normal levels and working together properly. Abnormal values will suggest the presence of hemophilia or liver disease. If the patient is taking Coumadin, an elevation in the results of these tests is expected; too high an elevation, however, would suggest that there is too high a level of Coumadin in the blood.

Complete blood count (CBC, p. 51): This test is done for two reasons: (1) The hematocrit will tell us how much bleeding has occurred, and (2) the platelet count will tell the doctor if there are sufficient numbers of these cells present for proper blood clotting.

Bleeding time (p. 80): Even if the platelets are present in normal numbers, it is possible that they are not working well. The bleeding time will determine if this is the case. Aspirin, as well as certain kinds of kidney disease, can cause an elevated bleeding time.

OTHER TESTS:
Test for blood in stool (p. 96).
Urinalysis (p. 87).
Liver function tests (LFTS, p. 77).
Kidney tests (p. 74).

BLOOD IN THE STOOL

BACKGROUND: Blood in the stool can take one of three forms: (1) bright red blood indicates bleeding from the large intestines or the rectum; (2) black stools indicate bleeding from the esophagus, stomach, or small intestine; and (3) occult blood—blood that is invisible to the naked eye but detectable by chemical tests—can occur with a small amount of bleeding from any of these sites. What is also confusing is that red or black stools can occur without any bleeding at all but as a result of eating certain foods. Eating spinach or other foods high in iron can cause the stool to appear black, while eating beets can result in bright red stools. The patient's age and medical history help us determine the cause for blood in the stool. For example, bright red blood in a 40-year-old woman will often be due to hemorrhoids, while black stool in a 30-year-old woman taking aspirin for rheumatoid arthritis would suggest gastritis (inflammation of the stomach due to the aspirin) as the cause. Finally, occult blood in a 70-year-old man who has recently lost weight suggests a cancer in the large intestine. Medical tests for patients with blood in the stool are often critical for making an accurate diagnosis. This is especially important since some of the problems that cause this symptom are not serious (hemorrhoids and anal fissure are some examples), while others, such as cancer, are very serious but potentially curable if detected early enough.

TESTS COMMONLY OBTAINED FOR A PATIENT WITH BLOOD IN THE STOOL
Complete blood count (CBC p. 51): The hematocrit does not reveal the cause of the bleeding but will indicate how severe the blood loss has been and how anemic the patient is. A low platelet count will often result in bleeding that may come from the intestines or stomach.

Sigmoidoscopy (p. 165): Bleeding from hemorrhoids, polyps, or tumors in that portion of the large intestine that is closest to the rectum can be seen using this technique.

Barium enema (p. 109): Polyps, tumors, and ulcerative colitis—all of which can cause red blood in the stool—can be diagnosed by this x-ray.

Upper GI series (UGI, p. 128): Ulcers, tumors, and inflammation in the esophagus, stomach, and small intestine—all of which can cause black stools—can be diagnosed by this x-ray technique.

OTHER TESTS:
Gastroscopy (p. 162).
Colonoscopy (p. 158).
Kidney function tests (p. 74).
Prothrombin time (PT, p. 80).
Partial thromboplastin time (PTT, p. 80).

BREATHING DIFFICULTY

BACKGROUND: Difficulty with breathing is usually perceived by patients as "shortness of breath." This sensation occurs when the body's demand for air is greater than the lung's capacity to respond. Regardless of whether the shortness of breath develops suddenly or over a period of months, medical tests are helpful to us in determining the cause of our patient's symptoms. Obstruction of the airway system can occur in patients who smoke or those with bronchitis, emphysema, or asthma. Fluid buildup in the lungs because of a pneumonia or congestive heart failure can also cause shortness of breath. In addition, a blockage of the arteries that supply the lung (pulmonary embolism) can also cause this sensation.

TESTS COMMONLY OBTAINED FOR A PATIENT WITH BREATHING DIFFI-CULTY

Chest x-ray (p. 113): This test will determine whether there is fluid in the lungs (pneumonia, congestive heart failure) or obstruction of the lungs from smoking, bronchitis, emphysema, or asthma.

Arterial blood gases (p. 183): This test measures the oxygen content of the blood but cannot diagnose the specific cause of the shortness of breath. It does, however, determine the severity of the disease causing the shortness of breath and the length of time that it has been present.

Pulmonary function tests (p. 216): Since these tests measure the patient's ability to inhale and exhale, they will be helpful in determining the severity of the lung disease. Asthma, bronchitis, and emphysema each have a different pattern of pulmonary function tests.

OTHER TESTS:
Complete blood count (CBC, p. 51).
Sputum culture (p. 173).
Lung scan (p. 142).
Electrocardiogram (EKG, p. 193).

CHEST PAIN

BACKGROUND: Chest pain is a frightening symptom because of the concern that it might be a heart attack or a sign of other heart disease. In fact, this is not always the case. Any organ or body structure within the chest or near it can cause chest pain. Vigorous exertion can result in strain and spasm of the muscles of the chest wall, causing pain. In addition, inflammation (from an infection or allergy) of the heart or lung as well as gallbladder disease can all cause chest pain. When the heart has insufficient oxygen for the demands that have been placed on it, a typical squeezing or pressure sensation develops, which sometimes radiates to the left shoulder or hand. Medical tests play an important part in distinguishing those patients who have pain from the heart and consequently require immediate medical attention from those who have pain due to some other cause.

TESTS COMMONLY OBTAINED FOR A PATIENT WITH CHEST PAIN
Electrocardiogram (EKG, p. 193): Changes in the EKG will indicate whether heart injury or damage is present as well as its exact location. Occasionally, the EKG will remain normal even when heart disease is present.
Chest x-ray (p. 113): Inflammation of the lung or its lining, such as that occurring with pneumonia or allergy, will appear as a whitened area on the x-ray.
Heart enzymes (p. 63): If a heart attack is the cause, these enzymes will be abnormal. Otherwise, they will appear normal.
Exercise tolerance test (p. 202): If heart disease is the cause of the chest pain, exercise will induce changes in the electrocardiogram. These changes will indicate how severe the heart disease is and what part of the heart is affected.

Heart scan (p. 138): A thallium scan of the heart will determine if the chest pain is caused by lack of oxygen in the heart muscle.

OTHER TESTS:
Cardiac catheterization (p. 111).
Echocardiogram (p. 150).
Erythrocyte sedimentation rate (ESR, p. 58).
Upper GI series (p. 128).
Complete blood count (CBC, p. 51).
Gallbladder x-rays (p. 119).

COUGH

BACKGROUND: Cough is your body's attempt to expel dust, fluid, mucus, or other substances from your lungs or throat; it may be present for only a few minutes or may last weeks or even months. Coughing can accompany a wide range of illnesses, from those that are of little consequence, like the common cold, to those that require immediate medical attention, like cancer. Therefore, when we see a patient complaining of a cough, it is necessary to do a series of tests to determine the specific cause.

TESTS COMMONLY OBTAINED FOR A PATIENT WITH A COUGH
Chest x-ray (p. 113): A chest x-ray is useful to detect those causes of cough that are due to disease in the lungs, including pneumonia, congestive heart failure, lung cancer, bronchitis, or emphysema.

Sputum culture (p. 173): Many infections of the respiratory tract (throat, larynx, trachea, and lungs) will produce phlegm or sputum. Culture of the sputum might determine if bacteria are present.

Cytology (p. 192): Examination of the phlegm or sputum for abnormal cells—sputum cytology—will help determine if lung cancer is present.

Complete blood count (CBC, p. 51): If the cough is due to a bacterial infection, the white blood cell count will be elevated.

Tuberculosis skin test (p. 224): This test will screen for the presence of tuberculosis.

OTHER TESTS:
Pulmonary function tests (p. 216).
Erythrocyte sedimentation rate (ESR, p. 58).
Infectious disease antibody titers (p. 72).
Lung scan (p. 142).

Diarrhea

BACKGROUND: In most instances diarrhea is a self-limited disease that lasts only a few days and does not require medical attention. These brief illnesses, known as a "stomach flu" or "stomach virus," are usually due to a viral infection, but occasionally bacteria, parasites, medications, or even stress can cause a bout of diarrhea. If the diarrhea persists, however, a physician should be seen to establish the specific diagnosis. When we see a patient with diarrhea, we will use a variety of medical tests to help determine the exact cause of the problem. In addition, certain symptoms, such as abdominal pain or blood in the stool—if present—will be helpful in narrowing down the likely possibilities.

TESTS COMMONLY OBTAINED FOR A PATIENT WITH DIARRHEA
Stool culture and Gram stain (p. 173): This test determines whether bacteria are causing the diarrhea.

Stool for ovum and parasites (p. 96): This test determines whether parasites are the cause of the diarrhea. The parasites or their eggs can frequently be seen under the microscope.

Sigmoidoscopy (p. 165): Direct observation of the intestinal lining enables the doctor to diagnose inflammation, infection, or cancer.

Barium enema (p. 109): A barium enema permits detailed evaluation of the large intestines as the source of the diarrhea. Cancers, polyps, ulcerative colitis, and other causes of bowel inflammation can be seen on the x-ray.

OTHER TESTS:
Colonoscopy (p. 158).
Stool fat (p. 95).
Complete blood count (CBC, p. 51).
Amylase (p. 44).
Liver function tests (LFTS, p. 77).
Vitamin B12 (p. 84).
Prothrombin time (PT, p. 80).
Electrolytes (p. 58).

Dizziness

BACKGROUND: Dizziness can be caused by problems in several different parts of the body. Symptoms that are frequently associated with dizziness include faintness, light-headedness, sensation of the room spinning around (vertigo), weakness, and hallucination of movement. The presence of each of these symptoms will suggest a different cause of dizziness. Vertigo is often associated with problems in the brain or middle ear, while faintness is often caused by anemia or heart disease. During our examination of the patient with dizziness, we will move the patient into different positions, trying to reproduce the dizzy feeling. This frequently pinpoints the cause and avoids the need for additional tests.

TESTS COMMONLY OBTAINED FOR A PATIENT WITH DIZZINESS

Electrocardiogram (EKG, p. 193): An EKG shows if there are irregular heart beats. If present, these irregular beats may cause decreased blood flow to the brain and result in dizziness.

Complete blood count (CBC, p. 51): The red blood cells carry the oxygen needed to supply the brain. Severe anemia will result in decreased oxygen flow to the brain and cause dizziness.

Audiogram (p. 185): Patterns of hearing at high and low frequencies are detected by the audiogram. Some causes of dizziness in adults are often associated with low-frequency hearing loss.

Skull x-ray (p. 98): Brain tumors—especially those that are located near the auditory (hearing) nerve—can cause dizziness.

OTHER TESTS:

Electroencephalogram (EEG, p. 197).
Brain CT scan (p. 115).
Blood glucose (p. 61).
Test for blood in stool (p. 96).
Holter monitor (p. 206).

FAINTING

BACKGROUND: When the brain does not receive an adequate supply of blood for it to function properly, fainting occurs. It is usually not a sign of serious disease, especially when it happens in young people. Common situations of this kind include a person who faints after being startled by an unexpected noise or after seeing his blood spurt out from a cut, or the soldier who faints after standing at attention for a long time on a hot summer day. In each of these cases, the body has temporarily lost its ability to send sufficient blood flow to the brain. But these patients will recover quickly because the blood flow to the brain will be quickly reestablished. Moreover, in these people the cause of fainting is obvious, and no medical tests are necessary to diagnose the problem.

In other cases, however, fainting can be a more worrisome sign. It can signal an irregular heart beat (arrhythmia), which disrupts the flow of blood to the brain. It could also be a symptom of a narrowing of the heart valves (aortic stenosis), which prevents adequate blood flow from the heart. When it is not certain what caused the fainting episode—as is usually the case with the elderly—we will order medical tests to help determine the specific cause.

TESTS COMMONLY OBTAINED FOR FAINTING

Electrocardiogram (EKG, p. 193): Irregular heart beats or abnormal heart rhythms can result in an insufficient blood flow to the brain and cause fainting. This is an especially important diagnosis to make because many of these patients can be successfully treated by implantation of a heart pacemaker.

Holter monitor (p. 206): Even if abnormalities are not found on the routine EKG (which lasts for only a few minutes), analysis of a Holter monitor 24-hour cardiogram will increase the chance of finding an irregular heart beat if this was the cause of the fainting.

Blood glucose (p. 61): Low blood glucose levels (hypoglycemia) can also cause fainting.

OTHER TESTS:
Complete blood count (CBC, p. 51).
Echocardiogram (p. 150).
Arterial blood gases (p. 183).
Electroencephalogram (EEG, p. 197).

FATIGUE

BACKGROUND: Frequently, we see patients who complain that they have no energy and are always tired. In many of these cases emotional stress plays an important role, although serious diseases can be associated with these types of symptoms. Often, patients are convinced that vitamin deficiency or "iron-poor blood" is the cause, but it is unusual for these problems to result in fatigue unless severe deficiencies exist. Medications, as well as hormone imbalances, such as an underactive thyroid or adrenal gland, can also cause fatigue.

TESTS COMMONLY OBTAINED FOR A PATIENT WITH FATIGUE

Complete blood count (CBC, p. 51): Oxygen is transported through-out the body by the red blood cells and is needed to convert food into energy. Anemia—a deficiency of red blood cells—will result in a reduction in the amount of available oxygen, causing fatigue and weakness. The hematocrit will be able to detect the anemia if present.

Thyroid function tests (p. 69): These tests measure the function of the thyroid gland, the organ that regulates the body's metabo-lism. If the gland is underactive, the patient may feel chronically fatigued.

Electrolytes (p. 58): Potassium and other electrolytes control muscle function in the body. Consequently, unusually low sodium or potassium levels in the blood may be associated with fatigue.

Blood glucose (p. 61): Glucose is a major source of the body's energy. Consequently, hypoglycemia (low glucose levels) may cause fatigue.

OTHER TESTS:
Kidney tests (p. 74).
Liver function tests (LFTS, p. 77).
Cortisol (p. 68).
Calcium (p. 47).

FEVER

BACKGROUND: It is critical that your body maintain a constant tem-perature within a narrow, fixed range. This is regulated by a "thermostat" that is located in a part of the brain called the hypo-thalamus. Fever occurs when this thermostat sets the body tem-perature higher than normal. Although many people associate fever only with infectious illnesses, such as the common cold or pneu-monia, it is actually a nonspecific symptom that can accompany many other diseases, including cancer, arthritis, and allergies. Fever rarely occurs alone but is usually accompanied by other symp-toms, such as abdominal pain, cough, or fatigue. Fever is a very common symptom. Not every patient we see with fever will have similar tests done; some will not have any tests done at all for that matter. To determine if the fever deserves medical tests, we will use two important criteria: its duration and the amount of tem-perature elevation.

TESTS COMMONLY OBTAINED FOR A PATIENT WITH FEVER

Complete blood count (CBC, p. 51): An elevated white blood cell count suggests infection as the cause of the fever. The white blood cell differential will help determine whether the infection is caused by a virus or bacteria.

Cultures (p. 167): Cultures are used to determine if the fever is due to an infection. Although many different parts of the body can be "cultured" (blood, sputum, urine, throat, stool), the person with fever will usually have other symptoms, such as cough, pain with urination, and abdominal pain. These will aid us in deciding which cultures are necessary.

Erythrocyte sedimentation rate (ESR, p. 58): The ESR is a useful test to distinguish serious from nonserious causes of fever. Generally, high ESR values are associated with more serious problems such as cancer, serious infection, or rheumatoid arthritis.

Chest x-ray (p. 113): A frequent cause of fever is pneumonia. A chest x-ray will detect if pneumonia is present, although it does not determine the specific cause.

OTHER TESTS:
Liver function tests (LFTS, p. 77).
Hepatitis test (p. 65).
Mononucleosis test (p. 78).
Antinuclear antibody (ANA, p. 45).
Urinalysis (p. 87).

HEADACHE

BACKGROUND: Although everyone has a headache at some time in his or her life, it rarely necessitates an appointment with the doctor. Only if it is especially severe or persistent should medical attention be sought. When we see a patient with a headache, it is unusual for us to order tests to determine the cause. Usually, we can make a diagnosis based on the history and physical examination and prescribe medication to alleviate the pain. In fact, most of the common causes of headaches, including migraine, muscle spasm, and tension, will not even show up on routine medical tests. Occasionally, however, tests are necessary to exclude more serious causes of headache, such as brain tumor, infection, or bleeding into the brain.

TESTS COMMONLY OBTAINED FOR A PATIENT WITH A HEADACHE

Brain CT scan (p. 115): For patients with severe or persistent headaches, this is the most important test to perform. It has largely replaced a variety of x-ray tests that were done in the past. A CT scan permits visualization of the brain and can diagnose tumors, infection, and blood from hemorrhage or stroke.

Erythrocyte sedimentation rate (ESR, p. 58): An elevated ESR will suggest inflammation of the arteries supplying the brain as the cause of the headaches.

Electroencephalogram (EEG, p. 197): The brain produces electrical wave patterns that are seen on an EEG. Abnormal wave patterns may suggest a tumor, seizure (epilepsy), or stroke.

Lumbar puncture (p. 210): Infection of the lining of the brain (meningitis) can cause severe headaches. The presence of bacteria and white cells in the spinal fluid will confirm this diagnosis.

OTHER TESTS:
Skull x-rays (p. 98).
Blood glucose (p. 61).
Brain scan (p. 135).
Brain angiography (p. 106).
Pituitary hormone tests (p. 70).

INDIGESTION

BACKGROUND: At one time or another almost everyone suffers from indigestion. Symptoms that are associated with indigestion include abdominal bloating, excessive belching, heartburn, and upper abdominal discomfort. To determine the cause of the indigestion, we should know the following: the location of the symptoms, whether the discomfort radiates to other parts of the body, the pattern of pain, and factors that alleviate the pain. Even with these helpful clues, we often need to order laboratory tests to confirm the diagnosis and plan therapy.

TESTS COMMONLY OBTAINED FOR A PATIENT WITH INDIGESTION

Abdominal x-ray (p. 105): This x-ray technique will demonstrate whether excessive gas in the intestine is causing the indigestion. Gallstones, which occasionally are seen on this type of x-ray, would suggest gallbladder disease as the cause.

Upper GI series (UGI, p. 128): Since an ulcer or stomach cancer can create the symptoms of indigestion, an upper GI series is helpful to determine whether or not these diseases are the cause. If an ulcer is present, pinpointing its exact location will be helpful in determining the specific treatment.

Gastroscopy (p. 162): Occasionally, ulcers will be missed on UGI series but can be seen by gastroscopy. Biopsies of possible cancers can be obtained as well.

Abdominal ultrasound (p. 147): Gallbladder disease is a frequent cause of indigestion, especially when accompanied by pain in the upper right part of the abdomen. Ultrasound will reveal stones in the gallbladder.

Gallbladder x-rays (p. 119): These x-rays further investigate the gallbladder as a possible cause for the indigestion.

OTHER TESTS:
Liver function tests (LFTS, p. 77).
Test for blood in stool (p. 96).
Complete blood count (CBC, p. 51).

INFERTILITY

BACKGROUND: Estimates are that as many as 1 in 10 couples have difficulty conceiving. Generally, we do not consider infertility to be a medical problem until the couple has tried to conceive for 12 consecutive menstrual cycles without success. In approximately 40% of cases, infertility is due to the male partner; in the other 60%, the problem rests with the woman partner. Men may be impotent because of medications, anatomic abnormalities, chemical imbalances, or emotional problems. They may also have insufficient numbers of sperm or abnormal sperm that are unable to penetrate the egg. Common causes of infertility in women are: an irregular menstrual cycle without monthly ovulation; anatomic abnormalities of the cervix, uterus, or fallopian tubes; or pelvic infections that can prevent the sperm from gaining access to the egg.

TESTS COMMONLY OBTAINED FOR A PATIENT WITH INFERTILITY

Basal body temperature (for women; p. 338): Just prior to ovulation the woman's base-line temperature decreases slightly, followed by a rise in temperature indicating that ovulation has taken place. The absence of this temperature change indicates that the woman is not ovulating and cannot become pregnant.

Semen analysis (for men; p. 218): Semen analysis determines if there are an adequate number of healthy sperm present in the semen for conception to occur.

Pituitary hormone tests (for women; p. 70): The ovaries are controlled by hormones released by the pituitary gland. An abnormality in one of these hormones will suggest that ovarian dysfunction is the cause of infertility.

Ultrasound (for women; p. 147): With an ultrasound of the pelvis, anatomic abnormalities or infection in the ovary, uterus, or fallopian tubes can be seen.

Hysterosalpingogram (for women; p. 121): This test determines whether the fallopian tubes—which carry the eggs from the ovaries to the uterus—are blocked thereby preventing conception.

OTHER TESTS:
Laparoscopy (p. 163).
Testosterone (p. 69).
Blood glucose (p. 61).
Cervix culture (p. 167).
Kidney tests (p. 74).
Thyroid function tests (p. 69).

JAUNDICE

BACKGROUND: Jaundice is the yellow discoloration of the skin that results from an increase in the amount of bilirubin in the blood. Bilirubin (p. 45) is a by-product of the breakdown of old red blood cells. It is useful to think of jaundice (hyperbilirubinemia) as resulting from one of two major causes: either the body is making too much bilirubin (because it is destroying too many red cells), or it is making the usual amount but the liver is not able to excrete it properly. Most cases of jaundice in adults are due to liver and gallbladder diseases. In addition, the use of several medications can result in jaundice. Many newborn babies develop jaundice as well because their liver is not yet fully mature at the time of birth. Occasionally, jaundice in the newborn infant is due to a more serious cause, such as infection or a mismatch in blood groups between the baby and the mother.

TESTS COMMONLY OBTAINED FOR A PATIENT WITH JAUNDICE

Bilirubin (p. 45): This test is necessary to confirm that the yellow skin color is in fact due to an increase in the amount of bilirubin present in the blood and not due to another cause. A patient with

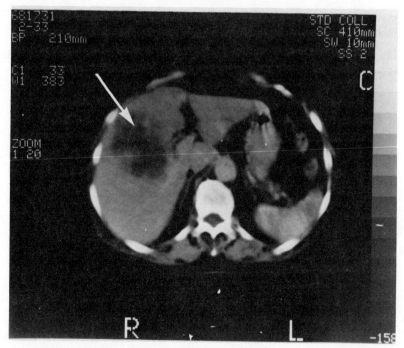

Abdominal CT scan in a 63-year-old man with cancer of the liver. Compare to the normal scan on page 29. The arrow points to the cancer.

jaundice may have this test done frequently so that the bilirubin level can be monitored over the course of his illness.

Liver function tests (LFTS, *p. 77*): Since the liver is critical to the excretion of bilirubin, these tests are also frequently obtained for the patient with jaundice because they provide the physician with key information about the status of that organ. If the liver function tests are abnormal, it usually means that disease in the liver or gallbladder—which drains the bilirubin from the liver—is the cause of the jaundice.

Complete blood count (CBC, *p. 51*) *and reticulocyte count* (*p. 81*): These tests are used to determine if excessive red blood cell destruction is the cause of the jaundice. In addition, some infectious causes of jaundice such as hepatitis may cause an elevation in the white blood cell count.

Prothrombin time (PT, *p. 80*): The various proteins involved in the clotting of blood are called clotting factors and are measured by this test. Since many of these clotting factors are made in the liver, it is a good test to determine if that organ is functioning properly.

Urinalysis (p. 87): The presence of bilirubin in the urine suggests certain kinds of liver or gallbladder disease as the cause of the jaundice. No bilirubin should be found in the urine if the jaundice is due to increased destruction of red blood cells.

Gallbladder x-rays (p. 119) and abdominal ultrasound (p. 147): These tests can be used to determine if gallstones are the cause of the jaundice.

Liver-spleen scan (p. 141): This is another test that helps to determine the presence of various kinds of liver disease.

OTHER TESTS:
Abdominal x-ray (KUB, p. 105).
Liver biopsy (p. 187).
Blood protein (p. 79).
Abdominal CT scan (p. 115).

LUMP IN THE BREAST

BACKGROUND: The thought of breast cancer is a frightening possibility for every woman—and with good reason. More than 100,000 new cases of breast cancer are discovered each year in the United States; in fact, 1 of 11 women will develop breast cancer in her lifetime. Furthermore, although new treatments are continually being developed, only 25% of patients with breast cancer are cured, and it remains the leading cause of death in the female population. Given these statistics, a breast lump requires prompt and careful investigation by the doctor even though all lumps are not malignant. Women less than 50 years old commonly have benign tumors called fibroadenoma and fibrocystic disease. When we order medical tests for a patient with a lump in her breast, the purpose is to distinguish between cancer and a benign condition. The specific tests we order will depend on a variety of factors, including the patient's age, any previous history of breast lumps, menstrual history, and family history of breast cancer.

TESTS COMMONLY OBTAINED FOR A PATIENT WITH A LUMP IN THE BREAST

Mammography and Xerography (p. 124): These x-ray techniques are able to detect cancer because of the difference on the picture between the tumor and the fatty tissue of the healthy breast. However, these tests are often not as helpful in examining the breasts of women under 50 because at that age there is less healthy fatty tissue present to contrast with a possible tumor.

Thermography (p. 221): Since cancer tissue has an increased blood flow, it is warmer than normal breast tissue. Any increase in breast temperature may be due to cancer. This test measures the temperature of the breasts and can be used to detect cancer. It is less accurate than mammography but does not have the radiation risk.

Breast self-exam (p. 345): When a lump is thought to be benign, we may ask the patient to observe it carefully over a period of time by doing frequent self-examinations. They will be useful to detect even small changes in the size and texture of the lump.

OTHER TESTS: These additional tests are performed once a breast lump has been determined to be cancerous in order to detect if the malignancy has spread to other parts of the body:
Bone scan (p. 133).
Liver-spleen scan (p. 141).
Chest x-ray (p. 113).
Calcium (p. 47).
Liver function tests (p. 77).
Brain scan (p. 135).
Brain CT scan (p. 115).

NAUSEA AND VOMITING

BACKGROUND: Vomiting is controlled by a specific region in the brain called the "vomiting center." Irritation within the abdomen, heart, gallbladder, and throat will send a message to this center, producing the sensation of nausea and resulting in vomiting. Medications and abnormalities in various body chemicals can also stimulate the "vomiting center."

TESTS COMMONLY OBTAINED FOR A PATIENT WITH NAUSEA OR VOMITING

Complete blood cell count (CBC, p. 51): Infections in the abdomen, ear, and brain, each of which can cause nausea and vomiting, will usually cause an elevation in the white blood cell count.

Pregnancy test (p. 214): The hormonal changes in a woman that accompany early pregnancy can cause stimulation of the "vomiting center."

Blood glucose (p. 61): A very high blood glucose can cause vomiting.

Liver function tests (LFTs, p. 77): When hepatitis is present, toxins are produced by the liver that can irritate the "vomiting center."

Electrolytes (p. 58): With prolonged vomiting, electrolytes (sodium, potassium, chloride) are lost from the body. This test is useful in ascertaining whether the blood levels of these electrolytes have become abnormal because of persistent vomiting.

Kidney tests (p. 74): The "vomiting center" can be stimulated by various toxins that accumulate in the body when the kidneys fail to function.

Upper GI series (UGI, p. 128): An ulcer or obstruction in the intestines irritates the abdomen and can lead to vomiting. This x-ray technique is useful in diagnosing these problems.

OTHER TESTS:
Gastroscopy (p. 162).
Hepatitis tests (p. 65).
Cortisol level (p. 68).
Arterial blood gases (p. 183).
Abdominal x-ray (KUB, p. 105).
Electrocardiogram (EKG, p. 193).
Brain CT scan (p. 115).
Lumbar puncture (p. 210).

SORE THROAT

BACKGROUND: There are many causes of a sore throat, including injury and irritation as well as infections caused by viruses or bacteria. The major aim we have in this situation is to diagnose the sore throat that is caused by infection with streptococcus bacteria ("strep throat") since, if left untreated, it can result in rheumatic fever. Unfortunately, simply examining the patient's throat does not enable us to distinguish between a sore throat caused by a virus and one caused by the strep bacteria since in both cases the throat appears red with pus covering the tonsils.

TESTS COMMONLY OBTAINED FOR A PATIENT WITH A SORE THROAT
Throat culture (p. 174): This test detects streptococcus bacteria as the cause of the sore throat.

Complete blood count (CBC, p. 51): A strep throat will usually cause an increase in the white blood cell count, while a sore throat from other causes (including viral infection) may not.

Mononucleosis test (p. 78): Occasionally, patients with a sore throat will have mononucleosis and a test for this illness will help to make that diagnosis. This test is usually done only if the throat culture is negative and the sore throat persists.

OTHER TESTS:
Chest x-ray (p. 113).
Gonorrhea culture (p. 172).

SWOLLEN GLANDS

BACKGROUND: Swollen glands—which are really enlarged lymph nodes—are composed of white blood cells. Since the main job of these cells is to protect the body against invading bacteria and viruses, swollen glands most frequently represent a temporary response of the body to a minor infection. Occasionally, however, swollen glands can be the first sign of more serious diseases, including tuberculosis, cancer, leukemia, lymphoma, rheumatoid arthritis, and acquired immunodeficiency syndrome (AIDS).

The major role of medical tests for the patient with swollen glands is to determine if they are due to a minor problem or to a more serious illness. The workup of the patient with swollen glands is a good example of where clear, logical thinking on the part of the health care team can have a significant impact on the proper use of medical tests. The issue basically comes down to this: Most patients with swollen glands do not have a serious illness; in fact, most would get better without medical treatment. On the other hand, a few patients may have swollen glands because of a very serious disease, like leukemia or cancer, and would benefit greatly from the correct diagnosis.

While a lymph node biopsy would quickly reveal the true nature of the swollen glands, it is an invasive test that carries with it some medical and psychological risk. What tests should be done before turning to a biopsy? Should some patients have a biopsy right away and others, only after a waiting period? The answers to these questions are complex and will vary among specific patients, based on their age, history, and physical examination. But for all patients with swollen glands, the following rule applies: before the workup starts, a clear order of testing should be determined as well as a plan of what to do based on each of the results.

TESTS COMMONLY OBTAINED FOR A PATIENT WITH SWOLLEN GLANDS
Complete blood count (CBC, p. 51): This is probably the most important test in the workup of a patient with swollen glands. It

will reveal the presence of infection (increased white blood cell count), inflammation, or allergies (increased eosinophil count) as well as malignancy (suggested by the presence of severe anemia).

Cultures (p. 167): Since infection is the most common cause of swollen glands, cultures are almost always obtained for a patient with this problem. The exact cultures that are done depend upon the specific site of the enlarged nodes within the body but frequently include throat culture (p. 174) and blood cultures (p. 170).

Erythrocyte sedimentation rate (ESR, p. 58): Inflammation and autoimmune diseases, such as rheumatoid arthritis and lupus erythematosus—which can cause swollen glands—are usually accompanied by an elevation in the sedimentation rate.

Mononucleosis test (p. 78): This test is done to determine if mononucleosis, a common cause of enlarged lymph nodes, is present.

Chest x-ray (p. 113): This test will be obtained if it is thought that the swollen glands might be due to cancer or tuberculosis.

Lymph node biopsy (p. 187): Ultimately, if all other medical tests have failed to reveal the specific cause for the enlarged lymph nodes, the patient will have a lymph node biopsy. This will enable the physician to see directly what is causing the nodes to be enlarged.

OTHER TESTS:
Antinuclear antibody (ANA, p. 45).
Rheumatoid factor (p. 45).
Allergy tests (p. 178).
Syphilis tests (p. 83).

WEIGHT LOSS

BACKGROUND: Although most everyone would love to be thinner, we always consider it a serious and worrisome sign when we see a patient who has lost weight without dieting. While the list of diseases causing weight loss is long, we divide patients with this problem into four categories. (1) *Decreased appetite* resulting in weight loss can be caused by medications, cancer, or psychological problems such as anorexia nervosa or depression. (2) *Difficulty in absorbing food* can be due to infection or diseases of the stomach or small intestines. (3) *Recurrent vomiting or diarrhea* results in weight loss because the patient is losing the necessary nutrients from the body. (4) *An overactive thyroid gland* will increase the body's metabolism and can also cause weight loss.

TESTS COMMONLY OBTAINED FOR A PATIENT WITH WEIGHT LOSS

Thyroid function tests (p. 69): An overactive thyroid gland causes the body to use more energy and will result in weight loss.

Digoxin level (p. 57): Excessive amounts of digoxin—a medicine commonly taken by patients with heart disease—cause a decrease in appetite resulting in weight loss.

Blood glucose (p. 61): Diabetes can also result in weight loss and can be determined by this test.

Stool fat (p. 95): Increased amounts of fat in the stool suggest poor intestinal absorption of food as the cause of the weight loss.

Complete blood count (CBC, p. 51): A low hematocrit frequently accompanies cancer and therefore might suggest that disease as the cause of the weight loss.

Erythrocyte sedimentation rate (ESR, p. 58): An increased ESR would indicate either cancer or an infection as the likely cause.

OTHER TESTS:
Liver funtion tests (LFTs, p. 77).
Kidney tests (p. 74).
Upper GI series (p. 128).
Barium enema (p. 109).
Calcium (p. 47).
Vitamin B12 and Schilling test (p. 84).

17

The Use of Medical Tests for Sixteen Common Diseases

ALLERGIES

BACKGROUND: The major purpose of your immune system is to react against anything in your body that should not be there. Your ability to fight off infections and reject transplanted organs are examples of the immune system at work. An allergy is a pathological reaction by the immune system to certain substances. Allergies are one of the oldest diseases ever recognized. The ancient Greeks recognized that some people would react to certain foods with hives and itching. But, in fact, allergies are not limited to food. People can develop allergies to almost anything with which they come into contact: chemicals, clothing, medicines, animals, molds, and insects. Allergic reactions can run the entire range from being very severe—as can occur with an anaphylactic allergic reaction to a bee sting—to being very mild. We use medical tests in the allergic patient for two reasons: to discover those substances (allergens) to which the patient is allergic, and to determine the severity of the allergy.

TESTS COMMONLY OBTAINED FOR A PATIENT WITH ALLERGIES

Allergy tests (p. 178): These tests are done to determine those specific substances to which the patient is allergic. There are two types of allergy tests:

Skin test (p. 179)—in which the potential allergens are tested on the patient's actual skin.

RAST (Radio-Allergo-Sorbent-Test) test (p. 179)—in which the test is conducted using the patient's blood.

Complete blood count (CBC, p. 51): Eosinophils are a type of white blood cell that are involved in certain allergic reactions. Therefore, these cells are measured in patients with allergies.

Pulmonary function tests (PFTS, p. 216): These tests are obtained since allergic reactions can lead to a lung problem or breathing difficulties like asthma.

OTHER TESTS:
Erythrocyte sedimentation rate (ESR, p. 58).

ANEMIA

BACKGROUND: Anemia is a decrease in the number of red cells in the blood. Since these red cells transport oxygen throughout the body, a patient who is anemic will often be tired easily. Anemia has many causes, some of which—like iron deficiency—are minor and easily treated, while others are life-threatening. For this reason, it is critical to discover the underlying cause of the anemia.

TESTS COMMONLY OBTAINED FOR A PATIENT WITH ANEMIA
When we first discover that a patient is anemic, we order these tests:

Complete blood count (CBC, p. 51): This test measures the number of red blood cells and, in addition, provides specific information concerning the size and shape of the red blood cells that will help determine the cause of the anemia.

Examination of the peripheral blood smear (p. 54): By looking at the red blood cells under the microscope, we can gain much information about their shape, which provides valuable clues about the cause of the anemia.

Bone marrow examination (p. 188): Like all blood cells, red blood cells are made in the bone marrow. Examination of the bone marrow will tell us if the anemia is present because of an abnormality in this "factory" where the cells are made. In addition, this test can be used to measure the amount of iron that is present in the body.

OTHER TESTS:
Based on the results from these first three tests, we may order some of the tests in the following table to determine a specific cause for the anemia.

Test	Possible Cause of the Anemia
Ferritin (p. 73).	Iron deficiency.
Serum iron (p. 73).	Iron deficiency.
Total iron binding capacity (p. 73).	Iron deficiency.
Hemoglobin electrophoresis (p. 82).	Thalassemia. Hemoglobinopathy. Sickle cell anemia.
Sickle cell test (p. 82).	Sickle cell anemia.
Red blood cell enzymes (p. 61).	Enzyme deficiencies.
Coombs' test (p. 55).	Immune hemolytic anemia.
Test for blood in stool (p. 96).	Gastrointestinal bleeding.
Urinalysis (p. 87).	Genitourinary bleeding. Intravascular hemolysis.
Folic acid (p. 84).	Megaloblastic anemia. Pernicious anemia. Folic acid deficiency.
Vitamin B12 (p. 84).	Megaloblastic anemia. Pernicious anemia. Vitamin B12 deficiency.
Schilling test (p. 84).	Megaloblastic anemia. Pernicious anemia.

Arthritis

BACKGROUND: Arthritis is not one illness but a group of more than one hundred different diseases, each of which causes damage in the joints of the body. Arthritis can affect young children as well as the elderly. Certain types of the disease tend to involve only one joint (infectious arthritis), while others can involve multiple joints (rheumatoid arthritis). Some arthritis is due to inflammation of the lining of the joint, which, in turn causes destruction of the underlying bone. In osteoarthritis—the most common type of arthritis—there is no inflammation but rather a "wear and tear" irritation of bones that have rubbed against each other over many years. This results in the roughening of the bony surfaces and leads to pain when the bones are moved. Because osteoarthritis is caused by this "wear and tear" process, it tends to occur in the elderly.

TESTS COMMONLY OBTAINED FOR A PATIENT WITH ARTHRITIS

Erythrocyte sedimentation rate (ESR, p. 58): Although an increase in the ESR does not help to diagnose the specific type of arthritis, it suggests inflammation (rheumatoid arthritis) and not "wear and tear" of the bone (osteoarthritis). Since the ESR will often decrease when rheumatoid arthritis is treated effectively, the test is also used to monitor therapy.

Rheumatoid factor (RF, p. 45): A positive test for the presence of rheumatoid factor suggests rheumatoid arthritis, although other causes of arthritis as well as nonarthritic diseases are associated with a positive result. In addition, some people with rheumatoid arthritis will have a negative rheumatoid factor.

Antinuclear antibody (ANA, p. 45): Although many types of arthritis are associated with elevated ANA titers, a high level will most often be due to lupus erythematosus, a form of arthritis that can also effect the lung, skin, heart, kidney, blood cells, and brain.

Bone x-rays (p. 98): X-rays will be used to reveal the extent and location of the bones damaged by the arthritis; they will also determine if treatment has been helpful in preventing further bone damage.

Arthrocentesis (p. 222): All of our joints are lubricated by a substance called synovial fluid. Certain types of arthritis that involve inflammation of the lining of the joint cause excessive production of synovial fluid resulting in swelling at the joint. Analysis of this synovial fluid will be useful in determining the specific type of arthritis that is present. A mild elevation in the synovial-fluid white blood cell count will suggest an inflammatory cause like rheumatoid arthritis, while an extremely high white blood cell count will suggest an infection. The synovial fluid is also sent for culture (p. 167) to see if an infection is present. The crystals of gout, another form of arthritis, can be seen in the fluid as well. After treatment of infectious arthritis, the synovial fluid will be analyzed to see if the white blood cell count has diminished and if the infection has been adequately treated. The synovial fluid is obtained by arthrocentesis.

OTHER TESTS:
Immune system tests (p. 71).
Bone scan (p. 133).

Complete blood count (CBC, p. 51).
HLA typing (p. 66).

ASTHMA

BACKGROUND: Asthma results from a narrowing of the airways (bronchi) in the lungs. This condition can be caused by infections, allergies, or emotional stress. In addition, a small number of patients develop asthma following vigorous exercise. Patients with asthma will usually have wheezing and whistling sounds during breathing (caused by the passage of air through the constricted airways), cough, excessive sputum, and shortness of breath. We use medical tests in a patient with asthma to determine the etiology and severity of the attack as well as to monitor the response to therapy.

TESTS COMMONLY OBTAINED FOR A PATIENT WITH ASTHMA

Pulmonary function tests (PFTS, p. 216): This test measures how well the lungs are working. Because patients with asthma generally have a more difficult time exhaling (breathing out) than inhaling (breathing in), two of these pulmonary function tests are used frequently: the peak flow rate, which measures the fastest rate of exhaling that a patient can achieve; and the FEV1, which measures the amount of air a person can exhale in one second.

Chest x-ray (p. 113): This is done to see if the asthma is caused by pneumonia.

Arterial blood gases (ABGS, p. 183): This test measures how well the lungs are working by determining the amount of oxygen and carbon dioxide that is carried by the blood as it travels through the arteries. It is difficult for a patient with asthma to exchange carbon dioxide for oxygen, so the carbon dioxide accumulates within the body. Consequently, if the asthma attack is very severe, the carbon dioxide level is higher than normal and the oxygen level lower than usual.

Complete blood count (CBC, p. 51): This test is used when an infection is suspected as the cause of the asthma. An elevation of the white blood cell count suggests that a bacterial infection is present. In addition, the eosinophil count may be higher than normal if the asthma is related to an allergic condition.

Theophylline level (p. 56): One of the most commonly used drugs in the treatment of patients with asthma is theophylline. If the level of the drug in the blood is too high, patients can experience a rapid heart rate, nausea, vomiting, and nervousness or restlessness. Most patients who take theophylline will have the level of the drug in their blood checked periodically to be sure that it is at a safe yet effective level.

OTHER TESTS:
Allergy tests (p. 178).
Sputum culture (p. 173).

CANCER

BACKGROUND: Cancer is not one disease but a collection of more than a hundred different diseases, all characterized by the uncontrollable growth of tumors. At the time that the diagnosis is first made, we will use medical tests to "stage" the patient's cancer. This process will measure the exact size and location of the tumor as well as determine if it has spread throughout the body. Following the staging process, a decision will be made as to the best therapy with which to treat the cancer. We will then use medical tests to monitor the therapy to see if it is working and if it is causing any serious side effects in the patient. Finally, if the patient is in remission and the tumor is no longer evident, medical tests will be used periodically to determine if the cancer has returned.

TESTS COMMONLY OBTAINED FOR A PATIENT WITH CANCER
Biopsy (p. 187): This test is done at some point with every cancer patient because it actually makes the specific diagnosis. It allows the physician to remove a piece of the tumor and examine it under the microscope to determine if it is cancerous, and, if so, the kind of malignancy.

One or more of the following tests are done—depending upon the symptoms—in an effort to find out where the cancer started as well as where it has spread. In addition, these tests monitor for the return of the cancer once the patient is in remission.
X-rays (p. 98).
CT scans (p. 115).
Ultrasound (p. 145).
Digital subtraction angiography (DSA, p. 118).
Nuclear medicine scans (p. 132).
Endoscopy (p. 153): These tests allow the physician to see the tumor directly; depending upon the site of the cancer, he could use one or several different kinds of scopes.

Complete blood count (CBC, p. 51): This test might be performed for a variety of reasons. Patients who are receiving chemotherapy might have the test done to ensure that the drugs haven't caused the patient to become anemic or develop a dangerously low white blood cell count. At other times a CBC might be obtained to see if the patient has developed an infection, which might be characterized by the presence of an elevated white blood cell count. Finally, in certain cases of cancer, the CBC will be done to ensure that the tumor has not spread into the bone marrow, causing abnormalities in the number and kind of blood cells that are present.

OTHER TESTS:
Urinalysis (p. 87).
Test for blood in stool (p. 96).
Liver function tests (LFTS, p. 77).
Carcinoembryonic antigen (CEA, p. 50).
Erythrocyte sedimentation rate (ESR, p. 58).
Cytology (p. 192).

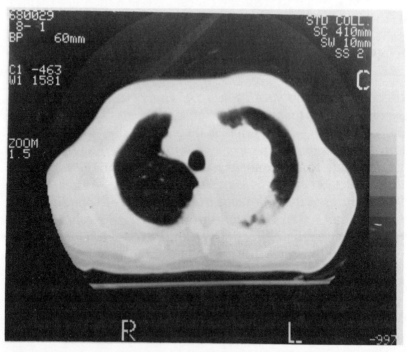

CT scan of the chest in a patient with lung cancer. The black area on the R side of the chest is normal lung. The white area growing into the lung on the L side is the cancer.

CHRONIC BRONCHITIS AND EMPHYSEMA

BACKGROUND: These diseases occur most frequently in people who have smoked cigarettes for many years. In chronic bronchitis, which is an inflammation of the airways in the lungs, the patient almost always has a chronic cough with phlegm production. In emphysema, a condition in which the delicate tissues of the lung degenerate, the person's major complaint is shortness of breath. In both of these diseases there is progressive destruction of healthy lung tissue. This makes it more difficult for the lung to carry out its normal function of exchanging carbon dioxide from the body for oxygen from the air. When we see a patient with these types of lung disease, we order medical tests both to diagnose the specific disease and to monitor its severity.

TESTS COMMONLY OBTAINED FOR A PATIENT WITH CHRONIC BRONCHITIS AND EMPHYSEMA

Chest x-ray (p. 113): A chest x-ray will reveal how much damage has occurred as a result of these diseases. In addition, since people with chronic bronchitis and emphysema frequently develop pneumonia, a chest x-ray will be obtained if these people become increasingly short of breath or develop fever.

Arterial blood gases (ABGS, p. 183): This test will monitor whether the lung is still capable of exchanging oxygen and carbon dioxide efficiently. In severe bronchitis or emphysema, carbon dioxide will accumulate in the body and the level will increase. The amount of oxygen in the blood will decrease as well.

Pulmonary function tests (PFTS, p. 216): Pulmonary function tests will also monitor the respiratory disability that occurs with these diseases. These tests might be repeated frequently to determine if the disease has improved or worsened.

OTHER TESTS:
Sputum culture (p. 173).
Complete blood count (CBC, p. 51).
Electrocardiogram (EKG, p. 193).
Lung scan (p. 142).

THE COMMON COLD AND FLU

BACKGROUND: The common cold is always caused by a virus. Because many different types of virus can cause the symptoms of running nose, sore throat, fever, and cough, the exact type of virus cannot be determined. Most of these episodes, commonly called URIS (upper respiratory infections), resolve in a few days and rarely require a visit to the doctor. The symptoms of the common cold, however, are sometimes difficult to distinguish from pneumonia, strep throat, and ear infections, which require different treatments. When we see a person with a cold that has persisted for an unusually long period of time or that is very severe, we sometimes do tests to exclude these other possible diseases. In addition, a viral URI that persists makes a person more susceptible to bacterial infections, such as pneumonia, sinusitis, or ear infections.

TESTS COMMONLY OBTAINED FOR A PATIENT WITH THE COMMON COLD AND FLU

Complete blood count (CBC, p. 51): An elevated white blood cell count will suggest an infection caused by bacteria, such as strep throat or bacterial pneumonia, rather than a viral URI.

Throat culture (p. 174). Frequently, a throat culture is obtained to exclude infection caused by the streptococcal bacteria.

Chest x-ray (p. 113): Because bacterial and viral pneumonias can cause symptoms similar to the common cold, a chest x-ray is sometimes helpful in detecting pneumonia. On the x-ray film, pneumonia would appear as a white area in the normally black region of the lung; a simple cold would not change the appearance of a chest x-ray.

Sinus x-ray (p. 98): An infection of the sinuses can cause symptoms similar to the common cold. Sinus x-rays will show signs of inflammation (white areas on the x-ray) if infection is present.

OTHER TESTS:

Tuberculosis skin test (p. 224).

DEMENTIA

BACKGROUND: Dementia is the slow but progressive loss of intellectual function that can affect a patient's judgement, speech, or memory. Though dementia may begin as short memory lapses, slight confusion, or difficulty articulating, in its final stages it can cause total disruption in the life of a patient as well as those in his family. Although most people think of severe dementia as afflicting only the elderly (a condition called senile dementia), it can occur in younger people as well. Unfortunately, most people under the age of 60 with dementia have Alzheimer's disease, an incurable form of dementia that is almost identical to the senile dementia of the elderly. There is no effective medical treatment available for either senile dementia or Alzheimer's disease. Some patients with dementia, however, do not have either of these diseases but rather have conditions that can be successfully treated. The purpose of medical tests for patients with dementia is to distinguish those with incurable forms of dementia (senile dementia and Alzheimer's disease) from those with treatable forms of the disease.

TESTS COMMONLY OBTAINED FOR A PATIENT WITH DEMENTIA

Thyroid function tests (p. 69): Elderly persons who have an underactive thyroid gland (hypothyroid) can develop a loss of memory, impairment in judgment, and inability to care for themselves.

Vitamin B12 (p. 84): Inadequate amounts of this vitamin in the diet can cause anemia (megaloblastic anemia) as well as symptoms of dementia.

Syphilis test (p. 83): Untreated syphilis can cause symptoms similar to dementia. Although the doctor's physical examination will often detect abnormalities suggestive of syphilis, this test should always be performed on patients of any age with symptoms of dementia because, if found, it is a treatable form.

Brain CT scan (p. 115): Old strokes, tumors in the brain, or shrinkage (atrophy) of brain tissue can be detected by this technique. Brain atrophy is commonly found in Alzheimer's disease.

Lumbar puncture (p. 210): Analysis of the spinal fluid will be able to check for syphilis, tumor cells, chronic infection, and abnormal brain pressures—all causes of dementia.

Electroencephalogram (EEG, p. 197): Although the EEG is usually normal in dementia, abnormal patterns suggest that a tumor, excessive medication, or epilepsy is the cause of the disease.

OTHER TESTS:

Complete blood count (CBC, p. 51).
Liver function tests (LFTs, p. 77).
Electrolytes (p. 58).
Kidney function tests (p. 74).
Calcium (p. 47).

Diabetes Mellitus

BACKGROUND: Your body's metabolism of glucose, the sugar most important for energy, is carefully regulated by the hormone insulin, which allows glucose to go from the blood into the cells of the body. When the regulation of glucose metabolism breaks down, diabetes develops. Clinical diabetes refers to people who are symptomatic from the disease, such as those who complain of thirst or excessive urination. Chemical diabetes, on the other hand, refers to people who are asymptomatic but have high blood sugar levels because of poor sugar and insulin regulation. Most of the medical tests that are used for a patient with diabetes are done to monitor the glucose level in the blood.

There is considerable controversy in the medical profession over how tightly controlled a diabetic's blood glucose level should be. Some doctors believe that the blood glucose level should be kept as close as possible to normal (100 mg / dl) so the diabetic will not develop the usual pattern of complications (blindness, kidney disease, circulation problems). Other doctors maintain that this approach is both unnecessary—in that the complications will develop regardless of the sugar level—and possibly even dangerous in that a patient may take so much insulin in an effort to keep the glucose level down that the sugar level will drop to dangerously low levels. All doctors agree, however, that frequent monitoring of sugar levels in the blood and urine, both by the doctor as well as by the diabetic at home (p. 342), is important in the management of this disease.

TESTS COMMONLY OBTAINED FOR A PATIENT WITH DIABETES MELLITUS

Blood glucose (p. 61): A blood glucose is obtained frequently in diabetics to monitor the effectiveness of their treatment and to make sure the blood sugar has not become too low from the insulin that is taken. A blood glucose level is also the usual method of screening patients for diabetes.

Glucose tolerance test (GTT, p. 61): People who have normal blood glucose levels can still have diabetes. The glucose tolerance test stresses the body's ability to release maximal amounts of insulin and will detect diabetes even before any symptoms appear.

Hemoglobin (A1C, p. 64): A normal value indicates that the person's blood glucose has been well controlled during the previous three to four weeks. An abnormal value will indicate poor glucose control.

Urine glucose (p. 89): This simple urine test enables the individual to monitor the glucose level at home. A high value indicates poor glucose control, while the absence of glucose in the urine indicates good glucose control.

OTHER TESTS:
Arterial blood gases (ABGS, p. 183).
Electrolytes (p. 58).
Home blood glucose monitoring (p. 342).

HEART ATTACK

BACKGROUND: In order for your heart to work properly, it needs oxygen. When the blood vessels that carry blood to the heart muscle do not supply the amount of oxygen that is needed, a person will experience a suffocating-like chest pain called angina pectoris. This decreased oxygen supply to the heart can be caused by a blockage in the blood vessels by fatty deposits (atherosclerosis) or by a temporary clamping (spasm) of the vessels. When the lack of oxygen to the heart persists, actual death of heart muscle can result. This is what is known as a heart attack (myocardial infarction). If the patient survives the heart attack, scar tissue will develop in place of the dead heart muscle. Although not every patient with chest pain is having a heart attack, it is the disease with which we are most concerned. The purpose of tests for a patient with a presumed heart attack is to document that the heart attack has actually happened and to determine how much heart muscle has died.

TESTS COMMONLY OBTAINED FOR A PATIENT WITH A HEART ATTACK
Electrocardiogram (EKG, p. 193): Actual death of heart muscle (myocardial infarction) gives a different pattern on the cardiogram than does a temporary decrease in the oxygen supply to the heart muscle (ischemia). Therefore, the cardiogram can be used to distinguish both these problems. In addition, if it has been determined that a heart attack has occurred, the EKG will locate the specific area involved and help measure how much muscle has died.

Heart enzymes (p. 63): Certain enzymes (SGOT, CPK, LDH) are found in normal heart muscle. When the heart muscle fibers are damaged, these enzymes, which are normally found only in low concentrations in the blood, leak out of the muscle and are then found in large quantities in the blood. These blood tests can help determine whether the actual death of heart muscle has occurred. They are also useful in determining how much heart muscle has been destroyed as well as when heart muscle damage stops.

Chest x-ray (p. 113): A heart attack can be accompanied by serious complications such as fluid in the lung from an inability of the heart to pump blood efficiently (congestive heart failure). The chest x-ray is obtained to see if any of these complications has occurred.

Exercise tolerance test (p. 202): This is frequently obtained several weeks after the heart attack and will help determine how much exercise the patient can safely do in the future.

OTHER TESTS:
Cardiac catheterization (p. 111).
Heart scans (p. 138).
Serum lipids (p. 76).

HYPERTENSION

BACKGROUND: Blood pressure is the measurement of the force with which your heart pumps blood throughout your body. Hypertension is present when the blood pressure is elevated above the normal range. Over fifteen million people in this country are being treated for hypertension, and it is believed that there are just as many people with the disease who have not yet been diagnosed. Most patients with hypertension do not complain of symptoms, although if left untreated hypertension can cause heart attacks, strokes, and kidney damage. When we see a patient with hypertension, we generally do not discover a specific cause although occasionally a disturbance in hormones or anatomy is diagnosed. Obesity, stress, and excessive salt in the diet may also contribute to the development of high blood pressure.

TESTS COMMONLY OBTAINED FOR A PATIENT WITH HYPERTENSION
Electrocardiogram (EKG, p. 193): With severe hypertension the walls of the heart become thicker and it cannot pump efficiently. The EKG can measure how thick the walls of the heart have become (a condition called hypertrophy) as well as whether any permanent heart damage has occurred.

Electrolytes (p. 58): Certain hormonal disturbances that cause hypertension can also result in abnormalities in the blood potassium level. Therefore low potassium levels will suggest one of these causes of hypertension. Also, many diuretics that are used to treat hypertension will cause a decrease in potassium levels. Consequently, it is important to monitor the blood potassium level once diuretic therapy has been started.

Kidney Tests (p. 74): The elevated blood pressures seen in patients with hypertension can damage the kidney as the blood flows through that delicate organ. These tests will be used to evaluate whether this has occurred. They will also be used when the patient is being treated with diuretics, which can also alter kidney function.

Chest x-ray (p. 113): Hypertension can also be caused by a narrowing in the aorta, the largest artery in the body. Although this narrowing is not itself evident on an x-ray, it can cause irregularities in the rib cage, which can be seen on a regular chest x-ray. A chest x-ray is of value, therefore, to see if this anatomical cause of hypertension is present. Also, since the size of the heart can be measured by chest x-ray, it is useful in determining if the hypertension has caused any heart damage.

Intravenous pyelogram (IVP, p. 121): A narrowing of the artery that supplies the kidney is another cause of hypertension. This test will detect this abnormality.

OTHER TESTS:
Cortisol (p. 68).
Urine vanillylmandelic acid (VMA, p. 93).
Kidney Scan (p. 140).
Urinalysis (p. 87).

PNEUMONIA

BACKGROUND: Pneumonia means an inflammation of the lungs. Although most people think pneumonia results from infection, the inflammation can be caused by many different factors, including inhalation of certain irritants, such as smoke or fumes from chemicals. Pneumonia due to infection can be caused by bacteria, viruses, or mycoplasma, another type of disease-producing organism. Mild pneumonia—usually due to infection with viruses or mycoplasma—is sometimes called walking pneumonia. Pneumonia can range in severity from mild to life-threatening. When we see a patient with pneumonia, we use medical tests to answer three questions:

1. What is the cause of the pneumonia?
2. How extensive is the pneumonia?
3. Is the patient responding to treatment and getting better?

TESTS COMMONLY OBTAINED FOR A PATIENT WITH PNEUMONIA

Chest x-ray (p. 113): The chest x-ray enables the physician to "see" the inflammation in the lung. Since a normal lung contains mostly air, it will appear black on a chest x-ray. When a patient has pneumonia, the inflammation that is present appears white. By looking at a chest x-ray, we can both pinpoint the location of the pneumonia as well as see how large an area of lung is affected. After a patient has been on treatment, we will usually repeat the chest x-ray to see if the pneumonia is getting better.

Complete blood count (CBC, p. 51): The white blood cell count and differential, obtained as part of a CBC, help the physician determine the specific cause of the pneumonia. This is because each of the various causes of pneumonia is associated with a different white blood cell pattern. Since the blood count will return to normal as the patient improves, this test is also useful in evaluating the response to treatment.

Culture and Gram stain of sputum (p. 173): This test also provides information concerning the specific cause of the pneumonia. If the disease is due to a bacterial infection, culture and Gram stain of the sputum will demonstrate its presence. If bacteria are not found in the sputum, it is likely that the pneumonia has another cause.

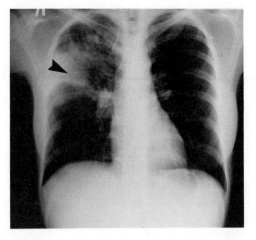

Chest x-ray from a patient with pneumonia. Compare to the normal chest x-ray on page 115. The arrow points to the white area of pneumonia.

OTHER TESTS:
Arterial blood gases (ABGS p. 183).
Tuberculosis skin test (p. 224).
Infectious disease antibody titers (p. 72).

Sexually Transmitted Disease (STD) or Venereal Disease

BACKGROUND: Until recently, when one thought of venereal disease, only syphilis and gonorrhea were considered. It is now known that many other types of infections, such as hepatitis and herpes, are transmitted through sexual contact. Often the patient with a sexually transmitted disease complains of symptoms such as a discharge (vaginal or penile) or irritation, but occasionally there are no symptoms at all. Infection with many other organisms can also cause venereal disease: chlamydia, which produces a discharge from the penis in men; herpes, which results in small ulcers on the penis or vagina; and other viruses that cause warts found on the genitalia. Most of these viruses are not routinely identified by tests that are presently available.

Unlike gonorrhea and syphilis, which are easily treated with antibiotics, these sexually-transmitted viruses are much more difficult to treat. Other diseases, such as hepatitis or acquired immunodeficiency syndrome (AIDS), can also be transmitted through sexual contact, but the symptoms occur in parts of the body other than the genitalia. AIDS, which occurs primarily in male homosexuals (although other people such as drug abusers, hemophiliacs, and Haitians also appear to be at increased risk), results in an inability of the body to fight infection. In addition to developing cancer, many people suffering from AIDS will contract life-threatening infections. The death rate from the disease is approaching 75%.

TESTS COMMONLY OBTAINED FOR A PATIENT WITH A VENEREAL DISEASE

Syphilis test (p. 83): A positive test usually indicates the presence of syphilis. Occasionally, however, other diseases such as lupus erythematosus can cause a false-positive test. After the patient is treated for syphilis, the test is repeated to be sure the treatment has been adequate.

Culture for gonorrhea (p. 172): If gonorrhea is present in the genital area, throat, or rectum, a properly prepared culture (Thayer-

Martin type) will grow the bacteria that cause the disease. This special culture medium is necessary because these bacteria—Neisseria gonorrhoeae—die quickly and will not grow in regular cultures.

Immune system tests (p. 71): Patients in whom the diagnosis of AIDS is being considered will have various tests done to monitor the status of their immune system. These people appear to have too many of the white cells that suppress the immune system (suppressor T-cells) and not enough of the type that stimulates the immune system (helper T-cells).

OTHER TESTS:
Hepatitis test (p. 65).
Liver function tests (LFTS, p. 77).
Vaginal culture (p. 167).
Pap smear (p. 212).

STROKE

BACKGROUND: A stroke (cerebral vascular accident or CVA) is usually caused by the sudden blockage of the blood vessels that supply the brain, resulting in the death of brain tissue. In some instances the blood vessel is not blocked but ruptures instead, and bleeding occurs within the brain. In either case the location of the damaged vessel in the brain will determine the symptoms that result. Occasionally, only temporary slurring of speech will occur, while other times there is loss of consciousness and even death. This blockage of the brain's blood vessels can be caused by fatty deposits in the vessel wall or by blood clots that break loose from the heart or elsewhere in the body. We use medical tests for a patient who has had a stroke to determine where the stroke has occurred and how large an area of the brain has been affected.

TESTS COMMONLY OBTAINED FOR A PATIENT WITH A STROKE
Brain CT scan (p. 115): This technique helps determine the site of the brain injury caused by the stroke as well as whether there has been bleeding associated with it.

Angiography (p. 106) and Digital Subtraction Angiography (DSA) (p. 118).: These procedures will determine the site of the damaged artery in the brain.

Echocardiography (p. 150): This test will be used to see if there are blood clots in the heart that may have dislodged and caused the stroke.

OTHER TESTS:
Doppler ultrasound (p. 149).
Blood cultures (p. 170).
Holter monitor (p. 206).
Brain scan (p. 135).
Electroencephalogram (EEG, p. 197).

ULCERS

BACKGROUND: An ulcer is a sore in the lining of the stomach or the first portion of the small intestine (duodenum). This damage usually results from increased amounts of stomach acids, although it can also be caused by certain drugs, such as aspirin or steroids. Frequently, ulcer pain is worse on an empty stomach and disappears after a meal is eaten. The initial treatment for ulcers is usually a combination of antacids and drugs called H2 blockers (e.g., Tagamet and Zantac), which decrease stomach acid production. In addition, patients who smoke will be urged to stop. With this therapy most ulcers disappear in a few weeks. Surgery may be necessary if the ulcers recur, especially if associated with bleeding. Although most ulcers are benign, ulcers in the stomach can occasionally be a sign of cancer. Tests are performed in the patient with ulcers to see the location and size of the ulcer and to determine if the ulcer is bleeding. After treatment many patients will have some of these tests repeated to check that the ulcer has resolved.

TESTS COMMONLY OBTAINED FOR A PATIENT WITH ULCERS
Complete blood count (CBC, p. 51): A hematocrit will indicate whether bleeding from the ulcer has occurred.
Upper GI series (p. 128): The location and size of the ulcer can be seen with this x-ray technique. Frequently, this test is repeated after treatment to check if the ulcer has disappeared.
Gastroscopy (p. 162): The ulcer itself can be seen by the doctor with endoscopy. This will enable him to do a biopsy, if necessary, to determine whether the ulcer is benign or malignant. Endoscopy is also used to ascertain if the treatment has been successful and the ulcer has healed.
Test for blood in stool (p. 96): The stool is checked to see if bleeding from the ulcer is taking place.

OTHER TESTS:
Gastric fluid analysis (p. 205).

URINARY TRACT INFECTION

BACKGROUND: The urinary tract refers to the kidneys, ureters (tubes between the kidneys and the bladder), bladder, and urethra (tube between the bladder and the outside)—those organs that are involved in the making and passing of urine. An infection in any part of the tract will often result in frequent urination (polyuria) as well as burning and itching with urination (dysuria). Urinary tract infections occur more commonly in women that in men because their urethra is shorter, allowing bacteria and viruses on the skin surface to enter and grow in the urinary tract.

TESTS COMMONLY OBTAINED FOR A PATIENT WITH A URINARY TRACT INFECTION

Urine culture and sensitivity (p. 175): A urine culture is the best way to diagnose a bacterial infection in the urinary tract. It will also identify which bacteria are present and which antibiotics will work to kill the bacteria. Once a person has taken antibiotics, the urine culture will be repeated to check that the bacteria have been eliminated.

Urinalysis (p. 87): The presence in the urine of white and red blood cells suggests an infection. If bacteria are seen during the urinalysis, a Gram stain (p. 167) may be done to better identify them, although only a culture and not a urinalysis can pinpoint the specific bacteria that are causing the infection. After a urine infection has been treated, the doctor may repeat the urinalysis to see if the white and red cells have disappeared, suggesting that the infection is gone.

Complete blood count (CBC, p. 51): A bacterial infection in the urinary tract will often cause an elevation in the white blood cell count.

Intravenous pyelogram (IVP, p. 121): If a urinary tract infection is not eliminated with antibiotic treatment or if a person has recurrent infections, it suggests to us that there may be an anatomic abnormality in the urinary tract that will predispose the patient to infection. An IVP will be used to determine if this is the case.

OTHER TESTS:
Ultrasound (p. 145).
Kidney tests (p. 74).

PART VI

Medical Tests You Can Do Yourself

18

Medical Tests You Can Do Yourself

Why Do Medical Tests Yourself?

In Chapter 1 of this book we took you on rounds with us as we saw some of our patients. This time let's look in on some other patients in their homes. Mary K., a 64-year-old woman with diabetes, is testing her urine for the presence of sugar. She takes two injections of insulin a day—one in the morning and another before supper. The amount of insulin she uses in this second injection will vary, depending upon how much glucose she finds in her urine.

Two blocks away from her lives Ed O., a 42-year-old dentist. Ed suffered a heart attack three years ago. Since that time he has been on a vigorous aerobic exercise program. At this moment he is using an exercise bicycle and intermittently checking his pulse to be sure it is at the optimal rate—fast enough to stress his body but not so fast as to be a danger.

Next door to him lives Faye G., a 39-year-old housewife. Faye's latest menstrual period stopped one week ago. This morning during her shower she performed a careful breast self-examination, looking for any unusual lumps or other abnormalities.

What we have successfully taught these three patients is that concern with your health cannot end once you leave your doctor's office. Health maintenance is a full-time job that only you can perform. Furthermore, there are many things you can do at home that will provide important information necessary to monitor your well-being. This information will assist your doctor in giving you the best care possible. The number of medical tests that can be performed at home has increased in recent years, and it is likely that many more will become available in the near future. It is important that any unusual or unexpected results from these tests be shared with your physician, who is best able to interpret them and decide whether further testing is necessary. This can avoid misinterpretation as well as needless worry. We want to emphasize that performing tests at home is not a substitute for having a good relationship with a physician. Rather, home tests will improve the care your doctor can give to you.

In this chapter we will describe the most important tests that can be performed at home. In addition, we have included several aspects of self-examination, which serve an important screening function. These self-examination tests can be performed more frequently than your routine physical examination with your doctor and are helpful both in diagnosing new diseases and in monitoring the treatment of known diseases. This chapter is not meant to provide detailed information on how to examine all the different parts of your body. Nor is it intended to reiterate tests previously discussed in this book that, although conducted in part at home, require laboratory analysis.

Remember that the single most important thing you can do at home to improve your health care is immediately report to your doctor any significant changes in your physical condition. This should include changes in your body (e.g., swollen glands, breast lumps, skin rashes, pains, or vision difficulties) as well as in bodily functions (such as blood in stool, abnormal menstrual cycle, shortness of breath). As we have said before, health maintenance is a full-time job and you are the only one who spends full-time with your body.

BLOOD PRESSURE

PURPOSE OF THE TEST: to check for hypertension and measure how hard the heart is working.

BACKGROUND: Hypertension is a silent killer. It most often does not cause early symptoms or indicate its presence. If left untreated, elevated blood pressure can cause stroke, heart disease, and kidney disease. It is important to screen carefully for elevated blood pressure so that appropriate treatment can be started immediately to prevent these complications. Once treatment has started, repeated blood pressure readings are important to monitor the results of therapy.

HOW THE TEST IS DONE: Many different devices have become available during the past several years to permit blood pressure to be

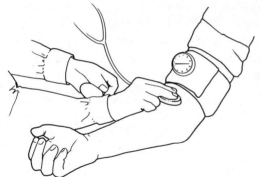

A wife taking her husband's blood pressure. Her left hand is squeezing the bulb that blows up the cuff, while her right hand is positioning the stethoscope over the brachial artery to listen to the flow of blood.

measured at home. In comparison to the conventional blood pressure equipment, the newer electronic blood pressure kits are easier to use (a stethoscope is not needed) but are also more expensive and more susceptible to problems in calibration. Before you use the blood pressure kit, read the details in the booklet that accompanies it because every device requires different instructions. Perhaps most importantly, your doctor should ensure that you are using the blood pressure device properly and that it provides an accurate reading. Blood pressure should be obtained while you are resting comfortably in a sitting position, with the device applied directly against your bare skin.

HOW TO INTERPRET THE RESULTS: The blood pressure reading consists of two numbers, the systolic and diastolic pressures. The systolic pressure—the higher number—measures how hard the heart is working when it contracts, while the diastolic pressure measures the efforts of the heart while it is resting between beats. A blood pressure reading is recorded as the systolic over diastolic pressures—for example, 120 / 80 (read as "one-twenty over eighty"). It is important to realize that the blood pressure varies during the day; one blood pressure reading that is elevated does not by itself indicate hypertension. Normal blood pressure depends on many factors, including a person's sex, age, weight, and state of health. Be sure to ask your doctor what he thinks is a normal blood pressure for you so that you can recognize when the pressures you take at home are elevated.

SYMPTOMS FOR WHICH THIS TEST SHOULD BE PERFORMED AT HOME: Headache (p. 297).

DISEASES FOR WHICH THIS TEST SHOULD BE PERFORMED AT HOME: Hypertension (p. 320)—When your doctor has diagnosed your disease as hypertension, you can measure the blood pressure at home to help him monitor therapy. But this home test should not be a substitute for physician care; instead, it should help your doctor manage your hypertension. Regular visits to him are important even if you use a blood pressure kit at home.

COST: approximately $75 for a standard blood pressure apparatus.

PULSE

PURPOSE OF THE TEST: to measure the heart rate.

BACKGROUND: Pulse is the measure of the number of heart beats that occurs in one minute. As your heart contracts with each beat, a wave of blood is sent through the arteries of your body. Those arteries located near the skin will transmit this wave as a pulse that can be felt. Veins, on the other hand, do not transmit pulse waves. Your pulse is not a constant number but varies greatly with the activity that is being performed and your overall health: your pulse might be 60 when resting and 160 when exercising. Even your resting pulse will vary from day to day.

HOW THE TEST IS DONE: The arteries located near the skin that permit the pulse to be obtained are shown in the illustration. They include the radial artery (on the thumb side of the underside of

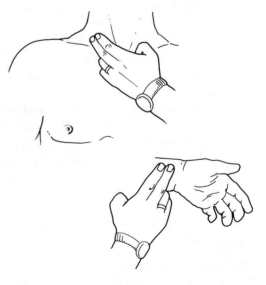

The bottom drawing shows the proper location of the fingers for obtaining a pulse rate from the radial artery in the wrist, while the top drawing shows where to take the pulse from the carotid artery in the neck.

the wrist), the carotid artery (next to the Adam's apple in the neck), and femoral artery (in the groin). The wrist artery is most commonly used. When you take your pulse, you should not use your own thumb to check it since the thumb has a pulse of its own that will interfere with the measurements. Place the first two fingers of one hand on the radial artery; count the number of beats in thirty seconds and multiply by two to get the pulse (heart beats per minute). In addition, note whether the rhythm of the beats is regular (the beats occurring at regular intervals) or irregular (the beats occurring at unevenly spaced intervals).

HOW TO INTERPRET THE RESULTS: A normal resting pulse is regular with the following rate:

Newborn infants—110–150.

Children under age 12—80–120.

Children over age 12 and adults—60–100.

As we explained in the chapter describing the effect of exercise on medical tests, a person who runs regularly or does other aerobic exercise may have a resting pulse in the 40s and 50s. With activity, the pulse rate can rise to a level of 150 to 195.

SYMPTOMS FOR WHICH THIS TEST SHOULD BE PERFORMED AT HOME:

Palpitations—Feeling the pulse will detect irregular heart beats that can cause palpitations. Your doctor may perform further tests to determine if these irregular beats are dangerous.

Exercise monitoring—The maximal benefit to a person's heart from vigorous exercise will occur only if the pulse achieves a fast heart rate. A patient's specific pulse goal must be determined after discussion with his physician, but a commonly used formula is:

$$(220 - \text{your age}) \times .75.$$

For example, a 20-year-old should strive to achieve a pulse of 150 during exercise ($220 - 20 = 200 \times .75 = 150$), while a 60-year-old should aim for 120 ($220 - 60 = 160 \times .75 = 120$). Once your goal has been determined, measuring the pulse during exercise can tell you if the desired heart rate has been obtained. Almost as important as the rate that your heart can achieve during exercise is how quickly it returns to its resting rate when exercise is stopped. Therefore, besides measuring the pulse during exercise to determine if it reaches the desired goal, you should measure your pulse two and five minutes after exercise is concluded. A healthy heart should return to its pre-exercise pulse two minutes and no later than five minutes after you are done exercising.

DISEASES FOR WHICH THIS TEST SHOULD BE PERFORMED AT HOME:
Heart disease—Two medications used to treat heart disease, digoxin and propranolol, will cause slowing of the heart rate. By taking the pulse periodically, a patient can monitor the medication's effect on his body and report unusual pulse changes to the doctor. It is important to remember that during an actual heart attack the patient's pulse will be normal or only slightly increased, and, therefore, checking the pulse cannot indicate if a heart attack has occurred.

RESPIRATORY RATE

PURPOSE OF THE TEST: to measure the number of breaths taken per minute.

BACKGROUND: The major function of your lungs is to exchange the carbon dioxide that has accumulated in your body for fresh oxygen from the air. The cycle of inspiration (bringing in oxygen) and expiration (removing carbon dioxide) constitutes one breath. Although counting the number of breaths seems simple to do, it is very difficult to obtain an accurate respiratory rate yourself since you will probably alter your regular breathing rate when you try to count it. It is best, therefore, to have someone else measure your respiratory rate.

HOW THE TEST IS DONE: The chest expands during inspiration and contracts during expiration. Have someone count the number of times the chest moves in 30 seconds, remembering that only a full cycle of inspiration and expiration counts as one breath. It is easier to count if the chest is uncovered. The number obtained in 30 seconds should be multiplied by two to get the respiratory rate per minute. For a child, a hand can be placed over the chest to feel and count the movement of the chest wall.

HOW TO INTERPRET THE RESULTS: The normal respiratory rate will vary with age and activity, but general guidelines are as follows:
Newborn infants—30–80 breaths / min.
Children age 1 through 12—23–30 breaths / min.
Children 12 or over and adults—15–18 breaths / min.

SYMPTOMS FOR WHICH THIS TEST SHOULD BE PERFORMED AT HOME:
Breathing difficulty (p. 290).
Fever (p. 296).

Cough (p. 292).
Anxiety.

DISEASES FOR WHICH THIS TEST SHOULD BE PERFORMED AT HOME:
This test will help to monitor the severity of the following diseases:
Asthma (p. 312).
Pneumonia (p. 321).
Common cold (p. 315).
Bronchitis and emphysema (p. 315).
Congestive heart failure.

TEMPERATURE

PURPOSE OF THE TEST: to measure the internal temperature of the body.

BACKGROUND: The temperature of your body is carefully regulated and varies little from day to day, although in most people it is slightly higher at night than in the morning. Increases or decreases in your temperature are significant and usually indicate inflammation or infection. There are many different types of thermometers available for measuring temperature. The old-fashioned glass thermometer is as good as any, but newer types have recently become available, including electronic thermometers that give the temperature on a digital readout and paper temperature strips that record the temperature by changes in the color of the paper. Like the outdoor temperature, body temperature can be expressed in Fahrenheit (F) or Celsius (C centigrade) degrees. Most physicians and patients are familiar with the Fahrenheit measurement, where 98.6° is "normal"—and for this reason we give that value first throughout this chapter.

HOW THE TEST IS DONE: Temperature can be measured from three places: mouth, axilla (armpit), and rectum. Although the rectal temperature is the most accurate, the oral temperature is more than adequate assuming that the person is able to cooperate. With all three locations it is important to shake down the thermometer to below 94°F (34.4°C). Failure to do this is the most common reason for an inaccurate temperature recording.

The rectal temperature, which is most often used in children under three years old, is obtained as follows: A special rectal thermometer is used and Vaseline is placed on the thermometer bulb.

The child lies face down on a flat surface. The person taking the temperature separates the buttocks with one hand and with the other hand places the bulb end of the thermometer about 1 inch into the anus. The thermometer is held in this position for two minutes.

The oral temperature is most often used for adults and older children. The thermometer is placed under the tongue and held there for two minutes. It is very important not to eat or drink very hot or cold foods or liquids and not to smoke for at least 20 minutes prior to taking your temperature as this will cause an invalid reading. In addition, do not talk during the time the thermometer is in the mouth for this will allow room air to flow in and out and cause an erroneous reading. Care must be taken—especially in children—that the thermometer is not swallowed or accidentally broken.

The axillary temperature is the easiest to perform but the least accurate. After shaking down the thermometer, place it under the arm against the skin. The arm is used to hold it in place for four minutes. Generally, we do not recommend that you take axillary temperatures unless your doctor specifically instructs you to do so.

HOW TO INTERPRET THE RESULTS: Normal temperatures are as follows:
  Rectal—99.6° F (37.6° C).
  Oral—98.6° F (37° C).
  Axillary—97.6° F (36.4° C).
  Fever is generally considered to be present if the oral temperature is greater than 100° F (37.8° C) or a rectal reading is more than 101° F (38.3° C).

SYMPTOMS FOR WHICH THIS TEST SHOULD BE PERFORMED AT HOME: Measuring the temperature will help determine the severity of these symptoms:
  Fever (p. 296).
  Cough (p. 292).
  Diarrhea (p. 293).
  Abdominal pain (p. 285).
  Earache.
  Headache (p. 297).
  Muscle aches.
  Vomiting (p. 303).

DISEASES FOR WHICH THIS TEST SHOULD BE PERFORMED AT HOME: Monitoring the temperature will help determine the success of treatment for these diseases:

Common cold (p. 315).
Pneumonia (p. 321).
Urinary tract infection (p. 326).
Mononucleosis (p. 78).
Otitis media (ear infection).
Bronchitis (p. 315).

COST: $5.

WEIGHT

PURPOSE OF THE TEST: to measure a person's weight.

BACKGROUND: Weighing yourself at home can provide much useful information. Most people weigh themselves to see if they have been eating too much and are in need of dieting, but unexpected changes in weight can be a sign of serious disease. In the United States as well as most countries in the British Commonwealth, weight is generally expressed in pounds. In the rest of the world it is measured in kilograms. There are 2.2 pounds per kilogram. Most older scales weigh in pounds only, but some newer versions give both units.

HOW THE TEST IS DONE: Although everyone has weighed himself countless times, most people have not done it as an accurate home medical test from which the results obtained one day can be compared with results obtained one week later. The most important requirement for accuracy is to do the weighing in a standardized manner. This means weighing yourself the same time of day, using the same scale, and wearing the same amount of clothes (preferably none). It makes little sense to compare a weight obtained Sunday morning when you were wearing only a towel with another done at a friend's home the following evening when you were fully clothed.

HOW TO INTERPRET THE RESULTS: Your normal weight will depend upon your age, sex, height, and build. Your doctor will always want to be informed about changes in your weight. As a guideline, an unexpected change (when you were not dieting in an attempt to lose) of greater than 5 pounds should be reported to your doctor.

SYMPTOMS FOR WHICH THIS TEST SHOULD BE PERFORMED AT HOME:
Obesity.
Prolonged fever.
Change in usual bowel habits.
Health maintenance.
Fatigue (p. 295).

DISEASES FOR WHICH THIS TEST SHOULD BE OBTAINED AT HOME:
Congestive heart failure—By weighing yourself regularly, you can detect a buildup of body fluids that might cause a worsening of this condition.
Cancer (p. 313)—When a patient has been treated for cancer, further unexpected weight loss will suggest recurrence of the disease.
Thyroid disease—Unexplained weight gain will occur when the thyroid gland is underactive, and weight loss will result when the thyroid is overactive.

BASAL BODY TEMPERATURE

PURPOSE OF THE TEST: to determine whether a woman is ovulating properly and predict the time of the month during which intercourse is most likely to result in pregnancy.

BACKGROUND: Your body temperature is partially controlled by hormones that are secreted by the pituitary gland in the brain. In a female during childbearing years, at the time of ovulation (when the egg is released from the ovary and can be fertilized by sperm) these hormones will cause a temporary drop, followed by a rise, in the body temperature. If this temperature change occurs, it is a good indication that a woman is ovulating and that this is the time when she is most likely to become pregnant. Infections, fatigue, and medications can alter the temperature results and make them difficult to interpret.

HOW THE TEST IS DONE: A special thermometer must be used that is very sensitive and records temperature in tenths of degrees (most usual thermometers measure only in fifths; i.e., two-tenths of a degree). These more accurate thermometers are needed to detect the subtle temperature changes that occur with ovulation. The

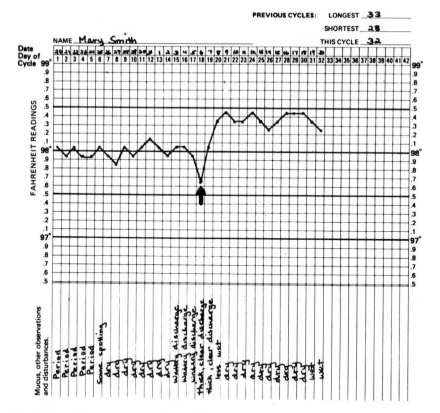

Typical basal temperature chart. The arrow marks the temperature changes that are associated with ovulation.

temperature can be taken orally or rectally (p. 355), but the same method should be used at the same time every day, preferably before rising from bed and before eating or drinking. The temperature results on each day of the menstrual cycle should be recorded on a graph or chart as illustrated

HOW TO INTERPRET THE RESULTS: Normally, the temperature drops 0.2° F just prior to ovulation. This is the time when intercourse will most likely result in pregnancy. One to three days after this drop, the temperature rises about 1.7°F above the lowest temperature, indicating that ovulation has taken place. If no temperature change occurs, ovulation did not take place.

SYMPTOMS FOR WHICH THIS TEST SHOULD BE PERFORMED AT HOME: Infertility (p. 299)—This test will detect if ovulation has taken place.

It will also determine the ideal time to have intercourse in order for pregnancy to occur.

Contraception—If pregnancy is not desired, the temperature chart will help determine a "safe" period when pregnancy is least likely to occur after intercourse. Although more accurate than simple "rhythm" methods, which only count the days between menstrual cycles, this method is not very effective when used as the only form of contraception.

TEST FOR BLOOD IN STOOL

PURPOSE OF THE TEST: to detect the presence in stool of small amounts of blood that cannot be seen with the naked eye.

BACKGROUND: The presence of bright red blood in the stool is always a cause for alarm. Similarly, we worry whenever a patient tells us that he or she is having black stools, an indication of bleeding from the stomach or small intestine. Frequently, however, serious conditions such as cancer or bleeding ulcers will "leak" only small amounts of blood into the stool that are of insufficient quantity to produce the red or black color change. This small amount of blood, called occult blood, is invisible to the naked eye and can be shown to exist only by a chemical test. Nevertheless, even though it is only a small amount of bleeding, its presence is highly significant and might allow for the early detection of a malignancy when it will still be possible to cure the patient. For this reason we will often want to screen for the presence of occult blood in the stool. This screening test will frequently be conducted at home as well as in the physician's office as part of the routine physical examination (p. 246).

HOW THE TEST IS DONE: The most commonly used technique is the Hemoccult II test in which three cards impregnated with chemicals are given to the patient by the doctor. The patient should not eat red meats for two days prior to the test because even the small amount of blood from the meat may cause the test to be positive and result in needless worry. In addition, certain medications, including vitamin C, will also give misleading results. To perform the test, the patient uses an applicator to smear two different parts of three bowel movements onto the cards. A cardboard covering is then placed over the stool, and the entire kit is mailed immediately to the doctor for final processing and interpretation of the

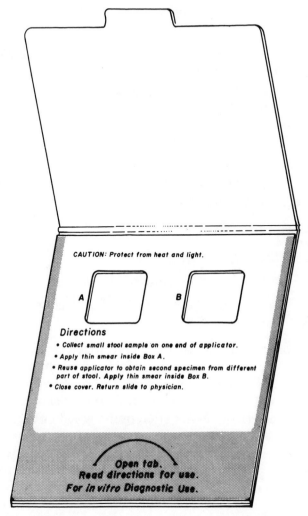

Hemoccult card used to test the stool for blood. Stool specimens are smeared on the card, which is then returned to the physician for final analysis.

test. Because these cards detect very small amounts of blood, this test should not be done when the patient is menstruating or when hemorrhoids are actively bleeding.

HOW TO INTERPRET THE RESULTS: Once the doctor obtains the cards, he will place a few drops of a chemical solution over the stool. If the paper turns blue, then blood is present in the stool. In the absence of blood, no color change will occur. The doctor will notify you if the test is positive (blood was present) or negative (no blood was detected).

SYMPTOMS FOR WHICH THIS TEST SHOULD BE PERFORMED AT HOME: All of these symptoms may be associated with colon cancer, and, if any is present, this test should be conducted:

Change in bowel habits.
Weight loss (p. 306).
Fever (p. 296).

DISEASES FOR WHICH THIS TEST SHOULD BE PERFORMED AT HOME: Cancer (p. 313)—This test will monitor whether a colon cancer that has been treated is recurring.

COST: approximately $5.

HOME DIABETES TESTING

PURPOSE OF THE TEST: to monitor the level of glucose in the blood and urine.

BACKGROUND: Diabetes, a disease characterized by elevated levels of glucose in the blood, can cause damage to many body organs if it is not well controlled. Once someone is known to have diabetes, it is essential to monitor carefully the level of sugar in his blood and urine. This will help determine whether the treatment (diet, insulin, or pills) has been successful in controlling the disease or whether additional treatment is necessary. If the glucose levels can be kept near normal, many of the complications of diabetes may be avoided. In addition to the risk from too much glucose, a diabetic patient must be careful not to take too much insulin, which can decrease the glucose to levels so low that dizziness, light-headedness, and even coma can result. The diabetic can also test for low glucose levels at home. We ask our patients with diabetes to check their urine and blood at home at different times of the day to determine how successful therapy has been.

HOW THE TEST IS DONE: Tests are available to measure the glucose in both the urine and blood. Urine tests are done by either of two methods: With Clinistix (a small 4-inch by $1/4$-inch strip of paper impregnated with chemicals), which is dipped into the urine and the color change that results is used to determine sugar content; or with Clinitest, a chemical tablet that will cause a color change

in urine depending upon the sugar content. Although the Clinitest tablets are more accurate, they are less convenient to use.
When a patient's glucose levels become very high, ketones may
also be present in the urine. Another kind of dipstick (Keto-Diastix)
will measure both glucose and ketones.

Blood glucose levels can be measured at home with the use of
dipsticks (Chemstrip bG). A drop of blood—obtained by pricking
the tip of the finger—is placed on a chemically coated dipstick and
the color change noted. This test will give an accurate measure of
the levels of blood glucose.

Each of these tests has specific instructions that should be read
in detail before the test is performed. Your doctor will advise you
as to which of these tests to use.

HOW TO INTERPRET THE RESULTS: The level of glucose in the urine
or blood is determined by comparing the color with a color chart
that comes with each test kit. Each patient must discuss individually with his or her doctor the optimal glucose levels in the blood
or urine that he wants maintained.

SYMPTOMS FOR WHICH THIS TEST SHOULD BE PERFORMED AT HOME:
All of these symptoms are associated with diabetes, which can be
screened by this test:

Frequent urination.
Excessive thirst and appetite.
Fatigue (p. 295).
Weight loss (p. 306).
Change in vision.

DISEASES FOR WHICH THIS TEST SHOULD BE PERFORMED AT HOME:
Diabetes (p. 318).

COST: approximately $1.

HOME PREGNANCY TEST

PURPOSE OF THE TEST: to determine if a woman is pregnant.

BACKGROUND: Women who are anxious to know if they are pregnant often do not wish to wait for a doctor's appointment to find
out. In addition, if pregnancy is unexpected or unwanted, the
woman may be embarrassed to go to a doctor who knows her.
For these reasons more and more women prefer testing for a pos-

sible pregnancy without delay in the privacy of their own homes. In response to this need, in recent years reliable pregnancy tests have become available for home use. These do not require a doctor's prescription and can be purchased over-the-counter in most drugstores. These tests, based on the identical principle as the standard pregnancy test (p. 214) done in the hospital or medical laboratory, measure whether human chorionic gonadotropin (HCG), a hormone secreted by the placenta and found in the urine during pregnancy, is present.

HOW THE TEST IS DONE: The test should be performed at least 10 days after the last menstrual period was expected. The first urine that is voided in the morning should be used because it will contain the highest concentration of HCG, if it is present. Since there are several different tests available on the market, it is important that the specific instructions for a particular kit be read carefully before use. In general, a few drops of urine are mixed with a few drops of the chemical that comes with the kit. This chemical consists of tiny, nearly microscopic, rubber beads that are coated with an antibody directed against HCG. The pattern that the beads take when they settle to the bottom will vary depending upon whether HCG is present or absent in the urine to be tested.

HOW TO INTERPRET THE RESULTS: If the result is positive, you should go to your doctor to have this confirmed. If the test is negative, however, it may be that it was performed too soon after the missed menstrual cycle—before the HCG level had a chance to become very high—and you might want to repeat the test after a few days. Even though the woman is pregnant, there may be other reasons for negative results: failure to test a first morning urine (the concentration of HCG may be too low for detection on urines voided later in the day), exposure of the test to heat, or the presence of a urinary tract infection.

SYMPTOMS FOR WHICH THIS TEST SHOULD BE PERFORMED AT HOME:
Missed menstrual period.
Nausea and vomiting.
Tender breasts.
Increase in abdominal size.

COST: approximately $10.

BREAST SELF-EXAMINATION

PURPOSE OF THE TEST: to examine the breasts in order to detect lumps and possible cancers.

BACKGROUND: Breast cancer is the most common malignancy in women. Yet, despite all the publicity in the news media about the need for early detection of this disease, many women first come to the doctor when the breast cancer has already spread to other parts of the body. Although the doctor's routine physical examination is important and can detect breast lesions, even if done on an annual basis, it is not frequent enough to detect most breast cancers before they have spread to other parts of the body. In addition, the doctor—no matter how skillful—is not as familiar with the patient's breasts as the patient herself is and consequently, may miss lumps that the woman would discover herself. For these reasons a monthly breast self-exam by every woman over the age of 20 is essential to detect cancer early and offer the best chance for a cure. Many women have not been taught how to examine their breasts; others who do know are reluctant or unwilling to do so. Still other patients who do examine their breasts do it incorrectly or do not perform the examination monthly. There is no acceptable excuse for a woman not to examine her breasts monthly.

HOW THE TEST IS DONE: The first time, the woman should examine her breasts in front of her doctor to make sure that she is using the correct technique. She can then ask him about anything unusual that she feels as she does the exam. Afterwards, she should be able to do subsequent examinations on her own. The exam should be performed every month, one week after the end of the woman's period.

Step I: It is easier to examine the breasts in the shower or bath because your hands glide more easily over wet skin. With your fingers flat, move them over every part of the breast. Use your left hand for the right breast and the right hand for the left breast. Check for lumps, knots, or thickening.

Step II: In front of the mirror inspect your breast with arms at your sides. Next, raise your hands over your head to look for swelling, dimpling of the skin, or changes in the nipple. Next, rest your palms on your hips and press down firmly to flex your

chest muscles. Remember, even with normal breasts, the left and
right breasts frequently do not match exactly.

Step III: While lying down, to examine the right breast, place a
pillow under your right shoulder. Place the right hand behind the
head. Using the left hand, with fingers flat, press gently in small
circular motions around an imaginary clock face. Begin at the out-
ermost top of the right breast and move in a clockwise fashion. A
ridge of firm tissue in the lower curve of each breast is normal.
Then move an inch towards the nipple while circling the breast
and making sure that each part of the breast including the nipple
is examined. The procedure is now repeated for the left breast,
with the pillow under the left shoulder and the left hand behind
the head. Finally, squeeze the nipple of each breast between the
thumb and index finger while looking for a discharge.

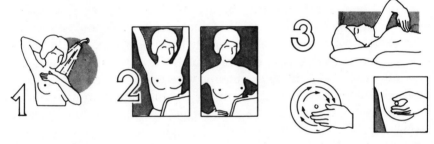

Proper procedure for monthly breast self-examination. See text for detailed
instructions. (Reprinted by permission of the American Cancer Society.)

HOW TO INTERPRET THE RESULTS: The presence of any abnormal
lumps or other warning signs should be reported to your doctor
immediately. Warning signs of cancer to be noted during the breast
exam include new hard lumps in the breast or under the arm,
changes in the color or texture of the skin over the breast, bloody
nipple discharge, and inversion of the nipple. Several changes in
the breast that are normal can also occur. Each month, at the time
of menstruation, the breasts become enlarged. There is increased
tenderness and occasional lumps may be felt that disappear later
in the menstrual cycle. During pregnancy, or when a woman is
taking birth control pills, the breasts become tender and increase
in size.

SYMPTOMS FOR WHICH THIS TEST SHOULD BE PERFORMED AT HOME:
Breast lumps (p. 302)—Sometimes a physician may ask the patient

to examine a particular lump for a period of a few months before deciding to investigate it further.

DISEASES FOR WHICH THIS TEST SHOULD BE PERFORMED AT HOME: Breast cancer—This test is used to monitor people who have had previous breast cancer in order to detect recurrence.

TESTICULAR SELF-EXAMINATION

PURPOSE OF THE TEST: to detect any lumps or other abnormalities in the testicles.

BACKGROUND: Testicular cancer is a common cause of cancer in men under 35 years of age. When detected early, the chance for complete recovery is very high. If detected late, the cancer rapidly spreads to other parts of the body and becomes more difficult to treat. Although there is much publicity in the media about the importance of breast self-exams, much less attenton is given to testicular self-exams. This test is easy to perform at home and should be done by all men age 20 and over on a monthly basis.

HOW THE TEST IS DONE: The test should be performed after a shower or bath when the skin overlying the scrotum and testicles is soft and relaxed. The scrotum should be gently squeezed to determine the location of one of the testicles. The testicle should be held between the thumb and fingers of one hand while the thumb and fingers of the other hand should be used to feel for lumps or unusual bumps. The same procedure should be performed for the other testicle. At the same time, the epididymis (sperm collecting structure) can be felt as a cord-like structure towards the back of the testicle. The first time, the patient should do the exam at the doctor's office so that he can ask the physician about any abnormalities he feels.

HOW TO INTERPRET THE RESULTS: Any lumps on the testicle should be immediately reported to your doctor. It is important to realize that there are other noncancerous causes of scrotal and testicular lumps, including varicocele (swelling of the veins in the scrotum), hydrocele (swelling of the capsule around the testicle), inguinal hernia, and epididymitis (infection of the epididymis).

SYMPTOMS FOR WHICH THIS TEST SHOULD BE PERFORMED AT HOME:
Testicular pain.
Testicular swelling.

Drawing of testicle. See text
for detailed instructions of
examination.

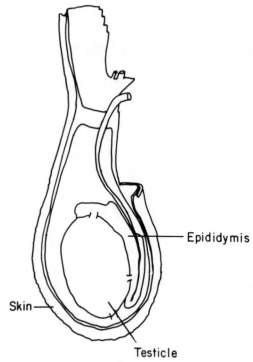

Epididymis

Skin

Testicle

DISEASES FOR WHICH THIS TEST SHOULD BE PERFORMED AT HOME:
Testicular cancer—This test will detect if a lump is present in the
testes.
Varicocele—Swelling of the veins in the scrotum will feel like a
"bag of worms."
Hydrocele—Swelling of the capsule around the testicle can become
large.
Inguinal hernia—A protrusion of parts of the abdomen will be felt
in the scrotal sac.

Recent Advances in Medical Testing

WE HAVE made the point often in this book that the field of medical testing is a constantly changing one. Tests that are routine today—such as CT scans—were experimental only a few years ago and wholly unknown a few years before that. Conversely, other tests, such as pneumoencephalography or thymol turbidity have fallen into disuse—either replaced by tests that are safer, less expensive, and more accurate or discarded because they are recognized as unreliable.

The tests we have listed throughout this book are referred to in medicine as "state of the art." They are what the world of medicine considers to be the best tests at this time with well-defined indications for their use and firmly established criteria for their interpretation. The tests described in this chapter are of a different nature. They are not yet routinely performed but represent, instead, recent advances in the field of medical testing. Some of the procedures or tests that we describe here are already being done on patients; the experimental aspect is not the technology but the specific circumstances and indications for their use. Other tests that we have included are better defined in regard to their medical application but are undergoing a period of continuing technological improvement. We have not included tests that are only hypothetical or that have not yet been used in actual patient testing.

Given the large amount of progress that is being made in the field of medical testing, it was difficult to select some of the tests for description here. Thus we have selected tests based on two criteria: the likelihood of their ultimate acceptance and wide-spread use; and the importance of such a test, when successful, on health care.

Positron Emission Tomography (PET Scanning)

PET scanning is a new technique for imaging and evaluating many body organs. It combines certain aspects of CT scanning and nuclear medicine scanning and is best applied to the study of the brain and related structures.

Like nuclear medicine scanning, PET uses radioactive isotopes or radionuclides. The actual type of radiation that is emitted in PET scanning is different, however. Instead of the gamma-like radiation that conventional radioisotopes emit, the isotopes used in PET emit a different radioactive particle called a positron—hence, the name of the procedure. As in nuclear medicine scans, the patient is injected with the isotope and after an appropriate duration a "camera" that can detect that kind of radiation measures the amount of emission from the organ to be studied. The procedure is like CT scanning—a computer is used to analyze "pictures" taken from numerous angles and from this data puts together a composite picture of the organ.

The real excitement about PET scanning is that these radioisotopes—unlike those used in conventional nuclear medicine scans—can be attached to a variety of chemicals—like glucose—that are found in the body and are involved in the body's metabolism. In this way the procedure not only can be used to detect the anatomy of a particular organ but, more importantly, can provide invaluable information about the biochemical status of that organ: is it working properly, is its metabolism normal, is it functioning as it should?

PET scanning offers the promise of answering those questions as well as giving information about simple structure and anatomy. The procedure, however, has two drawbacks. The first is the lack of experience in knowing the significance to the patient of abnormalities that are detected. For example, recent studies demonstrate that glucose use by the brain may be different in patients with schizophrenia than it is in healthy people. No one is certain yet of the practical importance of that difference. Can PET be used to screen for schizophrenia? Can it be used to monitor the treatment of that or other mental disorders? Can it be used to define different kinds of schizophrenics? No one knows, and until more information is forthcoming, PET will remain of uncertain real value. The other drawback is that the equipment necessary for PET scanning is very expensive—several million dollars at least for a complete machine. Given that cost, most hospitals have not been able to purchase the equipment, and even if they did, they would have to charge patients heavy fees for each test.

Nuclear Magnetic Resonance (NMR, Magnetic Resonance Imaging)

For over 25 years chemists and physicists have used a technique by which to study the internal structure of various molecules. Within the last five years this technique, nuclear magnetic resonance or NMR, has been applied with exciting results to the field of medicine as well. In NMR the patient is placed inside a gigantic hollow magnet that is so powerful it aligns in one direction some of the hydrogen atoms that are present in the various tissues of the body, in much the same way as a child's toy magnet from the local five-and-dime store will align iron filings. After the atoms are aligned, within seconds of turning on the magnet, a radio signal similar to that used in FM radio is directed at the part of the body being examined. This radio energy disrupts the perfect alignment that the magnet produced and temporarily energizes the hydrogen atoms. The radio signal is then stopped, and the hydrogen atoms will realign themselves, but not all at the same time. Slight differences in composition of the body—whether liquid or bone or fat tissue—will cause the atoms to align at a different rate.

A computer is used to measure this change in the realignment of the atoms and converts the data that is generated into picture form. The resultant image is similar, but not identical, to that produced by a CT scanner. NMR has been most widely used in imaging of the brain and related structures but is more recently being applied to the study of other parts of the body as well. The results indicate that it is a technique capable of producing images that are of equal or better quality than CT scanning. The apparent advantage to NMR scanning is that it does not involve radiation, the main risk associated with the use of CT scans. In fact, the only apparent problems that have resulted from NMR is that the magnets used are so powerful they have been known to stop watches, pull stethoscopes out of the ears of doctors standing nearby, and wreak havoc with cassette tapes.

A few other problems remain with NMR. First is the cost. Like PET equipment, the machinery necessary for a complete NMR setup will probably cost several million dollars, only adding to the burden of our expensive health care system. Second, while at the present time the risks in using NMR seem slight, only further testing and experience will tell if the strong magnetic fields that are used on the body are truly as safe as they currently appear to be.

MONOCLONAL ANTIBODIES

When any foreign material is injected into our body, or the body of any animal, antibodies are produced in response. Monoclonal antibodies result from a new method of producing antibodies and have two advantages over conventional antibodies. They are much more specific in their ability to recognize foreign material, and they can be produced in large quantities.

Monoclonal antibodies were first discovered in the late 1970s by Cesar Milstein and George Kohler, two immunologists working at the Imperial Cancer Research Center in London. They worked out a technique that fuses together a B-lymphocyte (the white cell that makes antibodies) with a myeloma cell (a cancer cell that can be grown in the laboratory in large quantities for long periods of time). The resultant fused cell, called a hybridoma, has the antibody-producing capability of the B-cell with the immortality and growth characteristics of the cancer cell, resulting in the continuing production of large quantities of powerful antibodies. Very recently, monoclonal antibodies have been used in the field of medical testing. While the list of applications is continually growing, here are two examples of the possible use of monoclonal antibodies for medical tests:

1. Monoclonal antibodies have been produced that are directed against tumor antigens, molecules on the surface of cancer cells. To these antitumor antibodies are attached a radioisotope, similar to the ones used in nuclear medicine scans (p. 132). When injected into the body of a person who has been treated for cancer, the antibodies will attach themselves to any cancer cells that are remaining. After a few hours the patient is scanned as he would be for a typical nuclear medicine scan, and the picture produced will demonstrate any remaining areas of cancer in the patient's body.

2. Currently, if a patient is suspected of having a strep throat, the doctor does a throat culture (p. 174). The results, however, are

not available for 36 to 48 hours; thus during that time it is unclear if the patient's sore throat is due to infection with strep and requires penicillin therapy or is due to some other bacteria or virus. Recently, scientists have produced monoclonal antibodies directed against the strep bacteria. Tests indicate that it may be possible to take a throat swab from a patient suspected of having a strep throat and, using the anti-strep monoclonal antibody, detect within minutes if strep bacteria are present on the swab. Similar monoclonal antibodies have been prepared against gonorrhea, and studies are underway in both of these diseases to see if monoclonal antibodies can provide "instant diagnosis" so that the physician does not have to wait days for the final culture report.

GENETIC SCREENING

Until recently, the only genetic diseases for which patients could be tested were sickle cell anemia (p. 82) and Tay-Sachs (p. 60). Today new tests have been developed that allow doctors to screen for over 200 genetic diseases. This screening can be done on cells obtained from the fetus during amniocentesis or, in some instances on the adult man or woman who, although not sick from the disease itself, is a "carrier" for the defective gene that may be transmitted to a fetus. Most recently, a screening test has been developed for carriers of cystic fibrosis, a very common genetic abnormality in man. The widening use of these new genetic screening tests poses several important ethical and moral questions. Who should have the screening done? Should two people carrying the gene for a disease be legally prevented from marrying each other so that their children won't contract the actual disease? Or, if they do marry, should amniocentesis be made compulsory and abortion performed on all fetuses with the defective genes? This is one example of recent advances in the world of medical testing that solves some problems while creating entirely new ones—with no easy solutions.

CHORIONIC VILLI SAMPLING (CVS)

The usual way in which fetal samples are obtained for genetic screening is amniocentesis. Recently, however, a new test has been developed that may revolutionize our ability to screen for genetic diseases. Chorionic villi sampling was developed nearly a decade ago in China and is currently being tested at several medical centers in the United States and Europe. In this test the doctor inserts a hollow tube (catheter) through the cervix and into the uterus, and while guided by ultrasound (p. 151), he takes biopsy samples from the chorionic villi. These are small protrusions from the chorion membrane, which surrounds the developing fetus and eventually will become part of the placenta. The cells that comprise the chorion reflect the genetic makeup of the fetus and not the mother. The tissue that is obtained is analyzed to determine if any genetic defects are present.

Chorionic villi sampling, or CVS, has three major advantages over amniocentesis:

1. It can be done much earlier in pregnancy. While amniocentesis cannot be performed before the 14th week of pregnancy, CVS is best performed at eight or nine weeks of pregnancy.

2. The amount of tissue obtained with CVS is much greater than that obtained with amniocentesis, allowing for the genetic analysis to be completed much more quickly.

3. The procedure appears to be much less risky. Although CVS requires the use of ultrasound—the risks of which are uncertain at this point—there seems to be little other danger involved. Like all new tests, it is still too early to know for sure, but it appears that chorionic villi sampling will have a dramatic impact on the field of genetic screening.

Screening for Mental Illness

Although mental illness is very common, there have been few tests available to detect these diseases or monitor them during treatment. This is changing. Recently, blood and urine tests have been described that detect the presence of certain chemicals (3-methoxy-4-hydroxyphenyl glycol, or MHG, as well as norepinephrine) that are found in abnormal concentration in patients with various mental illnesses, such as severe depression, schizophrenia, and manic-depression. The use of these tests will likely have a major impact on the diagnosis and treatment of these problems. Until now the psychiatrist has been forced to use his judgment only—without any laboratory confirmation—to make these diagnoses. If these blood and urine tests for mental disorders are as successful as they appear to be, psychiatrists may now have available a powerful new tool to assist them in caring for these patients.

"Do-It-Yourself Thermography"

Cancer tissue generally has more blood flow through it than does normal tissue. This principle led to the development of thermography (p. 221), a test useful in the diagnosis of breast cancer. Now a do-it-yourself version of this technique has been undergoing testing. The woman to be tested wears a garment that looks like a brassiere but is made out of a material containing chemical crystals that change color depending upon the temperature. The patient wears the test bra for a few hours and then compares the colors to a base-line color chart that was prepared in her physician's office. Any changes in color suggestive of a tumor would prompt her to call her physician for a careful physical examination and more testing.

Disease markers

It is now apparent that certain diseases will occur much more frequently in patients with a specific predisposition towards that illness. Here are a few examples:

Diabetes.

Rheumatic fever.

Certain kinds of arthritis.

Various forms of cancer.

The list could go on. The important point is that we now have certain ways of testing whether people are at increased risk for those diseases because they have unique body markers. Certain markers are HLA types (p. 66), while others are differences in the chromosomes that people carry in their cells. It is not yet certain what the optimal way is of using these tests for various disease markers. It is likely, however, that someday testing people for these disease markers will reveal which illnesses they are most prone to develop. Their doctor can then initiate the necessary precautions or treatment before the actual disease develops.

New Tests: How and When to Use Them

Advances in medical testing are a double-edged sword. Although new tests have the potential for improving the quality of health care, they can also be risky, costly, or just plain inaccurate. When should a new test be used and how does the patient find out about it? The rule here is the same that we have tried to stress throughout the book: frank discussion with your doctor is the best guide. If you read or hear about a new test, ask your doctor about it. He may be able to guide you, or if he is also uncertain about the current status of that test, he may want to speak first to some experts in the field before getting back to you. On the other hand, if your doctor suggests a test that is new, be sure to question him about it. Try to find out what this test offers that previous tests did not. If there were no previous tests that measured the same factor, try to find out what the possible risks and dangers are with the new test. Patients should never have tests done without knowing exactly why the doctor has ordered them, especially if the tests are new.

Appendices

Appendix 1

There are literally hundreds of medications that can interfere with test results. This can occur because the drug actually alters the level of the substance being measured in the body, or it interferes with the measurement of the substance causing a value that is not accurate. We have listed only commonly used drugs and their effect on some important blood tests and other procedures. Before your medical tests are done, be very sure to tell your doctor about *any* medicines that you are taking (even over-the-counter drugs).

The test is listed first, then the names of the common drugs that interfere with the results. First the generic name is listed, followed by its trade name in parentheses.

BLOOD TESTS

Antinuclear antibody: hydralazine (Apresoline), isoniazid (INH), procainamide (Pronestyl), gold, quinidine, chlorpromazine, imipramine (Tofranil).

Blood-urea-nitrogen (BUN): ibuprofen (Motrin), sulindac (Clinoril), furosemide (Lasix), gentamycin, lithium carbonate.

Calcium: hydrochlorothiazide (HydroDIURIL).

Coombs' test: isoniazid (INH), methyldopa (Aldomet), levodopa (Sinemet), phenytoin (Dilantin), tetracycline.

Creatinine: ibuprofen (Motrin), sulindac (Clinoril), furosemide (Lasix), gentamycin, lithium carbonate.

Glucose: furosemide (Lasix), hydrochlorothiazide (Hydro-DIURIL).

Platelet count: gold, quinidine, chlorpromazine, imipramine (Tofranil).

Potassium: spironolactone (Aldactone), furosemide (Lasix), hydrochlorothiazide (HydroDIURIL), laxatives.

Prothrombin time: Coumadin.

Serum glutamic-oxaloacetic transaminase (SGOT): hydralazine (Apresoline), isoniazid (INH), chlorpromazine, imipramine (Tofranil), aspirin.

Sodium: furosemide (Lasix), hydrochlorothiazide (Hydro-DIURIL), corticosteroids.

Uric acid: furosemide (Lasix), hydrochlorothiazide (Hydro-DIURIL), aspirin, allopurinol (Zyloprim), probenecid (Benemid).

URINE (EFFECT ON COLOR)

Rust-yellow or brown urine: nitrofurantoin (Furadantin).
Orange-red urine: phenazopyridine (Pyridium).

URINE (EXCRETION OF CHEMICALS IN URINE)

5-hydroxyindoleacetic acid (5-HIAA): guaifenesin, isoniazid (INH), imipramine (Tofranil).

OTHER TESTS

Test for blood in stool: Vitamin C.
Thyroid scan: chlortrimeton, lithium carbonate, propylthiouracil, cough medicines.

Appendix 2

One of the points we have tried to make in this book is that you must share the responsibility with the medical profession for the appropriate and effective use of medical tests. One of the most important ways in which you can aid in this regard is to keep an accurate and reliable medical test diary. This diary should be made available to your physician, especially when new medical tests are being considered. There are three ways in which this will help.

First, results of previous medical tests—even those from months and years in the past—will often help your doctor in his thinking about your case. Here is an example. Billy A. is a 13-year-old black boy whom we admitted to the hospital last month when he began passing red urine. We quickly came to the conclusion that this represented a hemolytic crisis due to a viral infection, a relatively common occurrence in patients with a genetic deficiency of G6PD, a red blood cell enzyme (p. 61). We were able to make that diagnosis rapidly because his medical test diary contained the information that in the nursery, when he was born, a screening test for this enzyme revealed it to be deficient. In this case the patient provided us with invaluable pieces of information from his medical test diary.

Second, the results from many medical tests are most useful in comparison to previous results from the same test. For example, last year we saw in the office a 28-year-old research assistant who works at the medical center. She came to us complaining of a chronic cough. A chest x-ray revealed an abnormal pattern in her lung. At first, we did not know if these changes were new—which would have been consistent with the diagnosis of pneumonia—or old and from some previous illness that was of no significance to the

361

current problem. Fortunately, the woman had kept a medical test diary that enabled us to recognize these abnormalities as old findings that were present on a chest x-ray from six years ago and were not evidence of a new pneumonia.

Another example of this is Linda F., a 42-year-old woman, who has a history of fibrocystic disease of the breast, a condition in which women frequently have benign tumors in the breast. Because of this problem, Linda had a mammogram done when she was 38. This past year, during her regular checkup, we felt a new lump in her breast and had another mammogram done that revealed an abnormal lesion. In comparison with her old mammogram, however, we were able to reassure her that the x-ray finding was nothing serious. Had the old mammogram result been unknown, we would have been forced to recommend a breast biopsy.

Third, having available the results from old medical tests will sometimes make it unnecessary to have new tests done. This happens many times. For example, Jeff P. has been having headaches and came to see us. We ordered a series of tests, including x-rays of the skull, CT scan of the brain and an electroencephalogram (EEG). We were unable to find the reason for his headaches and referred him to a neurologist who wanted to do the exact same three tests until Jeff showed him the results from the tests that we had just done.

Having hopefully convinced you that keeping a medical test diary is important and useful, the question is raised of what is the best way to do so. Any system of record-keeping that you devise is fine, as long as it fulfills two criteria: (1) It must be convenient, and (2) It must allow for enough accurate information as to be worthwhile.

On the next few pages we provide a sample diary. There is nothing "sacred" about it, however, and you should feel free to modify it to suit your own purposes.

MEDICAL TEST DIARY

The diary should consist of two parts. The first consists of the forms that follow. We have two suggestions as to the best way to store them: either as index cards in a filing box or as pages in a small (5 by 7 inches) loose-leaf notebook. The second part of the diary should consist of actual test reports that are made available to you. Most important are x-ray reports. Generally, physicians do not give patients their x-ray reports unless they ask for them.

Page #1

Name__John Smith__

Birthdate__4/3/47__   Place of Birth__Topeka, Kans.__

Blood Type__O, Rh+__   Allergies__bees__

Address__43 Pond St.__

_____Boston, MA._____

_____Telephone__617-555-3435__

Primary Physician__Dr. William Sloan__

Primary Physician Address__43 Beacon St.__

_____Boston, MA._____

_____Telephone__617-555-4534__

Major Illness or Surgery   and Date

__tonsillectomy__   __6/5/50 (Topeka General)__

__appendectomy__   __11/1/57 (Topeka General)__

__hypertension__   __Diagnosed: 3/2/77 (Dr. Sloan)__

_____   _____

_____   _____

_____   _____

_____   _____

Page #2

Hematology Tests

Test and Result

Date	Hematocrit	White Blood Cell Count	Platelet Count	Reason for Test
3/6/74	46%	7500	245,000	routine physical
3/2/77	44%	9600	323,000	routine physical
6/9/79	45%	8200	285,000	routine physical and hypertension monitoring
				"
11/3/82	43%	6700	345,000	

Page #3

Other Blood Tests

Date	Test	Result	Reason for Test
3/2/77	potassium	4.5	hyper-tension
''	sodium	143	''
''	BUN	14	''
''	glucose	98	''
6/4/83	potassium	4.3	monitoring of antihyper-tension drugs

Page #4

Urinalysis Tests

Date	Urinalysis Result	Reason for Test
3/6/74	all normal	routine physical
3/2/77	all normal	"
6/4/83	all normal	"

Page #5

X-Rays

Date	Part of Body X-Rayed	Result	Reason for X-Ray
7/3/53	clavicle	fractured	fall
3/9/77	chest x-ray	normal	hypertension

Page #6

Miscellaneous Tests

Date   Tuberculosis Test Result

3/6/74   negative

Date   Test   Result   Reason for Test

3/2/77   EKG   normal   hypertension

Appendix 3

REFERENCES FOR FURTHER READING

The following books all deal primarily with medical tests and their interpretation or their use in clinical medicine.

Fischbach, Frances. *A Manual of Laboratory Tests*, Philadelphia: J.B. Lippincott, 1984.

This is a very complete and comprehensive guide written as a quick reference for doctors and nurses and as a textbook for medical, dental, and nursing students. Its major strength is its completeness: it covers all the major kinds of medical tests—blood tests, urine tests, x-rays, endoscopy, etc. Numerous appendices provide information about normal values and the effect of various drugs on test results. Its major weaknesses are that it is written like a manual with little explanatory or background information, and it includes drug effects that are clinically irrelevant.

Garb, Solomon, M.D. *Laboratory Tests in Common Use*, New York: Springer, 1976.

This is a long-standing brief guide for the medical profession, yet it is written in relatively easy-to-understand terminology. Its major strength is that Dr. Garb writes from the perspective of a clinical physician who is in actual practice, thus the book has a very practical orientation. Its major weakness is that it concerns itself only with tests done on blood, urine, and stool and does not mention the numerous other procedures and tests (such as x-rays) that are used.

Kee, Joyce LeFever and Helen Liang Tang. *Laboratory and Diagnostic Tests with Nursing Implications*, East Norwalk, CT: Appleton-Century-Crofts, 1983.

This book is rapidly becoming an important text for nurses. A major strength is its timeliness. Also, it has very good sections written on what nurses should tell patients in preparation for medical tests. Although written for the nursing professional, this book provides excellent advice on side effects, risks, and patient anxieties. Its major weakness is that in an effort to be comprehensive it has included some material that is not really relevant to the common use of medical tests.

Berkow, Robert, ed. *Merck Manual of Diagnosis and Therapy*, Rahway, N.J.: Merck Sharpe and Dohme Research Laboratories, 1982.

This is the only book we have included that does not deal exclusively with medical tests. It is an excellent source of information about diseases and their treatments and the tests that are useful in their diagnosis and monitoring. There are many valuable tables and charts detailing the use of tests in the approach to various clinical problems. Although at one time written exclusively for the physician or health care provider, this book is becoming well-known among patients as well. A very good investment for the concerned health consumer.

Henry, John Bernard, M.D., and W.B. Saunders, *Todd-Sanford-Davidsohn: Clinical Diagnosis and Management by Laboratory Methods*, Philadelphia, 1979.

This is the standard medical school textbook on medical tests and their use in clinical medicine. This is a very good book if you want scientific, detailed, and sophisticated information on a particular test, but it is not useful for the patient as a cover-to-cover book. It is found in all medical school libraries, where it can be consulted when the need arises.

Appendix 4

ABBREVIATIONS COMMONLY USED IN MEDICAL TESTS

ABG	= Arterial blood gas
ANA	= Antinuclear antibodies
APTT	= Activated partial thromboplastin time
BUN	= Blood urea nitrogen
CAT or CT	= Computerized axial tomography
CBC	= Complete blood count
CEA	= Carcinoembryonic antigen
CO_2	= Carbon dioxide
CPK or CK	= Creatine phosphokinase
CSF	= Cerebrospinal fluid
dl.	= Deciliters
ECG or EKG	= Electrocardiogram
EEG	= Electroencephalogram
EMG	= Electromyography
ESR	= Erythrocyte sedimentation rate
FBS	= Fasting blood sugar
GI series	= Gastrointestinal series (upper)
Hct	= Hematocrit
Hg	= Mercury
IU	= International units
IVP	= Intravenous pyelography
K	= Potassium
kg.	= Kilogram
L.	= Liter
mcg.	= Microgram
MCH	= Mean corpuscular hemoglobin
MCHC	= Mean corpuscular hemoglobin concentration
MCV	= Mean corpuscular volume

mEq / L.	= Millequivalents per liter
mg.	= Milligrams
mIU	= Milli-International unit
ml.	= Milliliters
mm³	= Cubic milliliter
ng.	= Nanogram
NPO	= No food or water (literally, *nihil per os,* which is Latin for "nothing by mouth.")
pg.	= Picogram
PT	= Prothrombin time
PTT	= Partial thromboplastin time
RBC	= Red blood cell
RIA	= Radioimmunoassay
U	= Units
UA	= Urinalysis
VDRL	= Venereal disease research laboratory
WBC	= White blood cell (leukocyte)

Index